Sports Medicine Imaging

Editors

NICHOLAS C. NACEY
JENNIFER L. PIERCE

CLINICS IN
SPORTS MEDICINE

www.sportsmed.theclinics.com

Consulting Editor
MARK D. MILLER

October 2021 • Volume 40 • Number 4

ELSEVIER

1600 John F. Kennedy Boulevard • Suite 1800 • Philadelphia, Pennsylvania, 19103-2899

http://www.theclinics.com

CLINICS IN SPORTS MEDICINE Volume 40, Number 4
October 2021 ISSN 0278-5919, ISBN-13: 978-0-323-79163-2

Editor: Lauren Boyle
Developmental Editor: Diana Grace Ang

Clinics in Sports Medicine (ISSN 0278-5919) is published quarterly by Elsevier Inc., 360 Park Avenue South, New York, NY 10010-1710. Months of issue are January, April, July, and October. Business and Editorial Offices: 1600 John F. Kennedy Blvd., Ste. 1800, Philadelphia, PA 19103-2899. Customer Service Office: 3251 Riverport Lane, Maryland Heights, MO 63043. Periodicals postage paid at New York, NY and additional mailing offices. Subscription prices are $364.00 per year (US individuals), $931.00 per year (US institutions), $100.00 per year (US students), $405.00 per year (Canadian individuals), $964.00 per year (Canadian institutions), $100.00 (Canadian students), $475.00 per year (foreign individuals), $964.00 per year (foreign institutions), and $235.00 per year (foreign students). Foreign air speed delivery is included in all *Clinics* subscription prices. All prices are subject to change without notice. **POSTMASTER:** Send address changes to *Clinics in Sports Medicine*, Elsevier Health Sciences Division, Subscription Customer Service, 3251 Riverport Lane, Maryland Heights, MO 63043. Customer Service (orders, claims, online, change of address): Elsevier Health Sciences Division, Subscription Customer Service, 3251 Riverport Lane, Maryland Heights, MO 63043. **Tel: 1-800-654-2452 (U.S. and Canada); 314-447-8871 (outside U.S. and Canada). Fax: 314-447-8029. E-mail: journalscustomerservice-usa@elsevier.com** (for print support); journalsonlinesupport-usa@elsevier.com (for online support).

Reprints. For copies of 100 or more of articles in this publication, please contact the Commercial Reprints Department, Elsevier Inc., 360 Park Avenue South, New York, NY 10010-1710. Tel.: 212-633-3874; Fax: 212-633-3820; E-mail: reprints@elsevier.com.

Clinics in Sports Medicine is covered in *MEDLINE/PubMed (Index Medicus) Current Contents/Clinical Medicine, Excerpta Medica,* and *ISI/Biomed.*

Contributors

CONSULTING EDITOR

MARK D. MILLER, MD
S. Ward Casscells Professor, Department of Orthopaedic Surgery,
University of Virginia, Charlottesville, Virginia, USA

EDITORS

NICHOLAS C. NACEY, MD
Associate Professor, Department of Radiology and Medical Imaging, University of Virginia,
Charlottesville, Virginia, USA

JENNIFER L. PIERCE, MD
Associate Professor, Department of Radiology and Medical Imaging, University of Virginia,
Charlottesville, Virginia, USA

AUTHORS

ANTHONY BALZER, MD
Assistant Professor, Department of Radiology, Baylor College of Medicine, Houston,
Texas, USA

KATHERINE M. BOJICIC, MD
Diagnostic Radiology Resident, University of Michigan Medical Center, Ann Arbor,
Michigan, USA

MONICA KALUME BRIGIDO, MD
Associate Professor of Radiology, University of Michigan Medical Center, Ann Arbor,
Michigan, USA

MAJID CHALIAN, MD
Interim Section Head, Division of Musculoskeletal Imaging and Intervention, Department
of Radiology, University of Washington Medical Center, Assistant Professor of Radiology,
UW Radiology-Roosevelt Clinic, Seattle, Washington, USA

ERIC Y. CHANG, MD
Clinical Professor, Department of Radiology, UC San Diego Health, San Diego, California,
USA; Staff Physician, Radiology Service, Veterans Affairs San Diego Healthcare System,
San Diego, California, USA

KAREN Y. CHENG, MD
Department of Radiology, UC San Diego Health, San Diego, California, USA

FELIX CHEW, MD, MBA
Professor, Division of Musculoskeletal Imaging and Intervention, Department of
Radiology, University of Washington, Seattle, Washington, USA

CHRISTINE B. CHUNG, MD
Executive Vice Chair, Department of Radiology, UC San Diego Health, San Diego, California, USA; Staff Physician, Radiology Service, Veterans Affairs San Diego Healthcare System, San Diego, California, USA

KYLE COOPER, MD
Radiology Resident, Division of Musculoskeletal Imaging, Department of Radiology, Duke University Medical Center, Duke University Hospital, Durham, North Carolina, USA.

MARLEE CREWS, BS
Indiana University School of Medicine, Indianapolis, Indiana, USA

JULIA CRIM, MD
Professor of Clinical Radiology, Fellowship Program Director, Musculoskeletal Radiology, Department of Radiology, DC069.10, University of Missouri, Columbia, Missouri, USA

FILIPPO DEL GRANDE, MD
Assistant Professor, Clinica di Radiologia EOC, Instituto di Imaging della Svizzera Italiana, Lugano, Switzerland

CRISTY N. FRENCH, MD
Department of Radiology, Penn State Health, Milton S. Hershey Medical Center Hershey, Pennsylvania, USA

ROBERT J. FRENCH, MD
Assistant Professor, Division of Musculoskeletal Imaging, Department of Radiology, Duke University Medical Center, Duke University Hospital, Durham, North Carolina, USA

KARA GAETKE-UDAGER, MD
Assistant Professor of Radiology, University of Michigan Medical Center, Ann Arbor, Michigan, USA

ANDREW G. GEESLIN, MD
Assistant Professor, Department of Orthopedic Surgery, University of Vermont Medical Center, Burlington, Vermont, USA

MATTHEW G. GEESLIN, MD, MENG
Assistant Professor, Department of Radiology, University of Vermont Medical Center, Burlington, Vermont, USA

IMAN KHODARAHMI, MD, PhD
Assistant Professor, Division of Musculoskeletal Imaging, Department of Radiology, New York University Grossman School of Medicine, New York, New York, USA

PARISA KHOSHPOURI, MD
Postdoctoral Research Fellow, Division of Musculoskeletal Imaging and Intervention, Department of Radiology, University of Washington Medical Center, UW Radiology-Roosevelt Clinic, Seattle, Washington, USA

MAXINE ELLA KRESSE, MD
Assistant Professor, Department of Radiology and Medical Imaging, University of Virginia, Charlottesville, Virginia, USA

LAUREN M. LADD, MD
Assistant Professor of Clinical Radiology, Department of Radiology and Imaging Sciences, Indiana University School of Medicine, Indianapolis, Indiana, USA

DIEGO F. LEMOS, MD
Associate Professor, Radiology and Orthopedic Surgery, University of Vermont Medical Center, Department of Radiology, Burlington, Vermont, USA

JAYSON R. LOEFFERT, DO
Department of Family and Community Medicine, Penn State Health Medical Group Middletown, Middletown, Pennsylvania, USA

ALECIO F. LOMBARDI, MD
Department of Radiology, UC San Diego Health; Radiology Service, Veterans Affairs San Diego Healthcare System, San Diego, California, USA

NATHAN A. MAERTZ, MD
Assistant Professor of Clinical Radiology, Department of Radiology and Imaging Sciences, Indiana University School of Medicine, Indianapolis, Indiana, USA

ERIN MCCRUM, MD
Medical Instructor, Division of Musculoskeletal Imaging, Department of Radiology, Duke University Medical Center, Duke University Hospital, Durham, North Carolina, USA

NATHANIEL B. MEYER, MD
Assistant Professor of Radiology, University of Michigan Medical Center, Ann Arbor, Michigan, USA

NICHOLAS C. NACEY, MD
Associate Professor, Department of Radiology and Medical Imaging, University of Virginia, Charlottesville, Virginia, USA

ANDREW PALISCH, MD
Associate Professor, Department of Radiology, Baylor College of Medicine, Houston, Texas, USA

ASHISH PATEL, MD
Diagnostic Radiology Resident, Department of Radiology, Baylor College of Medicine, Houston, Texas, USA

MICHAEL T. PERRY, MD
Assistant Professor, Department of Radiology and Medical Imaging, University of Virginia, Charlottesville, Virginia, USA

PARHAM PEZESHK, MD
Assistant Professor, Division of Musculoskeletal Imaging, Department of Radiology, University of Texas Southwestern Medical Center, Dallas, Texas, USA

SHAWN F. PHILLIPS, MD
Department of Family and Community Medicine, Penn State Health Medical Group Mount Joy, Mount Joy, Pennsylvania, USA

JENNIFER L. PIERCE, MD
Associate Professor, Department of Radiology and Medical Imaging, University of Virginia, Charlottesville, Virginia, USA

LAUREN CLOUGH PRINGLE, MD
Assistant Professor of Clinical Radiology, Department of Radiology, DC069.10, University of Missouri, Columbia, Missouri, USA

CHRISTINE REHWALD, MD
Assistant Professor, Division of Musculoskeletal Imaging and Intervention, Department of Radiology, University of Washington, Seattle, Washington, USA

HUMBERTO ROSAS, MD
Associate Professor of Radiology, University of Wisconsin School of Medicine and Public Health, Madison, Wisconsin, USA

JONATHAN D. SAMET, MD
Assistant Professor of Radiology, Section Head, Musculoskeletal Radiology, Department of Medical Imaging, Ann and Robert H. Lurie Children's Hospital of Chicago, Northwestern University Feinberg School Medicine, Chicago, Illinois, USA

JAMES DEREK STENSBY, MD
Associate Professor of Clinical Radiology, Residency Program Director, Diagnostic Radiology, Department of Radiology, DC069.10, University of Missouri, Columbia, Missouri, USA

LINDSAY STRATCHKO, DO
Assistant Professor of Radiology, University of Wisconsin School of Medicine and Public Health, Madison, Wisconsin, USA

ERIC A. WALKER, MD
Department of Radiology, Penn State Health Milton S. Hershey Medical Center, Hershey, Pennsylvania, USA; Uniformed Services University of the Health Sciences, Bethesda, Maryland, USA

JOCELYN WITTSTEIN, MD
Division of Sports Medicine, Department of Orthopaedic Surgery, Duke University Medical Center, Durham, North Carolina, USA.

CORRIE M. YABLON, MD
Associate Professor of Radiology, University of Michigan Medical Center, Ann Arbor, Michigan, USA

Contents

The glenohumeral joint is intrinsically predisposed to instability because of the bony anatomy but maintained in alignment by many important structures, including the glenoid labrum, glenohumeral ligaments (GHLs), and muscles and tendons. Trauma and overuse can damage these stabilizers, which may then lead to subluxation or dislocation and eventually recurrent instability. This is most common in the anterior direction, which has several recognizable patterns of injury on advanced imaging, including humeral Hill Sachs deformities, bony Bankart lesion of the anteroinferior glenoid, soft tissue Bankart lesions, Bankart variant lesions (Perthes and ALPSA lesions), and HAGL/GAGL lesions. Similar reverse lesions are seen, as well as unique posterior lesions, such as Bennett and Kim's lesions. When symptoms of apprehension and instability in more than one direction are seen, one should consider multidirectional instability, which often presents with a patulous joint capsule. Finally, owing to significant impacts of daily activities and quality of life, surgical correction of labral tears, bony Bankart defects, Hill Sachs defects, and capsular laxity, may be considered.

Familiarity with throwing mechanics during elbow range of motion allows accurate diagnosis of sports-related elbow injuries, which occur in predictable patterns. In addition, repetitive stress-related injuries are often clinically apparent; however, imaging plays an important role in determining severity as well as associated injuries that may affect clinical management. A detailed understanding of elbow imaging regarding anatomy and mechanism of injury results in prompt and precise treatment.

Injuries to the wrist and hands occur frequently in athletes from the high forces applied during sporting events. The examples presented illustrate the important role imaging has in the diagnosis of wrist and hand injuries. In addition, different imaging modalities are complementary and various examinations may be needed to help guide the management of wrist and hand traumatic pathology.

The menisci of the knee are accurately evaluated by MRI. Knowledge of normal anatomy, imaging parameters, imaging appearance of the normal and torn meniscus, and common anatomic variants and pitfalls are essential in obtaining the correct imaging diagnosis. There are multiple imaging signs of meniscal tear, including linear signal intensity extending to an articular surface on at least 2 images, altered meniscal shape, displaced meniscal flap, ghost meniscus, meniscal extrusion, and parameniscal cyst. After surgery, granulation tissue may mimic tear. Diagnosis is improved by comparison to preoperative images, operative note, and intra-articular contrast administration.

Preoperative and postoperative imaging of knee ligament injury hinges on the appropriate use of available modalities. Knowledge of injury patterns as well as the surgical significance of certain image findings enhances injury detection and supports appropriate preoperative planning. The radiologist must be familiar with the strengths and weaknesses of each modality for evaluating specific aspects of ligamentous pathology. This article focuses on preoperative and postoperative imaging of knee ligament injury. Basic topics pertaining to preoperative image modality selection and isolated injury detection are addressed. More advanced areas including ligamentous injury patterns, surgical indications, and postoperative imaging are also discussed.

Articular cartilage injury and degeneration represent common causes of knee pain, which can be evaluated accurately and noninvasively using MRI. This review describes the structure of cartilage focusing on its histologic appearance to emphasize that structure will dictate patterns of tissue failure as well as MR appearance. In addition to identifying cartilage loss, MRI can demonstrate signal changes that correspond to intrinsic structural abnormalities, which place the cartilage at risk for subsequent more serious injury or premature degeneration, allowing for earlier intervention and treatment of important causes of pain and morbidity.

Patellar instability is a broad term that encompasses patellar dislocation, patellar subluxation, and patellar instability. Although both functional and anatomic considerations contribute to symptoms of patellar instability, the most important are thought to be patella alta, trochlear dysplasia, and lateralization of the tibial tubercle. In patients with a history suspicious for prior patellar dislocation, careful evaluation of MRI and radiographic studies can reveal characteristic findings. The most common methods to address patellofemoral instability are medial patellofemoral ligament reconstruction and tibial tubercle osteotomy with either anteromedialization or medialization. Less commonly trochleoplasty is indicated as well. Patients may be treated with one of or a combination of these techniques, each of which has specific indications and complications.

Hip pain is a common and complex clinical entity. The causes of hip injuries in athletes are many and diverse, requiring efficient, accurate diagnosis for proper management. Imaging is an important step in the clinical evaluation of hip pain, and familiarity with multiple imaging modalities as well as characteristic imaging findings is a helpful tool for sports medicine clinicians. This article discusses imaging recommendations and gives imaging examples of common causes of intra-articular and extra-articular hip pain including femoroacetabular impingement, labral tears, cartilage defects, ligamentum teres injuries, snapping hip syndrome, femoral stress injuries, thigh splints, athletic pubalgia, avulsion injuries, and hip dislocation.

Ankle sprain is the most common injury in athletic populations. Ligament and tendon pathologies of the ankle are common, ranging from traumatic injuries to degeneration leading to chronic pain and acquired foot deformities. MRI is the imaging modality of choice to evaluate tendon and ligament pathology of the ankle, specifically derangements of tendons and ligaments. 3-T MRI offers improved imaging characteristics relative to 1.5-T MRI, allowing for better delineation of anatomic detail and pathology. This article provides a review of the anatomy and common pathologies of the ankle ligaments and tendons using high-resolution 3-T MRI.

Turf toe is a common injury of the hallux metatarsophalangeal (MTP) joint in athletes which is the result of hyperdorsiflexion injury. While the term turf toe has been used to describe a variety of first MTP joint injuries, the term is now typically used in imaging to describe tearing or injury to the plantar plate complex. This review article will cover normal anatomy of the first MTP joint, mechanism of injury, typical imaging findings in normal individuals on MRI and ultrasound, as well as the most common patterns of injury.

CLINICS IN SPORTS MEDICINE

SERIES OF RELATED INTERESTED

Orthopedic Clinics
https://www.orthopedic.theclinics.com/
Foot and Ankle Clinics
https://www.foot.theclinics.com/
Hand Clinics
https://www.hand.theclinics.com/
Physical Medicine and Rehabilitation Clinics
https://www.pmr.theclinics.com/

THE CLINICS ARE AVAILABLE ONLINE!
Access your subscription at:
www.theclinics.com

CLINICS IN SPORTS MEDICINE

FORTHCOMING ISSUES

January 2022
Patellofemoral Instability Decision Making and Techniques
David Diduch, Editor

April 2022
Sports Anesthesia
Ashley Shilling, Editor

July 2022
Sports Cardiology
Dean Nelson Peter, Editor

RECENT ISSUES

July 2021
Sports Spine
Adam Shimer and Francis H Shen, Editors

April 2021
Athletic Injuries of the Hip
Dustin L Richter and F Winston Gwathmey, Editors

January 2021
Sport-Related Concussion
Peter K Kriz, Editor

SERIES OF RELATED INTEREST

Orthopedic Clinics
https://www.orthopedic.theclinics.com/
Foot and Ankle Clinics
https://www.foot.theclinics.com/
Hand Clinics
https://www.hand.theclinics.com/
Physical Medicine and Rehabilitation Clinics
https://www.pmr.theclinics.com/

THE CLINICS ARE AVAILABLE ONLINE!
Access your subscription at:
www.theclinics.com

Foreword

Sports Imaging: Plan Your Trip

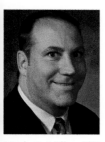

Mark D. Miller, MD
Consulting Editor

You wouldn't go on a road trip without first looking at a map (or the twenty-first century equivalent: GPS). Likewise, you shouldn't plan surgery without first obtaining and reviewing relevant imaging studies. This issue of *Clinics in Sports Medicine* should be considered map-reading 101. I asked two of our very talented University of Virginia (UVA) musculoskeletal radiology orienteers, Drs Nicholas Nacey and Jennifer Pierce, to help sports surgeons plan future trips. They elected to start North and head South, beginning with the shoulder and proceeding to the foot. They also have highlighted a few road hazards, stress imaging, pediatric imaging, and ultrasound to keep us on the highway. As the Guest Editors point out, surgeons and radiologists enjoy a tremendous collaborative relationship at UVA that benefits us all. In addition to the monthly MRI-Arthroscopy correlation conference, we visit the reading room on a regular basis and often send our fellows over for a "road trip" to gain a better understanding of what lies ahead. I would encourage you to do the same, and spend some time picking up a few orienteering skills offered in this issue. Happy Trails!

Mark D. Miller, MD
Division of Sports Medicine
Department of Orthopaedic Surgery
University of Virginia, Charlottesville
400 Ray C. Hunt Drive
Suite 330
Charlottesville, VA 22908-0159, USA

E-mail address:
MDM3P@hscmail.mcc.virginia.edu

Clin Sports Med 40 (2021) xiii
https://doi.org/10.1016/j.csm.2021.06.002
0278-5919/21/© 2021 Published by Elsevier Inc.

Preface

Intersection Between the Reading Room and the Operating Room

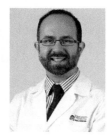
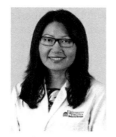

Nicholas C. Nacey, MD   Jennifer L. Pierce, MD
Editors

Orthopedic surgeons and musculoskeletal radiologists both interpret imaging studies as part of routine day-to-day practice. However, these 2 specialties approach image interpretation differently based on the perspective of their particular profession. Mutual understanding of each other's specialties is critical to providing the best patient care that we can. From the radiologist's perspective, we are always intrigued by seeing surgical correlations for the MRI findings that we see on a daily basis and can use knowledge that is gained about the surgical approaches undertaken by our colleagues to inform our understanding of expected postsurgical appearances. For orthopedists, knowledge about different imaging techniques as well as the normal and pathologic appearances of musculoskeletal structures can help to inform what you may be seeing in a patient in front of you in clinic or intraoperatively. We have always been exceedingly grateful for the collaboration we've had with our orthopedic colleagues and the insights we have gained, and as such, we hope to reciprocate by giving the readers a look inside the reading room with a group of leaders in the field of musculoskeletal radiology.

We have decided to take a shoulders-to-toes approach to sports medicine imaging, mixing bread-and-butter topics with others that tend to receive less attention in the literature but are still critical to managing patients with sports injuries. The first 3 articles deal with the upper extremity with focuses on shoulder instability, elbow injuries, and hand/wrist trauma. This is followed by a quartet of articles focusing on the knee with detailed imaging descriptions of the menisci, ligaments, cartilage, and patellofemoral instability. Understanding pathologic condition in the native knee is often only half the battle in image interpretation, and as such, these articles also describe some of the differences when evaluating imaging of postoperative patients. Articles on intraarticular and extraarticular causes of hip pain, tendon and ligament injuries in the ankle, and turf toe round out our tour of the lower extremity. Last are three articles

Clin Sports Med 40 (2021) xv–xvi
https://doi.org/10.1016/j.csm.2021.06.001
0278-5919/21/© 2021 Published by Elsevier Inc.

encompassing sports medicine imaging as a whole. The article on stress imaging describes findings on different modalities and classifies what particular findings are considered high risk. The next article on pediatric sports injuries highlights the unique pathologic condition found in the pediatric patient population. The final article on musculoskeletal ultrasound describes the growing importance of this modality as well as situations in which ultrasound should be considered for imaging evaluation.

We would like to thank Dr Miller for the opportunity to serve as guest editors, as well as Lauren Boyle, Donald Mumford, and Diana Ang at Elsevier for helping us to put this issue together. Last, we are extremely grateful to the many authors of this issue for contributing their extraordinary expertise; we could not have put this issue together without the assistance of these exceptional colleagues. We hope that the readers of the issue will find that the trip to the reading room was well spent.

Nicholas C. Nacey, MD
Department of Radiology and Medical Imaging
University of Virginia
1215 Lee Street
PO Box 800170
Charlottesville, VA 22903, USA

Jennifer L. Pierce, MD
Department of Radiology and Medical Imaging
University of Virginia
1215 Lee Street
PO Box 800170
Charlottesville, VA 22903, USA

E-mail addresses:
ncn5t@hscmail.mcc.virginia.edu (N.C. Nacey)
jp5aq@hscmail.mcc.virginia.edu (J.L. Pierce)

Glenohumeral Joint Instability

A Review of Anatomy, Clinical Presentation, and Imaging

Lauren M. Ladd, MD[a],*, Marlee Crews, BS[b],
Nathan A. Maertz, MD[a]

KEYWORDS

- Glenohumeral instability • MRI • Magnetic resonance arthrogram
- Computed tomography • Bankart lesion • Passive stabilizers

KEY POINTS

- Symptoms of pain and apprehension (or joint slipping) must be present with physical examination findings of joint laxity to diagnose recurrent glenohumeral instability.
- Osseous lesions are best depicted on CT imaging, whereas MRI is best for evaluating soft tissue injury due to its superior soft tissue contrast.
- MR arthrography has higher sensitivity and specificity for detecting Bankart and Bankart variant lesions, particularly in the subacute or chronic setting.
- Imaging plays an important role in accurately diagnosing the cause(s) of instability, helping to guide appropriate surgical management.

INTRODUCTION

The glenohumeral joint is a synovial ball-and-socket joint that is anatomically likened to a golf ball on a tee, with the rounded humeral head precariously balanced on the shallow glenoid fossa of the scapula. Although this provides the greatest range of motion of any joint in the body, it also creates inherent instability.[1–3] Thus, the glenohumeral joint depends on the synergy of bones, ligaments, muscles, and cartilage to provide stability both statically and dynamically.

Glenohumeral instability is defined as the loss of the ability to maintain normal joint alignment with associated symptoms of pain, apprehension, joint "slipping," and/or paresthesia.[1,4–6] Although traumatic dislocation is the commonest cause of chronic

[a] Department of Radiology & Imaging Sciences, Indiana University School of Medicine, 1701 N. Senate Boulevard, Indianapolis, IN 46202, USA; [b] Indiana University School of Medicine, 340 W 10th St, Indianapolis, IN 46202, USA
* Corresponding author.
E-mail address: LMLadd@iupui.edu

Clin Sports Med 40 (2021) 585–599
https://doi.org/10.1016/j.csm.2021.05.001
0278-5919/21/© 2021 Elsevier Inc. All rights reserved.

instability, one dislocation does not constitute "instability." Instability is defined as recurrent and symptomatic dislocation or subluxation and can lead to significant morbidity, including pain, loss of function, limited participation in occupational or recreational activities, and possibly progressive bone loss, joint damage, and early osteoarthritis.[4]

As will be discussed, there are many contributing factors to stability and instability of the glenohumeral joint, from the underlying anatomy, to congenital factors, to superimposed injury. For the purposes of this review, we will focus on instability characterized by directionality, as well as basic anatomy and causes, and imaging appearance.

DISCUSSION
Anatomy

As previously noted, the glenohumeral joint anatomy predisposes the shoulder to instability with relatively little osseous contact and heavy reliance on supporting soft tissue structures. The primary static stabilizers include glenohumeral congruency, the glenoid labrum, GHLs, and negative intra-articular pressure of the joint capsule.[1] The glenohumeral congruency, involving the articular surfaces of the humeral head

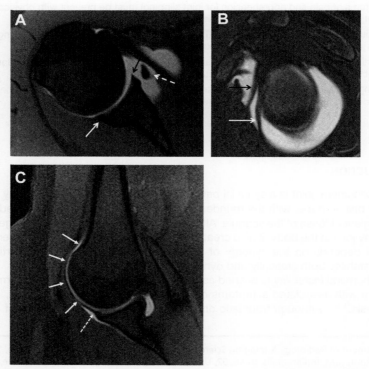

Fig. 1. Fat-suppressed T1-weighted MR arthrogram images of the glenohumeral joint. (*A*) Axial image through the mid joint exhibits normal anterior labrum (*black arrow*), middle glenohumeral ligament (white dashed *arrow*), and posterior labrum (*white arrow*). (*B*) Sagittal image through the glenoid demonstrates normal middle glenohumeral ligament (*black arrow*) and aIGHL (*white arrow*). (*C*) Abduction external rotation (ABER position) image shows a normal aIGHL (*solid arrows*) and anteroinferior labrum (*dashed arrow*).

and the glenoid fossa, provides compressive stability. This is crucial in midrange motion when the ligaments are slack, thus contributes less to stability.[2]

The labrum is a fibrocartilaginous structure that courses along and covers the margin of the glenoid fossa (**Fig. 1**). It augments the size of the socket, increasing the depth by one-third, which increases contact with the humeral head. This helps prevent displacement while also allowing for flexibility.[1,7,8] The labrum also serves as an attachment site for the GHLs.[1] As described below, these ligaments are also important stabilizers; therefore, injury of the labrum may contribute two-fold to instability.

The GHLs are the most important passive stabilizers of the glenohumeral joint (see **Fig. 1**B). Three anterior GHLs have been described: superior, middle, and inferior. Each of the ligaments assumes primary significance at different positions of the humeral head, becoming taut at the extremes of motion. When the shoulder is adducted or neutral, the superior GHL, which extends from the superior glenoid rim to just superior to the lesser tuberosity, is the main resistor against inferior and posterior subluxation.[9] Moving through abduction, the responsibility shifts to the middle GHL, which begins at the superior glenoid rim and inserts at the capsular component of the subscapularis tendon. At 45 degrees of abduction, it is the primary structure resisting anterior subluxation. However, wide anatomic variation of its configuration without consequence on stability suggests it is the least important GHL.[10] As abduction continues, the inferior GHL (IGHL) becomes the most important stabilizer of the ligaments. The IGHL is a complex composed of anterior and posterior bundles and an axillary pouch, coursing from the anteroinferior and posteroinferior glenoid, respectively, to the medial humeral head/neck. The anterior bundle of the IGHL is responsible for preventing anterior subluxation when the shoulder is abducted to 90° and externally rotated (ABER position) (see **Fig. 1**C).[11] This is the position often assumed during a fall on an outstretched hand, which is the most common cause of anterior glenohumeral dislocation. Thus, trauma most commonly exposes the IGHL to injury.[12]

The dynamic stabilizers are primarily muscular, including the rotator cuff muscles, pectoralis major, latissimus dorsi, periscapular muscles, as well as the tendon of the long head of the biceps.[1] The rotator cuff muscles are of primary importance as muscle contraction compresses the humeral head into the glenoid, both centering it and increasing the force necessary to shift the humeral head from this position. The midrange of motion depends heavily on dynamic stabilizers as the GHLs are lax in this range.[2]

Causes of Instability

As demonstrated by the relatively extensive anatomy contributing to glenohumeral stability, there are many sources for potential instability. Trauma is the most prevalent inciting cause of instability. The glenohumeral joint is the most commonly dislocated joint in the body, occurring in 2% of the general population.[1] Fall on an outstretched hand (anterior dislocation) or forceful adduction with internal rotation (posterior dislocation) may disrupt bony or labroligamentous anatomy, affecting the primary static and dynamic stabilizers in such a way that predisposes the joint to recurrent dislocation or subluxation. Fractures of the glenoid (bony Bankart or reverse bony Bankart lesion) and humeral head (Hill Sachs or reverse Hill Sachs fractures) may leave osseous voids that result in recurrent slippage into the same position as the original dislocation (**Fig. 2**). Tears of the labrum (soft tissue Bankart or Bankart variant lesions) (**Figs. 3–5**), GHLs (**Figs. 6 and 7**), and/or muscles, also leave an unbalanced stability of the joint, rendering it at risk for recurrent injury and/or malalignment.

Congenital configuration of the bony and soft tissue anatomy also plays an important role in chronic instability, including those without a history of trauma. These

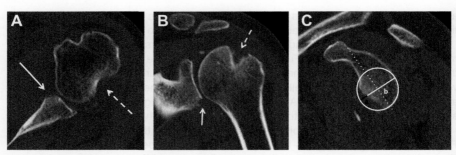

Fig. 2. CT image of the shoulder shows an acute bony Bankart lesion of the anterior glenoid (*solid arrow*) and Hill-Sachs deformity of the posterior humeral head (*dashed arrow*) on axial (*A*) and coronal (*B*) images. Sagittal (*C*) image shows the bony defect of the anterior inferior glenoid measured by the "best-fit circle" method to determine the percent surface area loss, where the % loss = [a/(a+b)] × 100%.

include, most importantly, glenoid morphology and anterior capsular insertion. Congenital variations in the posterior glenoid configuration include the normal triangular shape, as well as rounded (J shaped) and delta-shaped posterior glenoid. The latter two result in loss of concavity of the inferior glenoid margin, predisposing to posterior glenohumeral instability.[13] For further detail, see Mulligan and Pontius's review as a detailed discussion of these components is beyond the scope of this review.[14] In addition, variations in the anterior capsular insertion may predispose one to anterior glenohumeral instability. Types I and II anterior capsular insertions attach at the anterior labrum and within 1 cm of the labral base, respectively. In type III, however, the attachment is >1 cm medial to the labrum/glenoid rim, rendering the glenohumeral joint more unstable.[7,15,16] A comprehensive analysis of these variants is provided by Chen and colleagues.[17]

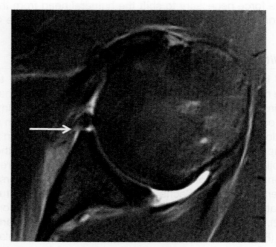

Fig. 3. Axial fat-suppressed T1-weighted MR image of the glenohumeral joint shows a fluid cleft traversing the anteroinferior glenoid labrum and the labrum is separated from the glenoid rim, consistent with an acute soft tissue Bankart lesion.

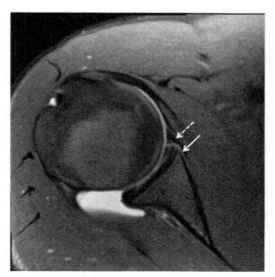

Fig. 4. Axial fat-suppressed T1-weighted MR image of the glenohumeral joint shows a fluid cleft separating a nondisplaced labrum from the anteroinferior glenoid (*dashed arrow*), as well as extension medially beneath a stripped periosteum that is, intact/attached more medially (*solid arrow*), consistent with a Perthes lesion.

IMAGING

Whether due to recent acute trauma, remote trauma, or no trauma, radiographs are the first-line test for imaging glenohumeral joint pain and/or instability.[18,19] The patient's age, history of injury, clinical examination, and radiographs, can often dictate whether the symptoms should be treated conservatively or surgically.[20] In the setting of acute trauma, a 3-view radiograph series, including a scapular Y or axillary view, will delineate malalignment and most fractures. The axillary view is particularly helpful in assessing bony injury (Bankart lesion) of the anterior inferior glenoid, and the AP

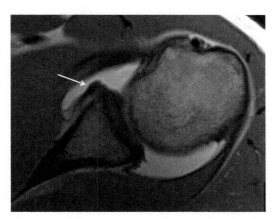

Fig. 5. Axial T1-weighted MR arthrogram image through the glenohumeral joint demonstrates a torn and medially displaced labrum (*arrow*) with subjacent periosteal irregularity, in keeping with a chronic ALPSA lesion.

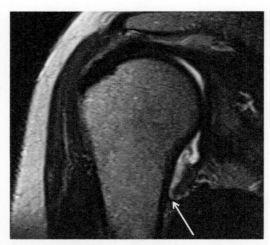

Fig. 6. Coronal T1 MR arthrogram image of the shoulder demonstrates loss of expected U-shaped axillary pouch and discontinuity at the humeral attachment with joint fluid extending inferior to the capsule (*arrow*), consistent with an HAGL lesion.

internal rotation is best to assess for the posterior superior humeral head impaction injury (Hill Sachs fracture).

After alignment and bony assessment with radiographs, MRI, with its superior soft tissue contrast, is the test of choice to determine if and how severe the dynamic and static glenohumeral stabilizers may be injured, consequently predisposing to recurrent instability. After acute injury or shortly after the traumatic event, noncontrast MRI can

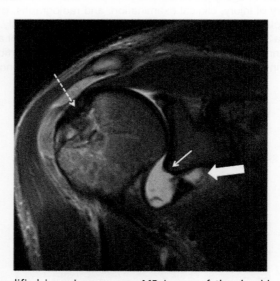

Fig. 7. Coronal-modified inversion recovery MR image of the shoulder shows extensive trauma, including a Hill Sachs impaction fracture of the humeral head (*dashed arrow*), tear of the anteroinferior glenoid labrum (*thin white arrow*), and discontinuity of the glenoid attachment of the inferior glenohumeral ligament (*block white arrow*) known as a GAGL lesion.

be considered, as a traumatic joint effusion may be present to outline intra-articular structures similar to intra-articular contrast of a magnetic resonance (MR) arthrogram.[2,21] As demonstrated by meta-analysis, MR arthrography is more helpful in the setting of chronic instability and/or pain, due to 98% specificity and 92% sensitivity in accurately detecting labroligamentous injury compared with 95% specificity but only 77% sensitivity of conventional, noncontrast MRI.[21]

Finally, computed tomography (CT) is a useful adjunct for the evaluation of bone loss. As detailed below, glenoid rim deficiency is an important factor of the likelihood of dislocation recurrence and need for/type of surgical management. With dedicated training, as is seen in the hands of experienced musculoskeletal radiologists, MRI may also be used to measure glenoid bone stock loss.[22,23] Generally, however, CT is the most accurate in providing assessment and measurements of bone loss.

Anterior Instability

Glenohumeral instability is characterized as anterior instability in 95% of cases.[6] Thus, most imaging findings discussed in this review will focus on bony and soft tissue injuries of the anterior inferior glenohumeral joint, including the following: bony Bankart lesion, Hill Sachs lesion, soft tissue Bankart and Bankart variant lesions, glenolabral articular disruption (GLAD) lesion, and humeral or glenoid avulsion of the glenohumeral ligament (HAGL or GAGL, respectively).

With anterior dislocation, there is impaction of the posterosuperior humeral head on the anteroinferior glenoid. If a fracture occurs at the anteroinferior glenoid, it is referred to as a bony Bankart lesion (see **Figs. 2 and 8**). Small fractures, which may be occult on MRI, are still important because of associated detachment of the anteroinferior labroligamentous complex. Larger bony Bankart lesions are also problematic as lack of sufficient glenoid surface area for centering of the humeral head contributes to chronic instability. Measurement of the osseous glenoid defects size helps determine if surgical treatment is necessary and, at times, what type of surgery will be necessary. This is most easily achieved using the "best-fit circle" method (seen in **Fig. 2**) with a circle fitted to the inferior 2/3 of the glenoid margin.[24,25] Measurement from the anterior circle to the new (fractured) margin of the glenoid is divided by the diameter of this best-fit circle, yielding the percentage of the surface area lost. If >20 to 30% deficient surface area, the patient is at risk for recurrent dislocation and bone augmentation may be indicated.[26,27]

Humeral head Hill Sachs defects (see **Figs. 2 and 8**) are more common than bony Bankart lesions and increase in incidence (up to 90%) with recurrent dislocations.[28]

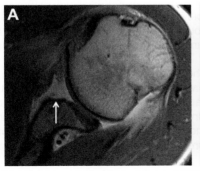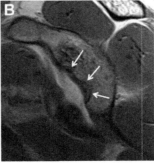

Fig. 8. Axial (*A*) and sagittal (*B*) T1-weighted MR images of the shoulder with a corticated bony defect of the anteroinferior glenoid, consistent with a chronic Bankart lesion (*arrows*).

These are identified on MR or CT images as a focal indentation of the posterior superior humeral head and maybe a helpful clue to seek other imaging evidence of instability. No imaging criteria accurately delineate which lesions will engage and/or need operative management. Rather, surgical treatment is reserved for those lesions that engages, or catch on, the anteroinferior glenoid (typically in abduction and external rotation), causing recurrent dislocation, and engaging Hills Sachs defects are diagnosed clinically.[2]

In addition to bony impaction, anterior dislocation of the humeral head may compress or cause excessive tension/tear of the anteroinferior labrum and attached anterior inferior glenohumeral ligament (aIGHL).[8] Tear of the anteroinferior labrum from the underlying glenoid is referred to as a soft tissue Bankart lesion—or simply a Bankart lesion—as described by the British orthopedic surgeon in 1923.[29] On MRI, which best depicts these soft tissue injuries, a Bankart lesion is identified by a cleft of joint fluid or contrast (if MR arthrogram) that separates the labrum from the underlying glenoid (see **Fig. 3**). This is the most common injury associated with instability and requires careful attention as it functionally destabilizes the anteroinferior capsulolabral complex.[6] Because there is minimal healing capacity of a Bankart lesion, surgical repair by reattachment of the labrum is required.[30]

Two important variants of the Bankart lesion are Perthes and anterior labroligamentous periosteal sleeve avulsion (ALPSA) lesions. Both involve a tear or separation of the anterior inferior labrum from the underlying glenoid; however, the periosteum is stripped from the glenoid yet remains attached medially. A Perthes lesion is a nondisplaced tear of the labrum with stripping of the periosteum. This is best identified on MRI with fluid or contrast extending beneath the labrum and medially along the anterior glenoid/scapula beneath the periosteum (**Fig. 4**).[2,8,31] Because this injury is nondisplaced, it may be occult on routine MRI with the arm in neutral position. However, diagnostic accuracy is improved with MR arthrography and use of the ABER position (see **Fig. 1C**), which stresses the anteroinferior capsule and accentuates pathology in this region.[31] Perthes lesions may heal on their own due to the nondisplaced position of the labrum and intact periosteum. However, with recurrent injury, the labrum may displace and convert to an ALPSA lesion.

ALPSA lesions are also tears of the anteroinferior labrum with stripping of the periosteum but differ from Perthes lesions in the position of the labral tissue, which is displaced and often scarred medially along the anterior scapula.[2] This is identified on MRI when the anteroinferior labrum is absent and soft tissue thickening is seen at the anterior glenoid neck (**Fig. 5**), 5 to 15 mm medial to the glenoid rim.[32] Because a smooth synovial surface develops over the lesion during scarring/healing, this may be difficult to identify during arthroscopy. Thus, accurate preoperative diagnosis on MRI is important for surgical planning and patient outcome. Surgically, ALPSA lesions must be converted to a Bankart lesion, the labrum then reduced, and anterior capsular tissue reconstructed for effective treatment.[33]

In addition to labroligamentous pathology, the adjacent cartilage may also be involved. The direct impaction of the humeral head on the glenoid may result in anteroinferior labral tear and associated adjacent chondral injury, which is referred to as a GLAD lesion (**Fig. 9**).[34] The chondral injury ranges from a chondral flap or delamination to an impaction or depressed osteochondral injury and is not generally unstable. Thus, pain associated with these lesions is more commonly due to the osteochondral lesion, rather than instability.[2]

Lastly, avulsion of the aIGHL is a traumatic injury and may contribute to chronic anterior glenohumeral instability. Avulsion of the IGHL may occur at the glenoid

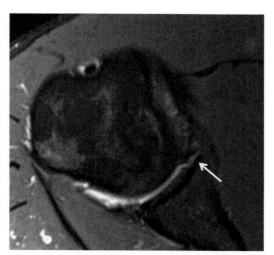

Fig. 9. Axial fat-suppressed proton density (PD) MR image of the glenohumeral joint shows a full-thickness defect of the anteroinferior glenoid cartilage (*arrow*) with adjacent anteroinferior labral tear, known as a GLAD lesion.

attachment (glenoid avulsion of the glenohumeral ligament or GAGL), at the midsubstance of the axillary pouch, or the humeral attachment (humeral avulsion of the glenohumeral ligament or HAGL). Despite biomechanical studies indicating that the glenoid is the most common site of tissue failure with strain, the HAGL lesion is commonest clinically with anterior dislocation.[35,36] On MRI, the HAGL lesion is identified most easily in the acute setting where joint fluid spills into the axillary soft tissues through a defect at the expected aIGHL humeral attachment (see **Fig. 6**). The inferior joint capsule, normally a "U" shape, becomes discontinuous near the humerus, and the inferior displaced/redundant aIGHL forms a "J" shape, hence described as the "J" sign on coronal MR images.[35] GAGL lesions were recognized in the literature much later than HAGL lesions but are characterized by a similar irregular fluid-filled gap near the anterior inferior glenoid capsule attachment (**Fig. 7**).[37] This may be present with an intact or torn labrum and either periosteal stripping or complete periosteal detachment. Similar to but opposite of the HAGL "J" sign, the appearance of GAGL lesions is referred to as the reverse "J" sign.[38] Both HAGL and GAGL lesions result in instability of the anteroinferior labroligamentous complex and must be repaired to restore stability.[6]

Posterior Instability

Posterior instability is much less common than anterior instability, accounting for 5% to 10% of shoulder instability, and is seen more commonly in men who participate in overhead throwing (ie, baseball pitchers) or contact (ie, football linemen) sports.[39–41] Posterior instability may result in limited abduction and a sense of apprehension, although the most common symptom is simply pain.[39,41] Posterior glenoid deficiency is seen in upwards of 90% of patients with posterior instability, which corresponds to a high incidence of posterior labral tearing (64%) and may be due to the previously described congenital posterior glenoid hypoplasia or as a consequence of traumatic injury to the posterior glenoid.[13] Care should be made on image interpretation, however, to ensure appropriate image slice and patient positioning to avoid overcalling the normal rounding of the caudal glenoid rim as glenoid deficiency.[12]

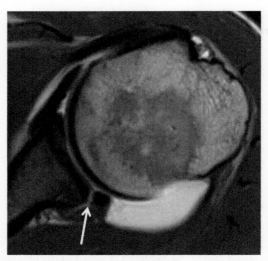

Fig. 10. Axial T1 MR arthrogram image of the glenohumeral joint shows a contrast-filled cleft separating the posteroinferior labrum from the underlying glenoid (*arrow*) and tear of the posterior periosteum, known as a reverse Bankart lesion.

Because the posterior capsule is a primary static stabilizer, injury to it results in posterior translation of the humeral head.[39] Imaging findings of posterior instability mirror anterior instability lesions, including a reverse bony Bankart lesion after posterior dislocation, reverse Hill Sachs deformity, reverse soft tissue Bankart lesion, posterior labroligamentous periosteal sleeve avulsion (reverse of ALPSA), and posterior humeral avulsion of the glenohumeral ligament (posterior HAGL). Comparison of **Fig. 3** (a Bankart lesion) and **Fig. 10** (a reverse Bankart lesion) highlight the similar but reversed appearance of the posterior instability lesions. An important clinical difference of the posterior HAGL, compared with its anterior counterpart, is the limited clinical significance. Thus, surgical treatment is not necessarily required but may be pursued based on clinical symptoms, rather than MRI findings.[42]

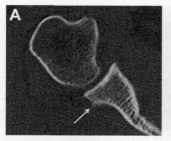 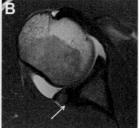 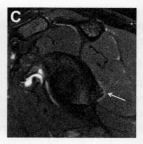

Fig. 11. (*A*) Axial CT of the glenohumeral joint reveals a small extra-articular, periosteal ossification at the posterior scapula near the posterior GHL attachment (*arrow*), consistent with a Bennett lesion. On MRI of a different patient, there is a more pronounced—but more difficult to delineate—osseous prominence at the posteroinferior glenoid at the site of posterior GHL attachment (*arrows*) on both (*B*) axial PD and (*C*) sagittal fat-suppressed T2-weighted images with associated labral hypertrophy and soft tissue, also consistent with a Bennett lesion.

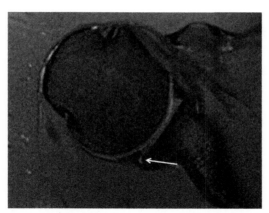

Fig. 12. Axial fat-suppressed PD MR image through the glenohumeral joint reveals a small cleft of fluid beneath the posterior labrum, extending from the chondrolabral junction, without complete detachment (*arrow*), also known as a Kim's lesion.

Two posterior-specific lesions that are seen in posterior glenohumeral instability include the Bennet lesion and Kim's lesion. The first is an extra-articular curvilinear calcification near the attachment of the posterior IGHL at the glenoid (**Fig. 11**), which is associated with posterior labral tear and posterior subluxation of the humeral head.[43] This is attributed to traction of the posterior IGHL and is often associated with pain on palpation and with the cocking phase of overhead throwing.[39] Because small calcifications may be difficult to identify on MRI, CT is considered most sensitive for the detection of these lesions. The Kim's lesion is a soft tissue lesion due to repetitive rim loading, best identified on MRI, defined as a tear, or cleft of fluid, between the posteroinferior labrum and glenoid articular cartilage without a complete detachment of the labrum (**Fig. 12**).[44] This is isolated to the posteroinferior quadrant in posterior instability but may extend through the entire inferior labrum with multidirectional instability (MDI). An accurate imaging diagnosis enables appropriate treatment, helping guide intraoperative identification. Once found, these lesions are treated by

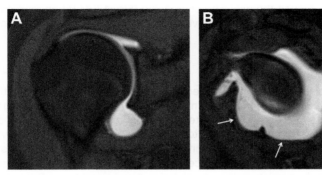

Fig. 13. Coronal (*A*) and Sagittal (*B*) fat-suppressed T1 MR arthrogram images of the glenohumeral joint that reveal a capacious joint capsule (*arrows*) without associated internal derangement, as per congenital laxity and causing symptomatic multidirectional instability in this patient.

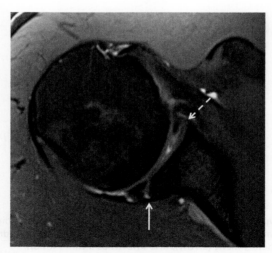

Fig. 14. Axial fat-suppressed PD MR image of the glenohumeral joint with evidence of a Bankart lesion (*dashed arrow*), adjacent chondral irregularity, mild posterior translation of the humeral head, and a tear of the posterior labrum (similar to a Perthes lesion) (*solid arrow*). Cranially (not shown here) were Hill Sachs and reverse Hill Sachs deformities. All these findings are indicative of recurrent post-traumatic multidirectional instability.

conversion to a complete tear, followed by reconstruction of the posterior IGHL attachment.[44]

Multidirectional Instability

MDI requires injury of multiple stabilizers of the shoulder and is generally defined as symptomatic instability in two or more directions.[5,45,46] This may be caused by congenital capsule laxity, microtrauma from overuse, and neuromuscular factors. Some athletes acquire hyperlaxity because of repetitive use during training, such as pitchers and swimmers, and associated pathology, such as rotator cuff impingement, may be seen in some individuals with MDI.[45,46]

Those with congenital laxity resulting in MDI often have little internal derangement. Rather, a patulous joint capsule, best seen on MR arthrogram with distention by intra-articular contrast, maybe the only sign on imaging (**Fig. 13**).[45] When repetitive injury has led to MDI, a combination of the above described anterior and posterior instability injuries may be seen (**Fig. 14**).

SUMMARY

The glenohumeral joint is intrinsically predisposed to instability because of the bony anatomy but maintained in alignment by many important structures, including the glenoid labrum, GHLs, and muscles and tendons. Trauma and overuse can damage these stabilizers, which may then lead to subluxation or dislocation and eventually recurrent instability. This is most common in the anterior direction, which has several recognizable patterns of injury on advanced imaging, including humeral Hill Sachs deformities, bony Bankart lesion of the anteroinferior glenoid, soft tissue Bankart lesions, Bankart variant lesions (Perthes and ALPSA lesions), and HAGL/GAGL lesions. Similar reverse lesions are seen, as well as unique posterior lesions, such as Bennett and Kim's lesions. When symptoms of apprehension and instability in more than one direction are seen, one should consider MDI, which often presents with a patulous joint capsule. Finally, owing to significant impacts of daily activities and quality of life, surgical correction of labral tears, bony Bankart defects, Hill Sachs defects, and capsular laxity, may be considered.

CLINICS CARE POINTS

- Symptoms of pain and apprehension (or joint slipping) must be present with physical examination findings of joint laxity to diagnose recurrent glenohumeral instability.
- Osseous lesions are best depicted on CT imaging, whereas MRI is best for evaluating soft tissue injury because of its superior soft tissue contrast.
- MR arthrography has higher sensitivity and specificity for detecting Bankart and Bankart variant lesions, particularly in the subacute or chronic setting.
- Imaging plays an important role in accurately diagnosing the cause(s) of instability, helping to guide appropriate surgical management.

DISCLOSURES

The authors have nothing to disclose.

REFERENCES

1. Dumont GD, Russell RD, Robertson WJ. Anterior shoulder instability: a review of pathoanatomy, diagnosis and treatment. Curr Rev Musculoskelet Med 2011;4(4): 200–7.
2. Bencardino J, Gyftopoulos S, Palmer W. Imaging in anterior glenohumeral insta-biilty. Radiology 2013;269(2):323–37.
3. Mutlu S, Mahıroğullari M, Güler O, et al. Anterior glenohumeral instability: classi-fication of pathologies of anteroinferior labroligamentous structures using MR ar-thrography. Adv Orthop 2013;2013:1–4.
4. Cameron KL, Mauntel TC, Owens BD. The epidemiology of glenohumeral joint instability: incidence, burden, and long-term consequences. Sports Med Ar-throsc Rev 2017;25(3):144–9.
5. Guerrero P, Busconi B, Deangelis N, et al. Congenital instability of the shoulder joint: assessment and treatment options. J Orthop Sports Phys Ther 2009; 39(2):124–34.
6. Ly JQ, Beall DP, Sanders TG. MR imaging of glenohumeral instability. Am J Roentgenol 2003;181(1):203–13.
7. Kadi R, Milants A, Shahabpour M. Shoulder anatomy and normal variants. J Belg Soc Radiol 2017;101(S2):3.
8. De Coninck T, Ngai SS, Tafur M, et al. Imaging the glenoid labrum and labral tears. RadioGraphics 2016;36(6):1628–47.
9. Burkart AC, Debski RE. Anatomy and function of the glenohumeral ligaments in anterior shoulder instability. Clin Orthop 2002;400:32–9.
10. Beltran J, Bencardino J, Padron M, et al. The middle glenohumeral ligament: normal anatomy, variants and pathology. Skeletal Radiol 2002;31(5):253–62.
11. Farrar NG, Malal JJG, Fischer J, et al. An overview of shoulder instability and its management. Open Orthop J 2013;7:338.
12. Omoumi P. Advanced imaging of glenohumeral instability: it may be less compli-cated than it seems. J Belg Soc Radiol 2016;100(1):97.

13. Harper KW, Helms CA, Haystead CM, et al. Glenoid dysplasia: incidence and association with posterior labral tears as evaluated on MRI. Am J Roentgenol 2005; 184(3):984–8.

14. Mulligan ME, Pontius CS. Posterior-inferior glenoid rim shapes by MR imaging. Surg Radiol Anat 2005;27(4):336–9.

15. Yoon JP, Oh JH, Choi JH, et al. Assessment of capsular insertion type and capsular redundancy in patients with anterior shoulder instability - quantitative assessment with CT arthrography. Arthrosc J Arthrosc Relat Surg 2013;29(10): e42–3.

16. Neumann CH, Petersen SA, Jahnke AH. MR imaging of the labral-capsular complex: normal variations. Am J Roentgenol 1991;157(5):1015–21.

17. Chen Q, Miller T, Padron M, et al. Normal Shoulder. In: Pope T, editor. Musculoskeletal imaging. 2nd edition. Philadelphia, PA: Elsevier Saunders; 2015.

18. Behrang A, Beckmann N, Beaman F, et al. ACR appropriateness criteria: shoulder pain-traumatic. J Am Coll Radiol 2018;15(5S):S171–88.

19. Small K, Adler R, Shah S, et al. ACR Appropriateness Criteria: Shoulder Pain-Atraumatic. J Am Coll Radiol 2018;15(11S):S388–402.

20. Cain EL, Ryan MK. Traumatic instability: treatment options and considerations for recurrent posttraumatic instability. Sports Med Arthrosc Rev 2018;26(3):102–12.

21. Liu F, Cheng X, Dong J, et al. Imaging modality for measuring the presence and extent of the labral lesions of the shoulder: a systematic review and meta-analysis. BMC Musculoskelet Disord 2019;20(1):487.

22. e Souza PM, Brandão BL, Brown E, et al. Recurrent anterior glenohumeral instability: the quantification of glenoid bone loss using magnetic resonance imaging. Skeletal Radiol 2014;43(8):1085–92.

23. Gyftopoulos S, Hasan S, Bencardino J, et al. Diagnostic accuracy of MRI in the measurement of glenoid bone loss. Am J Roentgenol 2012;199(4):873–8.

24. Nofsinger C, Browning B, Burkhart SS, et al. Objective preoperative measurement of anterior glenoid bone loss: a pilot study of a computer-based method using unilateral 3-dimensional computed tomography. Arthrosc J Arthrosc Relat Surg 2011;27(3):322–9.

25. Walter WR, Samim M, LaPolla FWZ, et al. Imaging quantification of glenoid bone loss in patients with glenohumeral instability: a systematic review. Am J Roentgenol 2019;212(5):1096–105.

26. Piasecki DP, Verma NN, Romeo AA, et al. Glenoid bone deficiency in recurrent anterior shoulder instability: diagnosis and management. J Am Acad Orthop Surg 2009;17(8):482–93.

27. Lo IKY, Parten PM, Burkhart SS. The inverted pear glenoid: an indicator of significant glenoid bone loss. Arthrosc J Arthrosc Relat Surg 2004;20(2):169–74.

28. Yiannakopoulos CK, Mataragas E, Antonogiannakis E. A comparison of the spectrum of intra-articular lesions in acute and chronic anterior shoulder instability. Arthrosc J Arthrosc Relat Surg 2007;23(9):985–90.

29. Bankart ASB. Recurrent or habitual dislocation of the shoulder-joint. BMJ 1923; 2(3285):1132–3.

30. Ozbaydar M, Elhassan B, Diller D, et al. Results of arthroscopic capsulolabral repair: bankart lesion versus anterior labroligamentous periosteal sleeve avulsion lesion. Arthrosc J Arthrosc Relat Surg 2008;24(11):1277–83.

31. Wischer TK, Bredella MA, Genant HK, et al. Perthes lesion (A Variant of the Bankart Lesion): MR imaging and MR arthrographic findings with surgical correlation. Am J Roentgenol 2002;178:233–7.

32. Waldt S, Burkart A, Imhoff AB, et al. Anterior shoulder instability: accuracy of MR arthrography in the classification of anteroinferior labroligamentous injuries. Radiology 2005;237(2):578–83.

33. Neviaser TJ. The anterior labroligamentous periosteal sleeve avulsion lesion: A cause of anterior instability of the shoulder. Arthrosc J Arthrosc Relat Surg 1993;9(1):17–21.

34. Sanders TG, Tirman PF, Linares R, et al. The glenolabral articular disruption lesion: MR arthrography with arthroscopic correlation. Am J Roentgenol 1999; 172(1):171–5.

35. Carlson CL. The "J" Sign. Radiology 2004;232(3):725–6.

36. Bigliani LU, Pollock RG, Soslowsky LJ, et al. Tensile properties of the inferior glenohumeral ligament. J Orthop Res 1992;10(2):187–97.

37. Wolf EM, Siparsky PN. Glenoid avulsion of the glenohumeral ligaments as a cause of recurrent anterior shoulder instability. Arthrosc J Arthrosc Relat Surg 2010;26(9):1263–7.

38. Mannem R, DuBois M, Koeberl M, et al. Glenoid avulsion of the glenohumeral ligament (GAGL): a case report and review of the anatomy. Skeletal Radiol 2016; 45(10):1443–8.

39. Shah N, Tung GA. Imaging signs of posterior glenohumeral instability. Am J Roentgenol 2009;192(3):730–5.

40. Tannenbaum E, Sekiya JK. Evaluation and management of posterior shoulder instability. Sports Health Multidiscip Approach 2011;3(3):253–63.

41. Antosh IJ, Tokish JM, Owens BD. Posterior shoulder instability: current surgical management. Sports Health Multidiscip Approach 2016;8(6):520–6.

42. Schoderbek RJ, Diduch D, Hart J, et al. Posterior humeral avulsion of the glenohumeral ligament lesions: correlation between MRI, clinical, and arthroscopic findings. J Arthrosc Relat Surg 2007;23:E4–5.

43. Ferrari JD, Ferrari DA, Coumas J, et al. Posterior ossification of the shoulder: the bennett lesion: etiology, diagnosis, and treatment. Am J Sports Med 1994;22(2): 171–6.

44. Kim S-H. Posterior instability: clinical history, examination, and surgical decision making. In: Shoulder instability: a comprehensive approach. Elsevier; 2012. p. 281–93.

45. Warby SA, Watson L, Ford JJ, et al. Multidirectional instability of the glenohumeral joint: etiology, classification, assessment, and management. J Hand Ther 2017; 30(2):175–81.

46. Saccomanno M, Fodale M, Capasso L, et al. Generalized joint laxity and multidirectional instability of the shoulder. Joints 2013;01(04):171–9.

Imaging of Elbow Injuries

Lindsay Stratchko, DO*, Humberto Rosas, MD

KEYWORDS

- Elbow dislocation • Elbow instability • Throwing injuries • Biceps rupture
- Nerve entrapment • Ulnar collateral ligament (UCL)

KEY POINTS

- The biomechanics in overhead throwing predispose athletes to valgus extension overload syndrome, resulting in a constellation of pathologies including UCL injuries, posteromedial impingement, medial epicondylosis, capitellar osteochondral injuries, and ulnar neuritis.
- Axial loading under valgus stress results in posterolateral rotatory instability, which produces a predictable pattern of elbow injuries and can result in progressive subluxation and dislocation.
- Posteromedial elbow instability (PMRI) results in fracture of the coronoid process anteromedial facet in combination with RCL and UCL tears. PMRI should be suspected when radiographs depict a coronoid process fracture in the absence of radial head abnormalities.

INTRODUCTION

Elbow pain is a common complaint in athletes, particularly those who participate in overhead throwing activities. Traumatic injuries in young patients generally present after high-velocity trauma, whereas elderly patients are susceptible after low-energy mechanisms. Either population is subject to overuse injuries related to occupational, recreational, or athletic activities. A thorough understanding of elbow anatomy and biomechanics aid in the identification of common injury patterns about the elbow.

Relevant Elbow Anatomy

Static and dynamic stabilizers provide support to the elbow joint throughout its range of motion. Static stabilizers consist of the osseous articulations, medial and lateral ligamentous complexes as well as the joint capsule. Muscles and tendons, particularly those that cross the elbow joint, provide dynamic stability to the elbow.

STATIC STABILIZERS

The elbow joint is composed of three articulations: the ulnohumeral, radiocapitellar, and proximal radioulnar joints. The ulnohumeral joint is principally a hinge joint

University of Wisconsin School of Medicine and Public Health, 600 Highland Avenue, Madison, WI 53792, USA
* Corresponding author.
E-mail address: LStratchko@uwhealth.org

Clin Sports Med 40 (2021) 601–623
https://doi.org/10.1016/j.csm.2021.05.002
0278-5919/21/Published by Elsevier Inc.

responsible for flexion and extension of the elbow with a functional range of motion between 30 and 130°. Primary stability is provided by the ulnohumeral joint in extreme flexion and extension (<20° and >120°), whereas soft tissues provide restraint in the interval range of motion.[1] Osseous stability in maximal range of motion is secondary to the conforming articulation between the trochlea of the distal humerus and the trochlear ridge of the olecranon. Joint stability is further strengthened by the configuration of the coronoid and olecranon processes, which inhibit subluxation of the elbow by engaging their corresponding fossae during full flexion and extension, respectively.[2,3]

The radiocapitellar joint is a pivot joint that allows pronation and supination of the forearm of approximately 50° in either direction during normal activities. There is a horizontal groove superior to the capitellum known as the radial fossa that accepts the radial head during elbow flexion, providing additional static stability.[4]

The proximal radioulnar joint is composed of the peripheral margin of the radial head and the semilunar notch of the proximal ulna, which is located distal and lateral to the coronoid process. The annular ligament attaches along the anterior and posterior margins of the semilunar notch providing circumferential restraint of the radial head.

The lateral collateral ligament (LCL) complex consists of the annular ligament (described earlier), radial collateral ligament (RCL) as well as the lateral ulnar collateral ligament (LUCL) (**Fig. 1**). The RCL originates from the lateral epicondyle (LE) of the

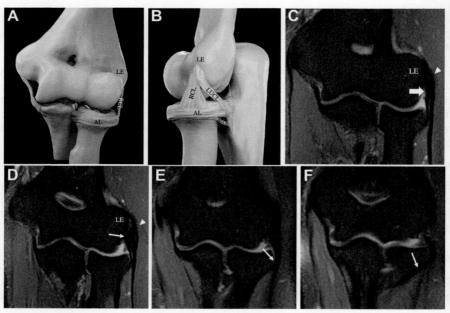

Fig. 1. Frontal (A) and lateral (B) illustrations of the lateral ligamentous complex show the annular ligament (AL) encircling the radial head and attaching to the margins of the lesser sigmoid notch. The RCL extends from the LE to the annular ligament. The LUCL extends from the LE to the supinator crest of the proximal ulna. The accessory lateral collateral ligament attaches to the supinator crest as well as the annular ligament. Coronal PD FS images (C–F) demonstrate the course of the common extensor tendon (*arrowhead*) superficial to the RCL (*thick arrow*) and LUCL (*thin arrow*). Note that the origin of the LUCL is thicker in comparison to the RCL and more posteriorly positioned. ([A, B] *Courtesy of* Aydin Rosas.)

humerus, forming a fan-shape as it blends with the annular ligament distally. The LUCL also arises from the LE, posterior to the RCL origin, inserting upon the supinator crest of the proximal ulna just distal to the annular ligament (see **Fig. 1**). The LUCL provides primary joint stability in varus stress and supination of the forearm.[5]

Three distinct bands form the medial collateral ligament complex, which provide resistance during valgus stress and inhibit posteromedial rotatory instability (**Fig. 2**). The anterior band of the ulnar collateral ligament (UCL) extends from the inferior aspect of the medial epicondyle to the sublime tubercle and UCL ridge of the proximal ulna.[6] Functionally, the anterior band consists of anterior and posterior portions that engage in extension and flexion, respectively; however, these components are not distinguishable on imaging. The anterior band is the strongest component of the UCL, playing the greatest role in valgus stability of the elbow between 30 and 120° of flexion.[7,8] The posterior band of the UCL forms a broad insertion at the medial olecranon, creating the floor of the cubital tunnel. Lastly, the transverse band extends from

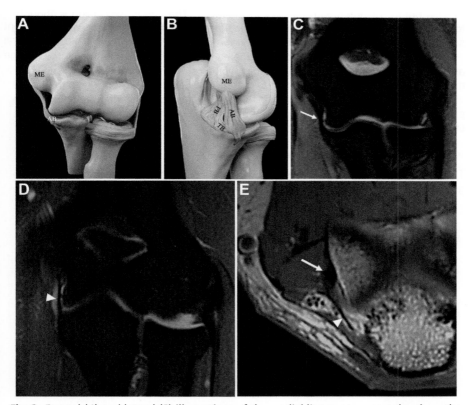

Fig. 2. Frontal (*A*) and lateral (*B*) illustrations of the medial ligamentous complex show the three components of the ulnar collateral ligament, including the anterior bundle (AB), which extends from the medial epicondyle (ME) to the sublime tubercle and ulnar ridge. The posterior bundle (PB) of the UCL forms the floor of the cubital tunnel by attaching to the medial epicondyle as well as the semilunar notch of the ulna. The transverse bundle (TB) travels along the semilunar notch. Coronal PD FS (*C, D*) and axial T1 (*E*) images show the anterior bundle (*arrow*) and posterior bundle (*arrowhead*) of the UCL. ([*A, B*] *Courtesy of* Aydin Rosas.)

the medial olecranon to the coronoid process and has minimal contribution to joint stability.

DYNAMIC STABILIZERS

The biceps brachii muscle consists of short and long heads. Proximal to the elbow joint, an aponeurosis known as the lacertus fibrosus originates from the myotendinous junction to incorporate with the proximal ulna and fascia overlying the flexor muscles (**Fig. 3**).[9] The lacertus fibrosus functions to protect the underlying brachial artery and median nerve, stabilize and augment the function of the biceps tendon, and limit the degree of tendon retraction in the event of complete rupture.[10]

The distal triceps tendon is composed of the long, lateral, and medial heads, which form superficial and deep layers at the olecranon insertion (**Fig. 4**). The deep layer consists of the muscular portion of the medial head with a short medial head tendon. The superficial layer is composed of the long and lateral heads, which form a combined central tendon as well as a broad lateral expansion that extends over the anconeus muscle before blending with the forearm fascia.[11] The lateral expansion is thought to be functionally analogous to the lacertus fibrosus, limiting retraction and providing some elbow extension in the setting of tendon rupture.[12]

The flexor-pronator muscle group originates from the medial epicondyle and plays an important role in dynamic stability during valgus stress while the extensor-supinator muscle groups arise at and adjacent to the LE, providing active support to the lateral elbow. The anconeus muscle also originates from the LE posteriorly, inserting at the posterior surface of the ulna. The anconeus muscle is a primary stabilizer during varus stress, inhibiting posterolateral rotatory instability.[5]

Valgus Extension Overload Syndrome

The late cocking and early acceleration phases of overhead throwing produce the greatest degree of valgus stress on the elbow. Repeated throwing results in tensile

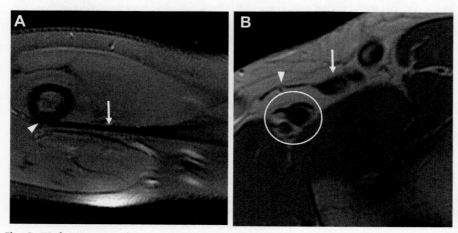

Fig. 3. T2 fat-suppressed image (*A*) in elbow flexion, abduction and forearm supination (FABS position) shows the entire distal biceps tendon (*arrow*) from the myotendinous junction to the radial tuberosity (*arrowhead*). Axial PD image above the level of the elbow joint (*B*) demonstrates the thin lacertus fibrosus (*arrowhead*) extending from the distal biceps tendon (*arrow*) medially over the brachial artery and median nerve (*circle*).

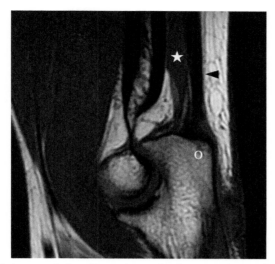

Fig. 4. Sagittal PD image of the elbow shows the low signal superficial triceps tendon (*arrowhead*), which is composed of the long and lateral heads and inserts distally at the olecranon (*O*). The medial head muscle (*star*) is seen deep to the superficial tendon.

force across the medial elbow, compression of the radiocapitellar joint, and shear stress of the posterior compartment.[13,14] Understanding the biomechanics of overhead throwing and the various forces on the static and dynamic stabilizers help characterize the injuries seen in valgus extension overload syndrome.

ULNAR COLLATERAL LIGAMENT INJURY

Repetitive tension on the UCL during overhead throwing causes inflammation, accelerated laxity, and eventual tearing of the anterior band. If osseous failure precedes ligamentous deficiency, an avulsion fracture of the sublime tubercle occurs. Low-grade sprains are characterized by intact ligament fibers surrounded by periligamentous edema. Computed tomography (CT) or MRI arthrography are reported to have higher sensitivity in detecting partial UCL tears compared with unenhanced MRI.[13] Partial fiber disruption and extension of intra-articular contrast into the substance of the UCL are diagnostic of partial tear, whereas ligament discontinuity, retraction, and extra-articular contrast spread at arthrography are consistent with complete tear. Partial UCL tears involving the undersurface fibers have a typical appearance of fluid or contrast interposed between the ligament and sublime tubercle, known as the "T-sign." It is important to evaluate the ligament fibers and surrounding soft tissues for evidence of injury rather than solely relying on the distance of the "T-sign" as normal UCL insertions can extend 3 to 4 mm beyond the articular cartilage (**Fig. 5**).[15] Heterotopic ossification is a secondary sign of UCL injury with approximately 75% of patients with ligamentous ossification demonstrating partial or complete tear at surgery.[16]

Ultrasound can aid in diagnosing UCL injury by the presence of UCL thickening, discontinuity, absence, or laxity during valgus stress; however, it is important to note that asymmetry in UCL thickness, appearance, and laxity has been noted in asymptomatic pitchers.[17,18] UCL thickness was found to be greater in asymptomatic dominant arms (6.2 vs 4.8 mm) and had higher incidences of hypoechoic foci and

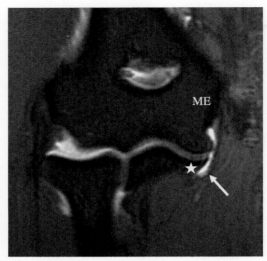

Fig. 5. Coronal T1 fat-suppressed arthrogram image shows contrast extension deep to the ulnar collateral ligament (*arrow*) along the sublime tubercle (*star*) consistent with a partial tear, which is also known as the "T-sign."

calcifications compared with nondominant arms (**Fig. 6**).[17] Dynamic ultrasound has a reported 96% sensitivity and 81% specificity in detecting UCL tear when relative medial joint gapping is greater than 1 mm compared with the contralateral arm. In addition, mean increase in joint gapping by 3.3 mm has been shown to correlate with full-thickness UCL tears.[19]

POSTEROMEDIAL IMPINGEMENT

Progressive UCL incompetence results in alteration of elbow contact area, increasing force on the posteromedial elbow joint causing localized joint degeneration, osteophyte formation, and synovitis.[20] Prolonged impingement and inflammation can lead to intra-articular body formation and mechanical symptoms. MRI is helpful in localizing cartilage degeneration or osteochondral injury in characteristic locations including the medial crista of the posterior trochlea and the medial olecranon fossa.[21] Additional findings associated with chondral wear are illustrated on MRI including osteophytosis, subchondral edema, sclerosis, and cystic change.[13] In the absence of a joint effusion, MR arthrography can help detect intra-articular bodies.

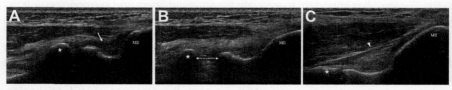

Fig. 6. Long axis image of the ulnotrochlear joint (*A*) demonstrates a redundant hypoechoic ulnar collateral ligament (*arrow*) that no longer attaches to the sublime tubercle (*star*). Valgus stress image (*B*) shows abnormal widening of the joint space (*dotted arrow*), which is a sign of UCL incompetence. Comparison long axis image (*C*) depicts an intact UCL (*arrowhead*).

FLEXOR-PRONATOR MASS INJURIES/MEDIAL EPICONDYLOSIS

Valgus stress during the early acceleration phase of throwing is dynamically opposed by the common flexor-pronator tendon. Acute or chronic tears, medial epicondyle avulsion fractures, as well as tendinopathy from repetitive overuse can result in medial elbow pain. MRI is a useful tool in distinguishing the etiology of medial elbow pain in throwing athletes as there is often overlap in symptoms. Tendinopathy (also referred to as medial epicondylosis) is depicted as thickening and intermediate signal within the common flexor tendon. Tendon tears are seen as fluid-signal on T2-weighted sequences within or traversing the tendon fibers and reactive edema can be present in the adjacent soft tissues (**Fig. 7**).

MEDIAL EPICONDYLE APOPHYSITIS

The medial epicondyle apophysis begins ossification at the age of 5 to 6 years and is typically the last to fuse at age 15 to 16 years. The early and late cocking phases of throwing produce significant compression on the lateral aspect of the elbow while distracting the medial structures, resulting in excessive tension on the immature medial epicondyle apophysis.[22] Patient age and skeletal maturity determines the radiographic and MRI findings encountered in valgus overload in the pediatric population. The apophysis is weakest during childhood and is prone to injury such as fragmentation or displacement. As children mature and the apophysis strengthens, avulsion fractures are common due to failure of the physeal cartilage. After skeletal maturity, UCL and flexor-pronator mass injuries predominate as elbow biomechanics more closely reflect those of the adult population.

Radiographs are often normal early in the pediatric throwing athlete presenting with elbow pain. Apophyseal displacement, fragmentation, and overgrowth can develop over time if repetitive trauma persists.[23] MRI may demonstrate bone marrow edema within the apophysis as well as widening and hyperintense signal of the physis on fluid-sensitive sequences. Increased signal and thickening of the common flexor tendon can accompany osseous changes of the medial epicondyle apophysis in keeping with the spectrum of medial elbow injuries encountered in valgus extension overload (**Fig. 8**).[24]

LATERAL RADIOCAPITELLAR COMPRESSION

Repeated compression of the lateral compartment of the elbow can lead to osteochondral injury involving the radiocapitellar joint. Although the exact etiology of

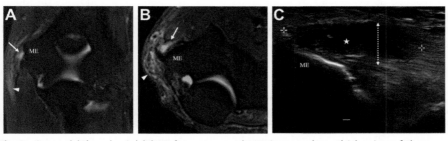

Fig. 7. Coronal (A) and axial (B) T2 fat-suppressed MRI images show thickening of the common flexor tendon with a fluid-signal intrasubstance tear (*arrow*) and superficial subcutaneous edema (*arrowhead*). Long axis ultrasound (C) image similarly demonstrates thickening (*dotted arrow*) and hypoechogenicity of the common flexor tendon origin with focal disruption of the superficial fibers (*star*).

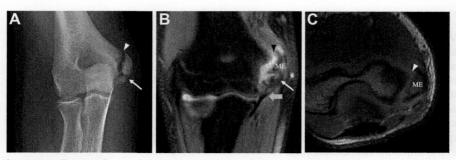

Fig. 8. AP elbow radiograph (*A*) and coronal T2 fat-suppressed MRI image (*B*) show fragmentation of the medial epicondyle apophysis (*arrow*) and widening of the physis (*arrowhead*). There is a fluid signal in the physis as well as marrow edema in the apophysis. The proximal attachment of the UCL is thickened and increased in signal compatible with partial tear (*thick arrow*). Axial PD image (*C*) demonstrates widening of the medial epicondyle physis (*arrowhead*).

capitellar osteochondritis dissecans (OCD) is unknown, it is a well-established injury pattern in adolescent overhead athletes. A detailed knowledge of elbow anatomy helps distinguish true pathology from normal osteochondral anatomy. For example, a pseudodefect of the capitellum has been well described of the articular cartilage along the posterolateral margin of the capitellum. This normal finding lacks underlying marrow edema or subchondral abnormalities and should not be mistaken for OCD.[25] In contrast, OCD involves the anterolateral capitellum and radiographs may show subtle subchondral lucency before the development of variable degrees of sclerosis, articular surface flattening, or fragmentation.[24] On T2-weighted MRI, a double-line sign consisting of a hyperintense inner line bordered by a hypointense rim of sclerosis denotes areas of osteonecrosis. Additional findings of OCD include cartilage defects, bone marrow abnormalities, cyst formation, subchondral flattening, fragmentation, and development of intra-articular bodies. Signs of lesion instability are associated with greater likelihood of nonoperative failure and include displacement, fluid, or contrast undermining the osteochondral fragment, and adjacent cyst formation (**Fig. 9**).[24,26]

Capitellar OCD must be distinguished from Panner disease as management and prognosis differ. Panner disease affects a younger age group (less than 10 years old) and is a self-limiting process. There is more diffuse capitellar involvement in Panner disease as evidenced by large areas of patchy sclerosis and lucency on radiographs and bone marrow edema on MRI (**Fig. 10**). Capitellar morphology is maintained and imaging findings typically normalize in 1 to 2 years without the need for surgical intervention.[27]

ULNAR NEURITIS

Traction of the ulnar nerve within the confines of the cubital tunnel during valgus stress predisposes it to injury, particularly if there is a failure of static restraint by the UCL. Posteromedial osteophyte formation can also result in extrinsic compression of the ulnar nerve. MRI and ultrasound are helpful in the evaluation of ulnar nerve course and caliber. Cross-sectional area of 0.08 cm^2 has an established 95% sensitivity and 80% specificity for detecting ulnar neuropathy. In addition, obliteration of perineural fat can be seen in combination with focal or diffuse nerve enlargement (**Fig. 11**). Subtle increase in ulnar nerve signal on fluid-sensitive MR sequences can be challenging to

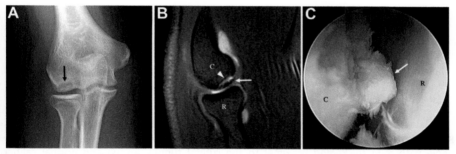

Fig. 9. AP elbow radiograph (*A*) shows subchondral lucency of the capitellum (*arrow*), cor-responding to an osteochondral lesion (*arrow*) on T2 fat-suppressed MRI (*B*). There is a fluid signal undermining the defect (*arrowhead*) suggesting instability, which was confirmed at arthroscopy (*C*) where a mobile osteochondral fragment was seen (*arrow*).

detect; however, the use of short-tau inversion recovery images or high spatial reso-lution neurography can provide a more accurate evaluation of the ulnar nerve.[28] Of note, increased ulnar nerve signal in isolation can be seen in asymptomatic individuals.[29]

Repetitive Trauma and Tendon Disorders

Overuse, improper mechanics, and direct injury can result in tendon injury about the elbow. Often, localized pain and weakness on physical examination is diagnostic, but imaging plays a role for potential surgical candidates as well as problem-solving in patients with refractory pain.

LATERAL EPICONDYLOSIS

Lateral epicondylosis (also known as tennis elbow) is the most common cause of elbow pain in the adult. During repetitive wrist extension, macroscopic or microscopic injury of the common extensor tendon occurs with subsequent incomplete healing and

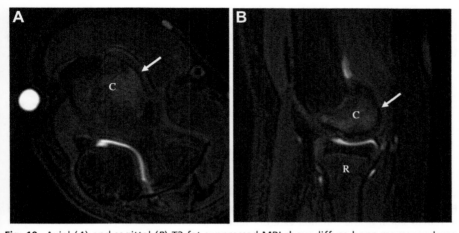

Fig. 10. Axial (*A*) and sagittal (*B*) T2 fat-suppressed MRI show diffuse bone marrow edema of the capitellum (*arrow*) without focal cartilage defect or fracture. Findings resolved on follow-up MRI 1 year later and are compatible with Panner disease.

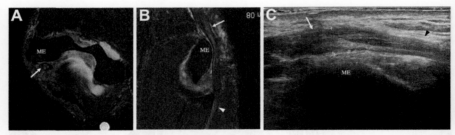

Fig. 11. Axial (*A*) and sagittal (*B*) T2 fat-suppressed MRI show increased signal of the ulnar nerve with mild thickening proximal to the cubital tunnel (*arrow*) and normal caliber distally (*arrowhead*). Long axis ultrasound (*C*) of the ulnar nerve at the cubital tunnel demonstrates thickening of the ulnar nerve proximal to the cubital tunnel (*arrow*) with normalization of caliber distally (*arrowhead*).

pain.[30] At ultrasound, typical appearance of LE is a focal hypoechoic region within the deep fibers of the thickened common extensor tendon corresponding to areas of collagen degeneration and fibroblast proliferation.[31] Similarly, MRI demonstrates thickening and increased T1-signal and T2-signal of the common extensor tendon. Fluid-signal on T2-weighted images within the common extensor tendon fibers corresponds with areas of tendon tears (**Fig. 12**). Bone marrow edema within the LE and increased signal on fluid-sensitive MRI sequences within the anconeus are secondary signs of LE on MRI.[32] Evaluation of the underlying LCL complex is necessary for patients with lateral epicondylosis as one study showed that 73% of patients with moderate and 100% of patients with severe LE were found to have LCL complex abnormalities.[33]

BICEPS TENDON

Distal tears of the biceps brachii tendon occur far less frequently than proximal tendon abnormalities, accounting for approximately 3% of all biceps tendon injuries.[34] Complete biceps tendon rupture often occurs as a result of forced extension of a flexed elbow. On examination, there is a palpable defect in the antecubital fossa accompanied by varying degrees of tendon retraction, often depending on the integrity of the lacertus fibrosus. At MRI, distal tendon disruption is accompanied by a fluid-filled tendon gap as well as increased signal intensity within the distal biceps muscle,

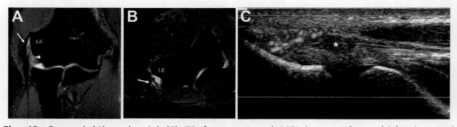

Fig. 12. Coronal (*A*) and axial (*B*) T2 fat-suppressed MRI images show thickening and increased signal of the common extensor tendon (*arrow*) as well as tear of the underlying RCL and LUCL (*arrowhead*). Long axis ultrasound (*C*) demonstrates thickening and decreased echogenicity (*star*) of the common extensor tendon with marked hyperemia on Power Doppler.

tendon, and adjacent soft tissues.[35] Sonographic evaluation of the distal biceps tendon can pose challenges due to anisotropy at the radial tuberosity, which can be corrected by imaging in the longitudinal plane or toggling the transducer over the tendon insertion (**Fig. 13**).[18] Posterior acoustic shadowing is a useful secondary sign to identify complete distal biceps tendon rupture.[36]

Partial biceps tendon rupture can pose diagnostic challenges on physical examination, requiring imaging to determine the location and severity of tendon involvement. Increased intratendinous signal accompanied by thinning or thickening of the distal tendon are common in partial biceps tendon rupture.[35] Secondary signs of partial tears include bicipitoradial bursitis as well as bone marrow edema within the radial tuberosity, seen in approximately 50% of cases.[34] The short and long heads of the distal biceps tendon are close to one another; however, have separate footprints at the radial tuberosity.[37] The short head is larger, superficial, and has a more ovoid footprint distally, whereas the long head is smaller, deeper, and along the proximal aspect of the tuberosity.[38] Given the anatomy of the distal biceps tendon with separate insertions of the short and long heads, it is crucial to differentiate an isolated rupture of the short or long head tendon from a partial rupture as the former may benefit from operative intervention while the latter is commonly managed conservatively (**Fig. 14**).[39]

TRICEPS TENDON

Triceps tendon ruptures are rare and often occur after inciting trauma such as a fall on an outstretched hand, direct blow, or forced eccentric contraction. Local and systemic factors may weaken the triceps tendon, predisposing it to injury with minimal force.[40] MRI or ultrasound can be used to differentiate complete versus partial distal triceps tendon rupture. Complete ruptures are far less common (less than 1%) than partial triceps tendon rupture.[12] Complete rupture frequently occurs at the olecranon process insertion site and radiographs can aid in the detection of distal triceps tendon rupture by the presence of an avulsed fracture fragment or enthesophyte. Sagittal MRI images are useful in identifying the torn tendon defect, degree of retraction, as well as osseous avulsion fragments (**Fig. 15**). In the acute setting, edema and hemorrhage is seen within the triceps muscle bellies as well as the posterior elbow soft tissues.

Instability

Posterolateral rotatory instability
Posterolateral rotatory instability (PLRI) results from axial loading in the setting of valgus force and supination of the forearm. This mechanism produces a characteristic pattern of capsuloligamentous injuries, progressing from lateral to medial, termed the "circle of Horii." Stage I involves isolated LUCL tear, allowing posterolateral subluxation of the radial head. Progression of injury leads to disruption of the anterior and posterior joint capsule as well as the RCL complex (stage II). Lastly, the medial aspect of the elbow is affected with injury to the posterior band of the UCL (stage IIIA) followed by the anterior band (stage IIIB). A stage IIIC injury involves complete soft tissue stripping from the humerus with marked elbow instability (**Fig. 16**).[41] The constellation of injuries result in progressive posterior subluxation and eventual dislocation of the elbow with maintenance of the proximal radioulnar joint. In addition to the ligamentous and capsular deficiencies described, MRI can detect osteochondral impaction injuries involving the posterolateral capitellum known as the Osborne-Cotterill lesion in the setting of PLRI.[42] Radiographically, radial head subluxation, coronoid tip fractures, impaction fractures of the capitellum, and widening of the ulnohumeral distance (greater than 4 mm, known as the "drop sign") are indications of elbow instability.[43]

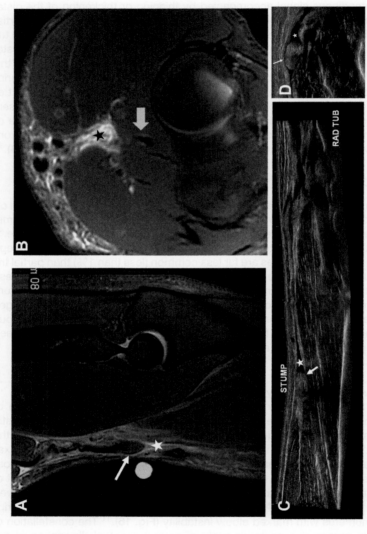

Fig. 13. Sagittal T2 fat-suppressed MRI (*A*) shows complete rupture of the distal biceps tendon with redundancy of the retracted tendon (*arrow*) and a fluid-filled tendon gap (*star*). Axial T2 fat-suppressed image (*B*) distal to the elbow joint demonstrates a fluid-filled tendon gap (*star*) superficial to the brachialis tendon (*thick arrow*). Long axis ultrasound image (*C*) shows the distal biceps tendon gap and short-axis image (*D*) shows fluid (*star*) surrounding the retracted tendon stump (*arrow*).

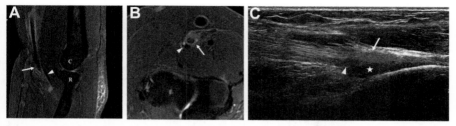

Fig. 14. Sagittal T2 fat-suppressed MRI (*A*) shows a torn and retracted short head biceps tendon (*arrow*) overlying an intact long head tendon (*arrowhead*). Axial T2 fat-suppressed MRI (*B*) shows thickening and increased signal of the superficial short head tendon (*arrow*) with normal long head tendon (*arrowhead*). Companion case with long axis (*C*) ultrasound image of the distal biceps tendon showing an intact short head tendon distally (*arrow*) and a torn and partially retracted long head tendon proximally (*arrowhead*) with a small tendon gap (*star*).

Posteromedial rotatory instability

Axial compression in combination with varus force and forearm pronation causes the spectrum of injuries seen in posteromedial rotatory instability (PMRI). PMRI results in anteromedial coronoid facet fracture, LCL injury, and tear of the posterior band of the MCL (**Fig. 17**). These injuries produce abnormally increased contact pressures often requiring fracture fixation and LCL repair to restore normal kinematics.[44] In patients after elbow dislocation, PMRI should be suspected when radiographs depict coronoid fracture in the absence of radial head trauma. MRI characterizes ligamentous abnormalities with LCL tears often occurring proximally while the location of MCL injuries are less predictable. Owing to the varus stress produced in PMRI, common extensor tendon tears are seen in approximately 70% of patients.[45]

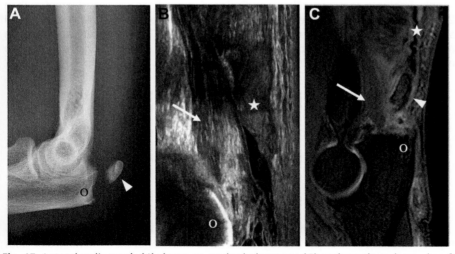

Fig. 15. Lateral radiograph (*A*) shows an avulsed olecranon (*O*) enthesophyte (*arrowhead*) attached to the superficial long and lateral head tendons (*star*), which are seen on long axis ultrasound (*B*) and sagittal MRI (*C*) images. Note the intact medial head muscle (*arrow*) fibers deep to the torn superficial tendons.

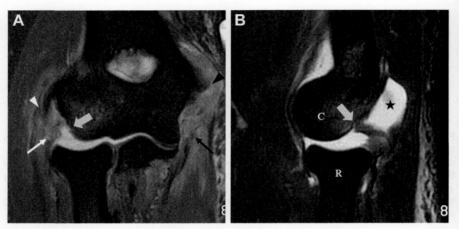

Fig. 16. Coronal PD FS (*A*) and sagittal T2 FS (*B*) images show stage IIIC PLRI injury with complete tears of the RCL and LUCL (*thin white arrow*) and rupture of the overlying common extensor tendon (*white arrowhead*). Medially, there is a complete tear of the anterior bundle of the UCL (*black arrow*) as well as rupture of the common flexor tendon (*black arrowhead*). There is an impaction fracture of the posterolateral capitellum (*thick white arrow*), known as an Osborne-Cotterill lesion, with adjacent bone marrow edema as well as a moderate joint effusion (*star*).

Fractures and Dislocations

Radial head and neck fractures

Radial head and neck fractures are the most common elbow fracture and typically result after a fall on an outstretched hand. Although several classification systems have been described, the Mason system is generally used and includes fracture comminution, displacement, and presence of dislocation. Type I and II fractures are simple fractures that are either nondisplaced (type I) or displaced greater than 2 mm (type II). These fractures are often managed nonoperatively unless mechanical symptoms accompany displacement in type II fractures. Type III radial head fractures are comminuted and displaced and frequently present with a mechanical block to movement, requiring fixation to restore unobstructed range of motion. Type IV

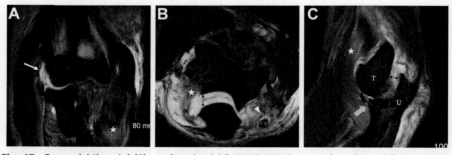

Fig. 17. Coronal (*A*), axial (*B*), and sagittal (*C*) T2 FS MRI images show lateral ligamentous injury with torn RCL and LUCL (*thin arrow*), injury to the posterior bundle of the UCL (*arrowhead*), muscular strain (*star*), and an anteromedial coronoid facet fracture (*thick arrow*). This constellation of injuries result in posterior subluxation and asymmetric widening of the posterior ulnotrochlear joint (*dotted line*).

fractures have associated elbow dislocation (**Fig. 18**).[46] Radiographs are useful in identifying radial head and neck fractures as well as joint effusions in the setting of subtle, nondisplaced fractures. MRI is useful in detecting radiographically occult fractures in adult patients with elbow effusion after trauma as well as additional fractures or ligamentous injuries.[47]

Ulnar and coronoid fractures

Different forces on the olecranon result in distinct fracture types. Triceps traction during throw deceleration or eccentric contraction characteristically produces transverse fractures. Repetitive contact with the olecranon fossa in valgus extension leads to oblique fractures while direct blow injuries typically cause comminuted olecranon fractures (**Fig. 19**). Identification of the degree of comminution and displacement is crucial because plate and screw fixation is required with comminuted fractures while tension bands or intramedullary fixation are preferred without comminution.[48] Nonoperative management is usually trialed in nondisplaced fractures or low-demand patients.

The coronoid process plays an important role in elbow stability, resisting posterior translation of the ulna. Loss of coronoid height is associated with instability and recurrent elbow dislocations.[49] Initially, Regan and Morrey classified coronoid fractures based on involvement in the horizontal plane: type I involved the tip, type II included 50% or less of the coronoid process height, and type III affected greater than 50% (**Fig. 20**).[50] More recently, the O'Driscoll system subdivides fractures according to location and number of fragments with an emphasis on the anteromedial facet and its known role in varus stability.[51] In addition, the anterior band of the UCL attaches to the anterior aspect of the sublime tubercle and functions to resist valgus force, which may be compromised in coronoid fractures. Type 1 fractures involve the coronoid tip; subtype 1 are less than 2 mm and subtype 2 are greater than 2 mm. The subtype 2 fractures typically involve the anterior joint capsule insertion and are often seen in terrible triad injuries (see below). Type 2 fractures include the anteromedial facet; subtype 1 involves the anterior half of the sublime tubercle (including the UCL anterior band insertion), subtype 2 extends into the tip, and subtype 3 comprises the entire sublime tubercle. Type 3 fractures involve the coronoid base in isolation (subtype 1)

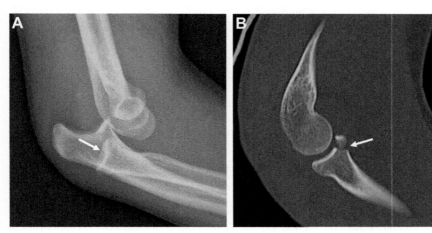

Fig. 18. Lateral radiograph (A) shows a posterior elbow dislocation. The intra-articular radial head fracture (*arrow*) is better demonstrated on postreduction CT (B).

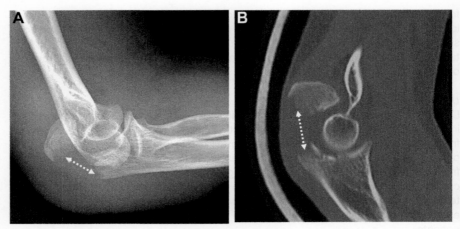

Fig. 19. Lateral radiograph (*A*) and sagittal CT (*B*) show an intra-articular olecranon fracture with significant displacement (*dotted line*) of the fracture fragments.

or occur with olecranon fractures (subtype 2).[52] Cross-sectional imaging plays a role in detailing anatomic involvement as well as defining associated capsuloligamentous injuries to help guide treatment.

Dislocations
Elbow dislocations are classified as either complex or simple based on the presence or absence of an associated fracture, respectively. Dislocations are named according to the direction of the olecranon in relation to the distal humerus or termed divergent when the distal humerus is interposed between the radius and ulna, forcing them in opposite directions.[53] The terrible triad injury is defined as a posterior elbow dislocation in combination with radial head and coronoid process fractures and is associated with extensive ligamentous injury (**Fig. 21**). The term terrible triad originated from the

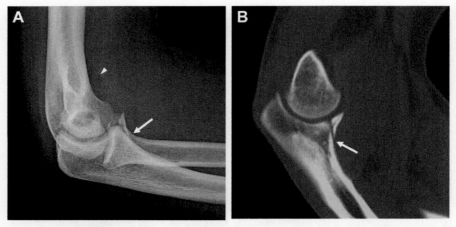

Fig. 20. Lateral radiograph (*A*) and sagittal CT (*B*) show a nondisplaced coronoid process fracture (*arrow*) involving less than 50% of the coronoid process height. There is an associated elbow joint effusion (*arrowhead*).

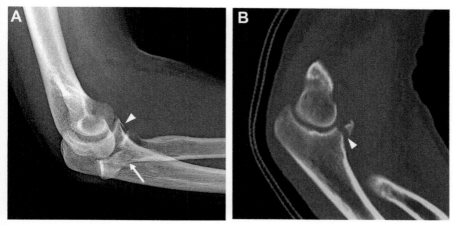

Fig. 21. Lateral radiograph (*A*) after reduction of posterior elbow dislocation shows a comminuted and impacted radial head fracture (*arrow*) as well as a minimally displaced fracture of the coronoid tip (*arrowhead*), which is confirmed on sagittal (*B*) CT image.

significant disability associated with this injury complex and the individual injuries must be taken into consideration during management.[54] CT often complements radiographs to aid in operative planning, allowing characterization of fracture patterns, degree of comminution and displacement, as well as identification of intra-articular fragments.

Radiohumeral Plica Syndrome

Plicae, or intra-articular synovial folds, are septal remnants resulting from synovial membrane development during the embryonal period. Although variably present and often asymptomatic, impingement of synovial folds may result in hypertrophy, inflammation, and chondral injury leading to pain and mechanical symptoms.[55] The radiohumeral plica is located along the proximal aspect of the annular ligament and may interpose between the radial head and the capitellum. Different portions of the radiohumeral plica are named for their anatomic location, including the anterior, lateral, posterolateral, and lateral olecranon folds (**Fig. 22**). The incidence of plicae in asymptomatic individuals range from 33% to 98% depending on location with the posterolateral plica being the most common. Thickness of synovial folds in asymptomatic individuals are often less than 2 mm, whereas those with mechanical symptoms average greater than 3 mm.[56,57]

Nerve Entrapment Syndromes

Ulnar nerve

Cubital tunnel syndrome is the second most common entrapment neuropathy of the upper extremity, after carpal tunnel syndrome. Symptoms include ring and small finger paresthesias as well as clawing in chronic cases. Repeated elbow flexion and ulnar nerve hypermobility are risk factors for ulnar neuropathy. Although the cubital tunnel is the most common location of nerve compression, the ulnar nerve may become confined at the arcade of Struthers (between the medial intermuscular septum to the medial head of the triceps), medial epicondyle, between the two heads of the flexor carpi ulnaris, or the deep flexor/pronator aponeurosis. Anatomic variations can play a role in ulnar neuropathy, including a thickened cubital tunnel retinaculum, anconeus epitrochlearis, and low-lying triceps medial head.[13] MRI and ultrasound depict ulnar

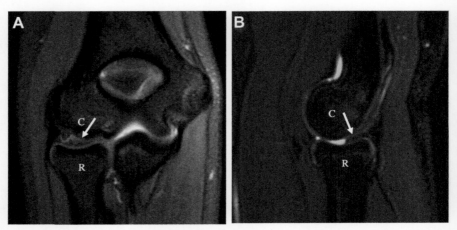

Fig. 22. Coronal (*A*) and sagittal (*B*) T2 fat-suppressed MRI images show an elongated and mildly thickened posterolateral synovial fold (*arrow*) that extends into the radiocapitellar joint.

nerve course and enlargement. MRI is helpful in identifying increased signal of the ulnar nerve as well as denervation edema or atrophy within the flexor carpi ulnaris and medial half of the flexor digitorum profundus muscles (**Fig. 23**). Ultrasound can dynamically reproduce ulnar nerve dislocation during flexion, which must be differentiated from snapping medial triceps that occurs during resisted extension.[58]

Median nerve
Pronator syndrome is caused by compression of the median nerve at the level of the elbow. The median nerve accompanies the brachial artery along the anterior

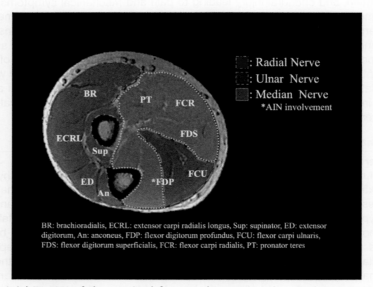

BR: brachioradialis, ECRL: extensor carpi radialis longus, Sup: supinator, ED: extensor digitorum, An: anconeus, FDP: flexor digitorum profundus, FCU: flexor carpi ulnaris, FDS: flexor digitorum superficialis, FCR: flexor carpi radialis, PT: pronator teres

Fig. 23. Axial T1 MRI of the proximal forearm shows motor innervation patterns of the radial, ulnar, and median nerves.

compartment of the arm. Known locations of entrapment include a supracondylar process, ligament of Struthers (from the supracondylar process to the medial epicondyle), lacertus fibrosus, between the heads of the pronator teres, and the flexor digitorum superficialis aponeurosis. Symptoms of pronator syndrome commonly overlap with carpal tunnel syndrome with differentiating features indicating more proximal compression such as forearm pain and positive Tinel sign at the proximal forearm.[58] Radiographs should be the initial imaging modality to evaluate patients with pronator syndrome to identify the presence of a supracondylar process. MRI may show denervation muscle changes in the anterior compartment of the forearm, excluding the flexor carpi ulnaris and medial half of the flexor digitorum profundus, which are innervated by the ulnar nerve.[59]

The anterior interosseous nerve (AIN) is a motor branch of the median nerve that arises approximately 5 cm distal to the elbow joint. The AIN passes between the two heads of the pronator teres before traveling distally along the volar margin of the interosseous membrane. Motor innervation is supplied to the deep forearm compartment including the pronator quadratus, flexor pollicus longus (FPL), and the radial half of the flexor digitorum profundus (FDP). Nerve entrapment resulting in AIN syndrome can be secondary to extrinsic compression, trauma from venous puncture, radial diaphysis fracture, weightlifting, and Gantzer muscle (an accessory head of the flexor pollicis longus muscle). Patients with AIN syndrome develop grip weakness due to flexor digitorum profundus and flexor pollicis longus paralysis.[59] Diffuse edema within the pronator quadratus muscle is the most predictable sign of AIN syndrome. MRI can also confirm integrity of the FPL and FDP tendons as tears can mimic AIN syndrome.[60]

Radial nerve

Posterior interosseous nerve (PIN) syndrome results from compression of the PIN, the deep motor branch of the radial nerve. Locations of compression include the radial tunnel, Leash of Henry (recurrent radial vessels that cross the PIN), extensor carpi radialis brevis tendon, the Arcade of Frohse (fibrous arch proximal to the supinator muscle), and the distal aspect of the supinator muscle.[58] PIN syndrome can result from overuse, trauma, mass-occupying lesions, or inflammatory processes. The course of the PIN directly superficial to the radial neck leaves it vulnerable to injury in the event of proximal radial fractures. Symptoms of PIN syndrome include pain as well as weakness with wrist extension due to PIN innervation of the common and deep extensors of the forearm (**Fig. 24**). PIN syndrome is often diagnosed clinically without the need for

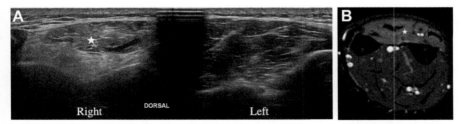

Fig. 24. Short axis ultrasound image at the dorsal forearm (*A*) shows volume loss and fatty replacement (*star*) of the right extensor compartment compatible with denervation changes in a posterior interosseous nerve distribution. Note normal volume and echogenicity of the contralateral asymptomatic left forearm. Axial STIR image (*B*) in a different patient shows increased signal in the extensor compartment muscles consistent with PIN syndrome.

imaging; however, MRI can be used to identify the level of nerve compression or for preoperative planning in the event of prolonged symptoms or the presence of a mass.[61]

SUMMARY

Familiarity with throwing mechanics during elbow range of motion allows accurate diagnosis of sports-related elbow injuries, which occur in predictable patterns. In addition, repetitive stress-related injuries are often clinically apparent; however, imaging plays an important role in determining severity as well as associated injuries that may affect clinical management. A detailed understanding of elbow imaging regarding anatomy and mechanism of injury results in prompt and precise treatment.

CLINICS CARE POINTS

- Overhead throwing athletes are subject to valgus extension overload syndrome, which can result in multiple medial elbow injuries including UCL tear, posteromedial impingement, medial epicondylosis, and ulnar neuritis. Lateral elbow compression during valgus force can also result in capitellar impaction injuries.

- Valgus stress results in posterolateral rotatory instability (PLRI), which results in progressive capsuloligamentous injuries leading to elbow subluxation and dislocation.

- Posteromedial elbow instability (PMRI) results in anteromedial coronoid process fracture as well as RCL and UCL tears.

DISCLOSURE

No authors have financial relationships with a commercial organization that may have a direct or indirect interest in the content of this article.

ACKNOWLEDGMENTS

The authors thank Aydin Rosas for the illustrations in **Figs. 1** and **2**.

REFERENCES

1. Cain EL, Dugas JR, Wolf RS, et al. Elbow injuries in throwing athletes: A current concepts review. Am J Sports Med 2003;31(4):621–35.
2. Rosas HG, Lee KS. Imaging acute trauma of the elbow. Semin Musculoskelet Radiol 2010;14(4):394–411.
3. Aquilina AL, Grazette AJ. Clinical Anatomy and Assessment of the Elbow. Open Orthop J 2017;11(1):1347–52.
4. Morrey BF. Anatomy of the elbow joint. The elbow and its disorders, 3rd Edition. W.B. Saunders, Philadelphia; 2000.
5. Bryce CD, Armstrong AD. Anatomy and Biomechanics of the Elbow. Orthop Clin North Am 2008;39(2):141–54.
6. Farrow LD, Mahoney AJ, Stefancin JJ, et al. Quantitative analysis of the medial ulnar collateral ligament ulnar footprint and its relationship to the ulnar sublime tubercle. Am J Sports Med 2011;39(9):1936–41.
7. Regan WD, Korinek SL, Morrey BF, et al. Biomechanical study of ligaments around the elbow joint. Clin Orthop Relat Res 1991;(271):170–9.

8. Callaway GH, Field LD, Deng XH, et al. Biomechanical evaluation of the medial collateral ligament of the elbow. J Bone Joint Surg Am 1997;79(8):1223–31.

9. Giuffrè BM, Moss MJ. Optimal Positioning for MRI of the Distal Biceps Brachii Tendon: Flexed Abducted Supinated View. Am J Roentgenol 2004;182(4):944–6.

10. Snoeck O, Lefèvre P, Sprio E, et al. The lacertus fibrosus of the biceps brachii muscle: An anatomical study. Surg Radiol Anat 2014;36(7):713–9.

11. Barco R, Sánchez P, Morrey ME, et al. The distal triceps tendon insertional anatomy—implications for surgery. JSES Open Access 2017;1(2):98–103.

12. Negrão JR, Mogami R, Ramirez Ruiz FA, et al. Distal insertional anatomy of the triceps brachii muscle: MRI assessment in cadaveric specimens employing histologic correlation and Play-doh® models of the anatomic findings. Skeletal Radiol 2020;49(7):1057–67.

13. Bucknor MD, Stevens KJ, Steinbach LS. Elbow imaging in sport: Sports imaging series. Radiology 2016;279(1):12–28.

14. Karbach LE, Elfar J. Elbow Instability: Anatomy, Biomechanics, Diagnostic Maneuvers, and Testing. J Hand Surg Am 2017;42(2):118–26.

15. Munshi M, Pretterklieber ML, Chung CB, et al. Anterior bundle of ulnar collateral ligament: Evaluation of anatomic relationships by using MR imaging, MR arthrography, and gross anatomic and histologic analysis. Radiology 2004;231(3):797–803.

16. Mulligan SA, Schwartz ML, Broussard MF, et al. Heterotopic calcification and tears of the ulnar collateral ligament: Radiographic and MR imaging findings. AJR Am J Roentgenol 2000;175:1099–102.

17. Ciccotti MG, Atanda A, Nazarian LN, et al. Stress sonography of the ulnar collateral ligament of the elbow in professional baseball pitchers: A 10-year study. Am J Sports Med 2014;42(3):544–51.

18. Miller TT, Adler RS. Sonography of tears of the distal biceps tendon. AJR Am J Roentgenol 2000;175:1081–6.

19. Roedl JB, Gonzalez FM, Zoga AC, et al. Potential Utility of a Combined Approach with US and MR Arthrography to Image Medial Elbow Pain in Baseball Players. Radiology 2016;279(3):827–37.

20. Ahmad CS, Park MC, Elattrache NS. Elbow medical ulnar collateral ligament insufficiency alters posteromedial olecranon contact. Am J Sports Med 2004;32(7):1607–12.

21. Osbahr DC, Dines JS, Breazeale NM, et al. Ulnohumeral chondral and ligamentous overload: Biomechanical correlation for posteromedial chondromalacia of the elbow in throwing athletes. Am J Sports Med 2010;38(12):2535–41.

22. Klingele KE, Kocher MS. Little league elbow: Valgus overload injury in the paediatric athlete. Sport Med 2002;32(15):1005–15.

23. Hang DW, Chao CM, Hang YS. A Clinical and Roentgenographic Study of Little League Elbow. Am J Sports Med 2004;32(1):79–84.

24. Iyer RS, Thapa MM, Khanna PC, et al. Pediatric bone imaging: Imaging elbow trauma in children - A review of acute and chronic injuries. Am J Roentgenol 2012;198(5):1053–68.

25. Rosenberg ZS, Blutreich SI, Schweitzer ME, et al. MRI features of posterior capitellar impaction injuries. Am J Roentgenol 2008;190(2):435–41.

26. Takahara M, Shundo M, Kondo M, et al. Early detection of osteochondritis dissecans of the capitellum in young baseball players: Report of three cases. J Bone Joint Surg Am 1998;80(6):892–7.

27. Stoane JM, Poplausky MR, Haller JO, et al. Panner's disease: X-ray, MR imaging findings and review of the literature. Comput Med Imaging Graph 1995;19(6): 473–6.

28. Keen NN, Chin CT, Engstrom JW, et al. Diagnosing ulnar neuropathy at the elbow using magnetic resonance neurography. Skeletal Radiol 2012;41(4):401–7.

29. Husarik DB, Saupe N, Pfirrmann CWA, et al. Elbow nerves: MR findings in 60 asymptomatic subjects–normal anatomy, variants, and pitfalls. Radiology 2009; 252(1):148–56.

30. Coonrad RW, Hooper WR. Tennis elbow: Its course, natural history, conservative and surgical management. J Bone Joint Surg Am 1973;55(6):1177–82.

31. Connell D, Burke F, Coombes P, et al. Sonographic examination of lateral epicon-dylitis. Am J Roentgenol 2001;176(3):777–82.

32. Coel M, Yamada CY, Ko J. MR imaging of patients with lateral epicondylitis of the elbow (tennis elbow): Importance of increased signal of the anconeus muscle. Am J Roentgenol 1993;161(5):1019–21.

33. Bredella MA, Tirman PFJ, Fritz RC, et al. MR imaging findings of lateral ulnar collateral ligament abnormalities in patients with lateral epicondylitis. Am J Roent-genol 1999;173(5):1379–82.

34. Williams BD, Schweitzer ME, Weishaupt D, et al. Partial tears of the distal biceps tendon: MR appearance and associated clinical findings. Skeletal Radiol 2001; 30(10):560–4.

35. Chew ML, Giuffrè BM. Disorders of the distal biceps brachii tendon. Radio-graphics 2005;25(5):1227–37.

36. Lobo LDG, Fessell DP, Miller BS, et al. The role of sonography in differentiating full versus partial distal biceps tendon tears: Correlation with surgical findings. Am J Roentgenol 2013;200(1):158–62.

37. Athwal GS, Steinmann SP, Rispoli DM. The Distal Biceps Tendon: Footprint and Relevant Clinical Anatomy. J Hand Surg Am 2007;32(8):1225–9.

38. Eames MHA, Bain GI, Fogg QA, et al. Distal biceps tendon anatomy: A cadaveric study. J Bone Joint Surg Am 2007;89(5):1044–9.

39. Koulouris G, Malone W, Omar IM, et al. Bifid insertion of the distal biceps brachii tendon with isolated rupture: Magnetic resonance findings. J Shoulder Elbow Surg 2009;18(6).

40. Van Riet RP, Morrey BF, Ho E, et al. Surgical treatment of distal triceps ruptures. J Bone Joint Surg Am 2003;85(10):1961–7.

41. O'Driscoll S, Morrey B, Korinek S, et al. Elbow subluxation and dislocation. A spectrum of instability - PubMed. Clin Orthop Relat Res 1992;(280):186–97. Avail-able at: https://pubmed.ncbi.nlm.nih.gov/1611741/. Accessed October 31, 2020.

42. Jeon IH, Micic ID, Yamamoto N, et al. Osborne-cotterill lesion: An osseous defect of the capitellum associated with instability of the elbow. Am J Roentgenol 2008; 191(3):727–9.

43. Coonrad RW, Roush TF, Major NM, et al. The drop sign, a radiographic warning sign of elbow instability. J Shoulder Elbow Surg 2005;14(3):312–7.

44. Bellato E, Kim Y, Fitzsimmons JS, et al. Role of the lateral collateral ligament in posteromedial rotatory instability of the elbow. J Shoulder Elbow Surg 2017; 26(9):1636–43.

45. McLean J, Kempston MP, Pike JM, et al. Varus Posteromedial Rotatory Instability of the Elbow: Injury Pattern and Surgical Experience of 27 Acute Consecutive Surgical Patients. J Orthop Trauma 2018;32:E469–74.

46. Mason ML. Some observations on fractures of the head of the radius with a review of one hundred cases. Br J Surg 1954;42(172):123–32.

47. Major NM, Crawford ST. Elbow effusions in trauma in adults and children: Is there an occult fracture? Am J Roentgenol 2002;178(2):413–8.

48. Hak DJ, Golladay GJ. Olecranon fractures: treatment options. J Am Acad Orthop Surg 2000;8(4):266–75.

49. Closkey RF, Goode JR, Kirschenbaum D, et al. The role of the coronoid process in elbow stability: A biomechanical analysis of axial loading. J Bone Joint Surg Am 2000;82(12):1749–53.

50. Regan W, Morrey B. Classification and treatment of coronoid process fractures - PubMed. Orthopedics. 1992. Available at: https://pubmed.ncbi.nlm.nih.gov/1630968/. Accessed October 31, 2020.

51. O'Driscoll S, Jupiter J, Cohen M, et al. Difficult elbow fractures: pearls and pitfalls - PubMed. Instr Course Lect. 2003. Available at: https://pubmed.ncbi.nlm.nih.gov/12690844/. Accessed October 31, 2020.

52. Ring D. Fractures of the Coronoid Process of the Ulna. J Hand Surg Am 2006; 31(10):1679–89.

53. Sheehan SE, Dyer GS, Sodickson AD, et al. Traumatic elbow injuries: What the orthopedic surgeon wants to know. Radiographics 2013;33(3):869–88.

54. O'Driscoll S, Jupiter J, King G, et al. The unstable elbow - PubMed. The Journal of Bone & Joint Surgery. 2000. Available at: https://pubmed.ncbi.nlm.nih.gov/11372363/. Accessed October 31, 2020.

55. Cerezal L, Rodriguez-Sammartino M, Canga A, et al. Elbow synovial fold syndrome. Am J Roentgenol 2013;201(1). https://doi.org/10.2214/AJR.12.8768.

56. Husarik DB, Saupe N, Pfirrmann CWA, et al. Ligaments and plicae of the elbow: Normal MR imaging variability in 60 asymptomatic subjects. Radiology 2010; 257(1):185–94.

57. Awaya H, Schweitzer ME, Feng SA, et al. Elbow synovial fold syndrome: MR imaging findings. Am J Roentgenol 2001;177(6):1377–81.

58. Miller TT, Reinus WR. Nerve entrapment syndromes of the elbow, forearm, and wrist. Am J Roentgenol 2010;195(3):585–94.

59. Linda DD, Harish S, Stewart BG, et al. Multimodality imaging of peripheral neuropathies of the upper limb and brachial plexus. Radiographics 2010;30(5): 1373–400.

60. Dunn AJ, Salonen DC, Anastakis DJ. MR imaging findings of anterior interosseous nerve lesions. Skeletal Radiol 2007;36(12):1155–62.

61. Kim S, Choi JY, Huh YM, et al. Role of magnetic resonance imaging in entrapment and compressive neuropathy - What, where, and how to see the peripheral nerves on the musculoskeletal magnetic resonance image: Part 2. Upper extremity. Eur Radiol 2007;17(2):509–22.

Wrist and Hand Trauma Imaging

Anthony Balzer, MD*, Ashish Patel, MD, Andrew Palisch, MD

KEYWORDS

• Wrist • Hand • Trauma • Imaging • Radiology

KEY POINTS

• Traumatic injuries of the wrist and hand are common in athletes and imaging plays a key role in diagnosis.
• Radiographs are the primary imaging examination for osseous injuries such as fractures and dislocations.
• Intrinsic and extrinsic ligaments of the wrist are crucial for stability of the carpal joints after traumatic injuries and best evaluated with MRI.
• MRI is also the best imaging study for evaluating soft tissue injuries in the hands such as tendons, volar plates, and flexor tendon pulleys.

INTRODUCTION

Athletes are at high risk for injuries to the wrist and hand with an estimated frequency from 3% to 9% of all injuries.[1] This is especially true for athletes playing sports involving rackets and clubs, given the physical stresses placed on the upper extremities.[2] Wrist and hand radiographs are commonly the first step in imaging evaluation of these injuries, given the ease of obtaining radiographs and the cost-effectiveness.[3] Radiographs are especially useful for suspected fractures and evaluation of osseous alignment. Further evaluation of osseous injuries, which may not be visualized on radiographs, can be achieved with computed tomography (CT). CT evaluation also plays a role in preoperative planning for complex fractures and dislocations. In the setting of wrist and hand soft tissue injuries, MRI is the primary imaging modality. Given the high contrast resolution, MRI can provide a detailed assessment of ligament and tendon integrity. In addition, MRI is used to evaluate cartilage abnormalities and underlying bone marrow pathology if prior imaging is inconclusive. Ultrasound (US) evaluation of the musculoskeletal system is becoming more common in wrist and hand injuries, especially with a dynamic assessment of soft tissue pathology. This article reviews imaging of common traumatic wrist and hand injuries.

Department of Radiology, Baylor College of Medicine, One Baylor Plaza, BCM 360, Houston, TX 77030, USA
* Corresponding author.
E-mail address: anthony.balzer@bcm.edu

Clin Sports Med 40 (2021) 625–639
https://doi.org/10.1016/j.csm.2021.05.003
0278-5919/21/© 2021 Elsevier Inc. All rights reserved.

DISCUSSION
Wrist Fractures

The scaphoid bone is the most commonly fractured carpal bone of the wrist, estimated to be up to 70% of carpal fractures.[1] Fractures are frequently associated with contact sports and falls on an outstretched hand resulting in hyperextension. Complete radiograph series with posteroanterior (PA), lateral, oblique, and additional views with ulnar deviation can help to evaluate poorly visualized fractures.[4] However, the sensitivity of radiographic examination is approximately 81% and fractures may not be visualized initially.[5] Alternatively, cross-sectional imaging with CT or MRI is more sensitive for scaphoid fractures after the initial trauma.[6] (**Fig. 1**) Fractures

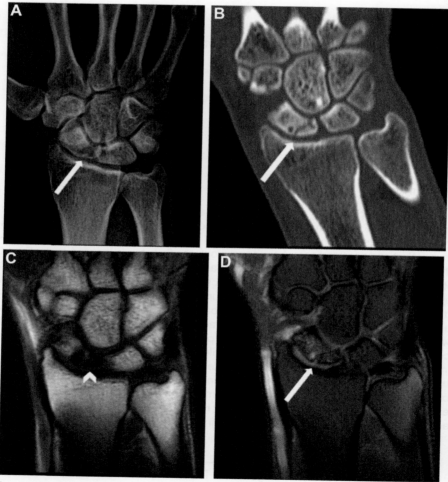

Fig. 1. PA radiograph (*A*) shows a nondisplaced fracture of the proximal pole of the scaphoid (*arrows*), which is more clearly visualized on coronal CT (*B*). Coronal T1-weighted (*C*) and STIR-weighted MRI (*D*) re-demonstrate the scaphoid fracture (*arrow*) with nonunion as indicated by well-corticated fracture line. Associated hypointense signal on T1-weighted image throughout the proximal scaphoid fragment (*arrowhead*) is consistent with avascular necrosis.

involving the proximal pole and scaphoid waist increase the risk of nonunion and subsequent avascular necrosis, given the tenuous retrograde blood supply of the scaphoid.[6] Follow-up MRI evaluation may be needed to monitor for osteonecrosis if healing does not progress as expected. Over time, long-standing nonunion of a scaphoid fracture can result in scaphoid nonunion advanced collapse arthropathy. The distal fracture fragment of the scaphoid rotates in a volar direction and causes an abnormal articulation with the radial styloid. Eventually, arthritis between the entire radius and scaphoid develops, and then the capitate migrates proximally, resulting in arthritis with the lunate.

The hook of the hamate may be fractured after a direct blow to the palm, which is more commonly associated with club and racket sports.[2] These fractures are frequently missed on initial radiographs, as findings may be subtle, such as lack of visualization of the hook of the hamate on PA view.[7] However, even with specialized positioning including the carpal tunnel view, sensitivity is estimated to be only 40% to 50%.[8] (**Fig. 2**) Accordingly, CT examination is usually required to confirm the diagnosis and further evaluate fracture characteristics to guide management.

Fractures of the ulnar styloid process can also occur from direct impact or fall on an outstretched hand. These fractures are easily visualized on wrist radiograph series, and cross-sectional imaging is not usually needed for initial fracture diagnosis (**Fig. 3**). Ulnar styloid fractures are rarely isolated injuries and greater than 40% of distal radius fractures have concurrent ulnar styloid fractures.[9] In addition, the incidence of ulnar styloid process fractures resulting in nonunion is up to 53%, which predisposes to ulnar-sided wrist disorders.[10] Given the triangular fibrocartilage complex (TFCC) attachments on the ulnar styloid process, these fractures can have a significant impact on the stability of the distal radioulnar joint. If fractures involve the base of the ulnar styloid or result in greater than 2 mm of displacement, there is a significant increased risk of distal radioulnar joint instability.[9] Wrist MRI may be required to further assess ulnar styloid process fractures for distal radioulnar instability and involvement of the TFCC, which is further described in later sections.

Fractures of the triquetral bone are the second most common isolated fracture of the carpal bones, behind the scaphoid.[11] Triquetral fractures can occur from hyperextension, ulnar styloid impaction, or forced flexion with avulsion from the dorsal-sided ligaments.[11] Radiographs can identify common fracture patterns of the triquetral bone with lateral views being especially helpful in visualizing dorsal avulsion type fractures (**Fig. 4**). For more complex fracture patterns, CT examination of the wrist may be required to demonstrate the full extent of injury and fracture characteristics.[12] In

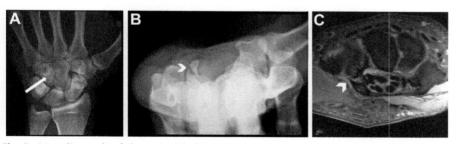

Fig. 2. PA radiograph of the wrist (*A*) demonstrates irregularity at the hook of the hamate (*arrow*) with mildly displaced fracture (*arrowhead*) easily seen on carpal tunnel view radiograph (*B*). Axial proton density-weighted FS MRI (*C*) in a different patient shows a mildly displaced fracture at the hook of the hamate (*arrowhead*).

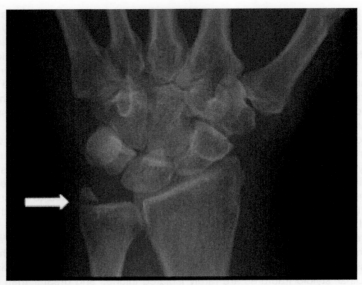

Fig. 3. PA radiograph of the wrist with a transverse fracture through the base of the ulnar styloid process (*arrow*). Fractures of the ulnar styloid process with greater than 2 mm displacement or involving the base have a significantly higher risk of concurrent ligament injury and distal radioulnar joint instability.

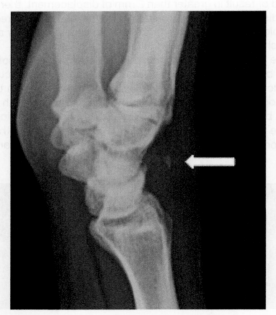

Fig. 4. Lateral radiograph of the wrist shows small ossific fragments overlying the dorsal aspect of the proximal carpal row (*arrow*), consistent with triquetral avulsion fracture. These avulsions usually arise from the dorsal extrinsic ligaments (dorsal intercarpal and dorsal radiotriquetral ligaments), which insert on the dorsal triquetrum.

addition, MRI examination can further evaluate injury of the lunotriquetral ligament or extrinsic carpal ligaments in the setting of triquetral fractures associated with carpal instability.

Intrinsic Carpal Ligament Injuries

The scapholunate ligament is commonly injured in sports-related activities due to hyperextension from falls and high-energy contact.[7] The ligament is composed of dorsal, central fibromembranous, and volar bands with the dorsal band being the strongest and most important for stability.[13] Injury of the scapholunate ligament is suspected when the scapholunate interval is widened, greater than 3 mm, on PA wrist radiographs and asymmetric widening is present compared with the contralateral wrist.[14] A clenched fist radiographic view may also be beneficial to illicit dynamic widening of the scapholunate interval.[14] Visualization of the injured scapholunate ligament is best seen on MRI evaluation. Increased signal and irregularity of the ligament is seen with a sprain, partial discontinuity with a partial tear, and complete discontinuity or nonvisualization with a complete tear.[7] (**Fig. 5**) Over time, chronic tear of the scapholunate ligament can result in scapholunate advanced collapse arthropathy. There is a volar rotation of the scaphoid, which creates an abnormal articulation with the radial styloid. Eventually, arthritis between the entire radius and scaphoid develops, and then the capitate migrates proximally leading to arthritis with the lunate.

The lunotriquetral ligament can also be injured in athletes after a fall on an outstretched hand.[1] Similar to the scapholunate ligament, the lunotriquetral ligament has three bands with the dorsal and volar bands representing true ligaments, while the interosseous portion is a thin membranous component. However, unlike the scapholunate ligament, the strongest band of the lunotriquetral ligament is the volar band, which is the most important for lunotriquetral stability.[13] Radiographs are commonly normal in the setting of lunotriquetral ligament injury and stress views may be required to elucidate diastasis of the lunotriquetral interval.[15] MRI can demonstrate increased signal with injury of the lunotriquetral ligament; however, partial or complete tears can be difficult to adequately visualize with lack of joint fluid or lunotriquetral widening[7] (**Fig. 6**). Accordingly, MR arthrography has been shown to increase the detection of lunotriquetral ligament tears, especially when using axial oblique imaging planes with a sensitivity and specificity up to 75% and 93%, respectively.[16]

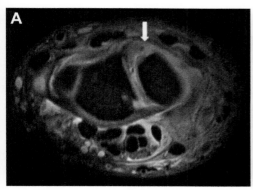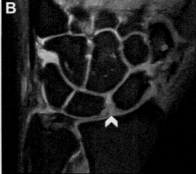

Fig. 5. Axial (*A*) and coronal (*B*) proton density-weighted FS MRI demonstrate an acute scapholunate ligament tear with discontinuity and increased signal of the dorsal (*arrow*) and interosseous bands (*arrowhead*). The dorsal band typically avulses from the scaphoid attachment.

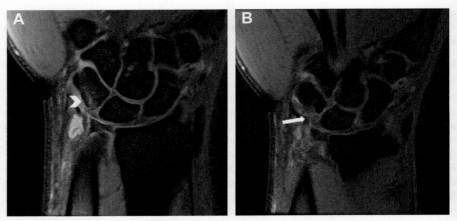

Fig. 6. Coronal proton density-weighted FS MRI (*A, B*) shows edema in the volar triquetrum (*arrowhead*) and linear tear of the volar lunotriquetral ligament from the triquetrum (*arrow*).

Extrinsic Carpal Ligament Injuries

In addition to the intrinsic scapholunate and lunotriquetral ligaments, the extrinsic carpal ligaments are a group of ligaments that extend along the volar and dorsal aspect of the wrist. Although many of these extrinsic ligaments are difficult to visualize individually, the most significant dorsal ligaments include the dorsal radiocarpal ligament from the radius to the triquetrum and the dorsal intercarpal ligament from the scaphoid to the triquetrum[17] (**Fig. 7**). The most frequently visualized volar ligaments include the radioscaphocapitate and the radiolunotriquetral (aka long radiolunate) ligaments.[17] Together, these extrinsic ligaments help maintain carpal stability and can be injured in isolation or associated with intrinsic ligament injuries.[18] Wrist radiographs do not directly identify ligament injuries; however, carpal misalignment patterns can suggest compromise of the extrinsic ligaments. Similar to MR assessment of intrinsic ligaments, sprains, partial tears, and complete tears can be visualized.

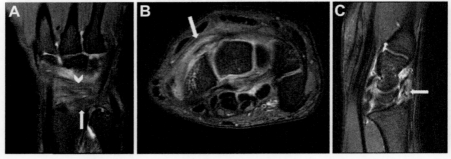

Fig. 7. Coronal (*A*), axial (*B*), and sagittal (*C*) proton density-weighted FS MRI. The dorsal radiotriquetral ligament (*arrow*) and dorsal intercarpal ligament (*arrowhead*) remain intact on the coronal image. However, an increased signal is present surrounding the ligaments on axial and sagittal images (*arrows*), compatible with sprain.

When injury occurs to the scapholunate ligament and the extrinsic ligaments, the scaphoid rotates in a volar direction and the lunate rotates dorsally, referred to as dorsal intercalated segmental instability (DISI). DISI deformity is best visualized in the sagittal plane with radiolunate angle greater than 10°, scapholunate angle greater than 70°, and capitolunate angle of greater than 30°.[7] Alternatively, volar intercalated segmental instability occurs when the lunotriquetral and extrinsic ligaments are injured.[19] VISI is defined as volar angulation of the lunate and dorsal rotation of the capitate and hamate resulting in scapholunate angle of less than 30° and capitolunate angle greater than 30°.[20]

Carpal Dislocations

In addition to these ligament injuries, dislocation of the carpal joints can occur from high-energy trauma with or without associated fractures. A common pattern of perilunate ligament injuries and dislocations has been referred to as "lesser arc" injuries classified by Mayfield.[15] These injuries are identified on wrist radiograph series by misalignment of the carpal arcs of Gilula. Gilula's arcs include arc I along the proximal surface of the scaphoid, lunate, and triquetrum; arc II along the distal concavity of the scaphoid, lunate, and triquetrum; and arc III along the proximal convex alignment of the capitate and hamate.[15] Stage I of the Mayfield classification involves injury of the scapholunate ligament described previously.[21] Stage II also involves disruption of the lunocapitate joint leading to perilunate dislocation with dislocation of the capitate bone, usually in the sagittal plane, while the lunate still articulates with the distal radius.[21] Stage III combines lunotriquetral disruption with the previous stages and results in midcarpal dislocation, with neither the lunate nor the capitate in appropriate sagittal alignment with the radius.[21] Finally, stage IV of the Mayfield classification completes the lesser arc injury with disruption of the radiolunate joint and dislocation of the lunate with usual volar displacement.[21] Lateral views of the wrist radiograph series are crucial for identifying these carpal misalignments (**Fig. 8**). Wrist MRI can provide more dedicated assessment of wrist ligaments; however, is usually not required for diagnosis in the setting of carpal dislocations.

Triangular Fibrocartilage Complex Injuries

The TFCC can be injured from a combination of forced axial load, such as a fall on an outstretched hand, or a torsional force associated with racket or club sports.[2] Wrist

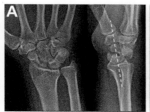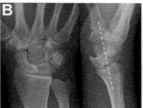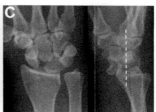

Fig. 8. PA and lateral wrist radiographs (*A*) with dorsal dislocation of the distal carpal row; however, anatomic alignment is maintained at the radiolunate articulation (reference line), which is consistent with perilunate dislocation. Similar dorsal subluxation of the distal carpal row is noted on PA and lateral wrist radiographs (*B*) with additional volar subluxation of the lunate in relation to the distal radius (reference line), which is compatible with midcarpal dislocation. Finally, lunate dislocation is demonstrated on PA and lateral wrist radiographs (*C*) with the volar displacement and angulation of the lunate while the sagittal plane of the radius and capitate is maintained (reference line).

radiographs provide little assessment of the TFCC besides identifying ulnar styloid avulsion fractures or widening of the distal radioulnar joint.[14] MRI provides the best visualization of the TFCC structures and MR arthrography may help identify smaller complete tears allowing communication of contrast between joint spaces.[22] **(Fig. 9)** Any structure of the TFCC can be injured, but typical injury patterns are described with the Palmer classification. Class 1A and 1B injuries are the most common, which refer to central perforation of the articular disc and avulsion of the ulnar-sided attachments, respectively.[23] Avulsion of the volar ulnocarpal ligaments (class 1C), radial-sided avulsion of the articular disc (class 1D), and horizontal tear of the articular disc (class 1E) are less frequently encountered.[23] In addition to the Palmer classification injuries, integrity of the dorsal and volar radioulnar ligaments is a crucial component of MRI evaluation as these ligaments play important roles in distal radioulnar joint stability.[23]

Hand Dislocations

Finger dislocations are a common occurrence in contact sports and can be acutely painful but also may lead to long-term joint deformity if not properly identified and managed. Proximal interphalangeal (PIP) joints are the most commonly dislocated joint of the fingers and may be described as dorsal, volar, or lateral depending on the direction of the middle phalanx in relation to the proximal phalanx.[24] Dorsal PIP joint dislocations, also known as 'Coach finger,' result from hyperextension with axial loading causing volar plate injury. Volar PIP joint dislocations are more rare, resulting from an axial force and rotation of a flexed joint, and are associated with injury to the

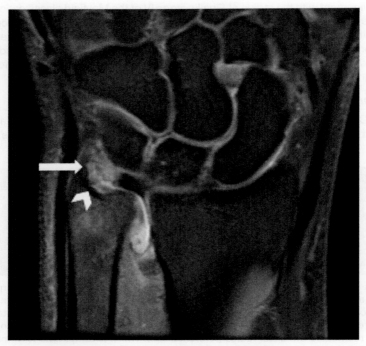

Fig. 9. Coronal proton density-weighted FS MRI with increased signal and tear at the styloid attachment (*arrow*) and foveal attachment (*arrowhead*) of the TFCC. Associated effusion of the distal radioulnar joint is also noted.

extensor tendon central slip (**Fig. 10**). Initial imaging evaluation consists of a standard finger series, including a PA view of the entire hand followed by oblique and lateral views of the injured finger. Postreduction imaging is beneficial to assess for persistent joint subluxation or other complication such as coexisting fracture. Irreducible dislocations and fracture dislocations with greater than 40% articular surface involvement may benefit from MRI evaluation to assess for additional soft tissue injury[25] (see **Fig. 10**).

Hand Ligament Injuries

Ulnar collateral ligament (UCL) tears are the most common injury to the first metacarpophalangeal (MCP) joint.[25] The UCL of the thumb MCP joint is composed of the proper ligament, which extends from the metacarpal head to the phalangeal base, and the accessory ligament, which extends from the metacarpal head to the ulnar sesamoid. The proper ligament is tight during thumb flexion and the accessory ligament is tight during thumb extension. Acute post-traumatic UCL tears, known as skier's thumb, result from thumb hyperabduction. UCL injury may be recognized clinically by pain, instability at the first MCP joint, or weakness with a thumb-index pinch grip and require multimodality imaging evaluation. Radiographs are useful to assess for avulsion fractures, which are present in 20% to 30% of cases, and maybe a surgical indication when displacement is greater than 5 mm or there is greater than 25% involvement of the articular surface.[26] It is advisable to avoid performing stress testing of the thumb before imaging, as the maneuver may further damage or displace the torn UCL. US provides a rapid, cost-effective method of diagnosis, with sensitivity and specificity of 83% and 75%, respectively. Proximally retracted UCL tears that displace superficial to the normally overlying adductor pollicis aponeurosis are known as Stener lesions. MRI is the gold standard examination with sensitivity of 96% to 100% and specificity of 95% to 100% for detecting UCL injuries, although in chronic UCL injuries, it can be more difficult to differentiate Stener lesions in the presence of excess scarring[27] (**Fig. 11**).

Hand Tendon Injuries

"Mallet finger" is the commonly known eponym for disruption of the terminal extensor tendon at the dorsal aspect of the distal phalanx base. This is the most common finger

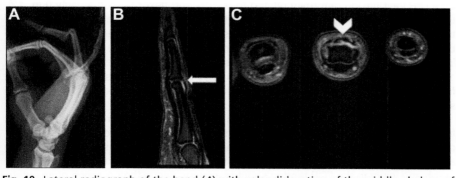

Fig. 10. Lateral radiograph of the hand (A) with volar dislocation of the middle phalanx of the third digit at the proximal interphalangeal joint. Postreduction sagittal (B) and axial (C) T2-weighted FS MRI shows tear of the central slip of the extensor tendon from the middle phalangeal base (arrow) with partially retracted irregular extensor tendon (arrowhead).

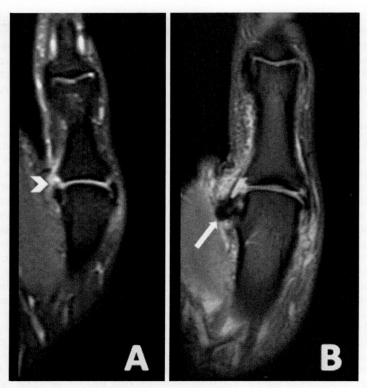

Fig. 11. Coronal proton density-weighted FS MRI (*A*) demonstrates tear of the ulnar collateral ligament at the metacarpophalangeal joint of the thumb (*arrowhead*). Additional coronal proton density-weighted FS MRI (*B*) from another injury, which shows the torn ulnar collateral ligament retracted (*arrow*) and interposition of partially visualized adductor pollicis aponeurosis (Stener lesion).

tendon injury seen in athletes and results from forced DIP hyperflexion or less commonly a direct axial force on the fingertip. Diagnosis may be suspected clinically by a DIP joint flexion deformity related to unopposed flexor tendon activity (**Fig. 12**). Initial radiographs may assist with identifying an associated fracture, most often of the distal phalanx base. Most cases present with isolated tendon injury and are best evaluated on MRI sagittal images.[25] Proper healing is usually achieved by splinting the DIP joint in extension for 6 to 8 weeks. Patients with persistent joint instability or associated fractures involving greater than 50% of the articular surface may benefit from surgical repair to restore joint congruity and minimize the risk of a chronic swan-neck joint deformity.[28]

"Jersey finger" refers to avulsion injuries of the flexor digitorum profundus tendon from its insertion at the volar aspect of the distal phalanx base. These injuries are secondary to forced DIP hyperextension during active DIP flexion, as occurs during the action of grabbing an opponent's jersey. Imaging evaluation should begin with a radiograph and injury to the FDP tendon should be suspected in the presence of an extension deformity at the DIP joint or a volar avulsion fracture of the distal phalanx base (**Fig. 13**). US or MRI can be used to definitively diagnose the soft tissue injury and for injury classification, per the Leddy–Packer classification. On MRI, the axial and

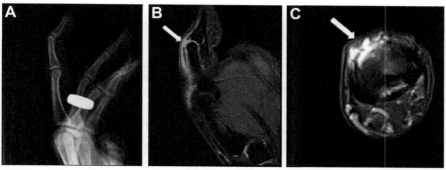

Fig. 12. Lateral radiograph of the middle finger (*A*) shows fixed flexion of the distal inter-phalangeal joint after injury, which is concerning for terminal extension tendon injury (Mallet finger). Sagittal (*B*) and axial (*C*) proton density-weighted FS MRI after a similar injury to the thumb demonstrates torn extensor pollicis longus tendon (*arrows*) at the base of the distal phalanx.

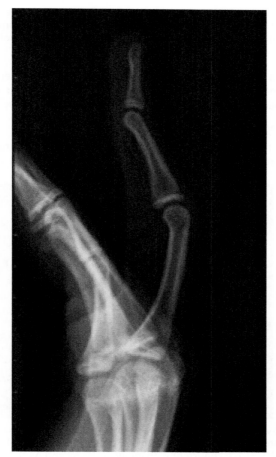

Fig. 13. Lateral radiograph of the middle finger after hyperextension injury displays fixed extension at the distal interphalangeal joint, which is suspicious for flexor tendon injury at the base of the distal phalanx (Jersey finger).

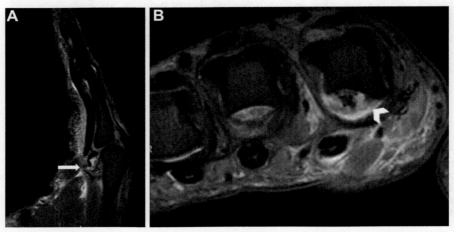

Fig. 14. Sagittal (*A*) and axial (*B*) proton density-weighted FS MRI demonstrates volar plate injury at the metacarpophalangeal joint of the index finger with displacement of the volar plate from the joint and tearing of the proximal fibers from the metacarpal head (*arrow*). Associated irregularity of the volar plate and edema in the surrounding soft tissues is noted (*arrowhead*).

sagittal sequences should be used to identify the degree of FDP tendon retraction. Greater degrees of tendon retraction increase the risk of vascular compromise to the tendon and result in greater necessity for prompt surgical repair.[28]

Hand Volar Plate and Flexor Pulley Injuries

The volar plate is found at the volar aspect of the MCP and IP joints, serving as a joint stabilizer along with the collateral ligaments to prevent joint hyperextension.

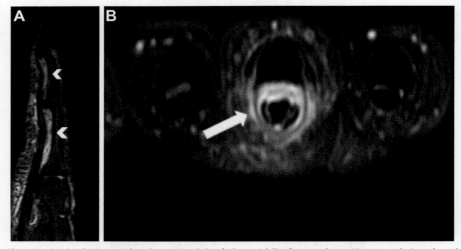

Fig. 15. Sagittal T2-weighted FS MRI (*A*) of the middle finger shows increased signal and widening of the interval between the flexor tendons and the proximal and middle phalanges (*arrowheads*), which is consistent with injury of the A2 and A4 flexor tendon pulleys. Axial T2-weighted FS MRI (*B*) with laxity of the annular A2 pulley and surrounding edema (*arrow*).

Volar plate injuries most commonly occur at the PIP joint, secondary to forced hyperextension or an axial compression force ("jammed finger"). Initial radiographic evaluation may be normal or show dislocation or fracture, depending on Eaton classification. Type 1 injuries include volar plate ruptures, usually distally, without an avulsion fracture. In type 2 injuries, dorsal subluxation or dislocation occurs at the PIP joint due to more extensive soft tissue injury involving the volar plate and collateral ligaments. Type 3 injuries are associated with fracture dislocation of the middle phalanx base.[29] MRI is the optimal modality to evaluate the volar plate and collateral ligaments (**Fig. 14**). Treatment is often conservative, although unstable type 3 injuries or irreducible dislocations secondary to volar plate entrapment may be an indication for surgical repair. In those injuries managed conservatively, dynamic US has shown to be a useful modality to assess volar plate stability when deciding on a return to full mobilization.[30]

The digital flexor tendons are housed by osteofibrous canals, lined with multiple fibrous annular and cruciform pulleys, which protect the tendons and allow for efficient flexor function. Pulley injuries occur with hyperflexion forces, which are common with rock climbers as various grips place significant stress on the flexor tendons and supporting pulleys. The A2 pulley often bears the greatest amount of stress during activity and is the most commonly injured pulley. MRI is paramount in the diagnosis of pulley injuries, which are demonstrated by direct signs of increased pulley intrasubstance signal intensity and fiber disruption. An additional indirect sign of pulley injury includes "tendon bowstringing" where the flexor tendon displaces greater than 2 mm from the underlying bone[28] (**Fig. 15**). Larger bone to flexor tendon gaps (>5 mm) are seen with simultaneous injury to multiple pulleys in the same digit.[31] US is often used to diagnose and perform therapeutic intervention for trigger finger, a condition causing thickening of the A1 pulley secondary to repetitive microtrauma.

SUMMARY

Injuries to the wrist and hands occur frequently in athletes from the high forces applied during sporting events. The examples presented above illustrate the important role imaging has in the diagnosis of wrist and hand injuries. In addition, different imaging modalities are complementary and various examinations may be needed to help guide the management of wrist and hand traumatic pathology.

CLINICS CARE POINTS

- Radiographs should be the first imaging study ordered for evaluation of wrist and hand trauma. Specialized views may be necessary depending on the location of expected osseous or soft tissue injury.

- CT is more sensitive for fractures when initial radiographs are negative and may be needed for preoperative planning in complex fractures or dislocation.

- Ligament and tendon injuries of the wrist and hand can be visualized with MRI. Occasionally, MR arthrography may provide higher sensitivity for these soft tissue injuries.

- US evaluation can be a useful tool for dynamic assessment of ligament or tendon injury after wrist and hand trauma.

DISCLOSURE

The authors have nothing to disclose.

REFERENCES

1. Rettig A. Athletic injuries of the wrist and hand part I: Traumatic injuries of the wrist. Am J Sports Med 2003;31(6):1038–48.
2. Werner SL, Plancher KD. Biomechanics of wrist injuries in sports. Clin Sports Med 1998;17(3):407–20.
3. Torabi M, Lenchik L, Beaman FD, et al. ACR appropriateness criteria acute hand and wrist trauma. J Am Coll Radiol 2019;16:S7–17.
4. Berber O, Ahmad I, Gidwani S. Fractures of the scaphoid. Br Med J 2020;369: m1908.
5. Welling RD, Jacobson JA, Jamadar DA, et al. MDCT and radiography of wrist fractures: Radiographic sensitivity and fracture patterns. AJR Am J Roentgenol 2008;190:10–6.
6. Fowler JR, Hughes TB. Scaphoid fractures. Clin Sports Med 2015;34:37–50.
7. Cockenpot E, Lefebvre G, Demondion X, et al. Imaging of sports-related hand and wrist injuries: sports imaging series. Radiology 2016;279(3):674–92.
8. Klausmeyer MA, Mudgal CS. Hook of hamate fractures. J Hand Surg Am 2013; 38:2457–60.
9. Logan AJ, Lindau TR. The management of distal ulnar fractures in adults: a review of the literature and recommendations for treatment. Strat Traum Limb Recon 2008;3:49–56.
10. Meyer H, Kramer S, O'Loughlin PF, et al. Union of the ulnar styloid fracture as a function of fracture morphology on conventional radiographs. Skeletal Radiol 2013;42:1135–41.
11. Hopkins AD, Bowman SRA, Preketes AP, et al. Triquetral fractures – a retrospective, multi-centre study of management and outcomes. Australas J Plast Surg 2020;3(1):11–5.
12. Oh E, Kim HJ, Hong A, et al. Evaluation for fracture patterns around the wrist on three-dimensional extremity computed tomography, especially focused on the triquetrum. J Med Imaging Rad Onc 2015;59:47–53.
13. Geissler WB, Burkett JL. Ligamentous sports injuries of the hand and wrist. Sports Med Arthrosc Rev 2014;22(1):39–44.
14. Tiegs-Heiden CA, Howe BM. Imaging of the hand and wrist. Clin Sports Med 2020;39:223–45.
15. Kani KK, Mulcahy H, Chew FS. Understanding carpal instability: a radiographic perspective. Skeletal Radiol 2016;45:1031–43.
16. Lee RKL, Griffith JF, Ng AWH, et al. Intrinsic carpal ligaments on MR and multidetector CT arthrograpy: comparision of axial and axial oblique planes. Eur Radiol 2017;27:1277–85.
17. Totterman SM, Miller R, Wasserman B, et al. Intrinsic and extrinsic carpal ligaments: Evaluations by three-dimension fourier transform MR imaging. Am J Rad 1993;160:117–23.
18. Theumann NH, Pfirrmann CW, Antonio GE, et al. Extrinsic carpal ligaments: Normal MR arthrographic appearance in cadavers. Radiology 2003;226:171–9.
19. Nicoson MC, Moran SL. Diagnosis and treatment of acute lunotriquetral ligament injuries. Hand Clin 2015;31:467–76.
20. Zanetti M, Hodler J, Gilula L. Assessment of dorsal or ventral intercalated segmental instability configuration of the wrist: Reliability of sagittal MR images. Radiology 1998;206:339–45.

21. Scalcione LR, Gimber LH, Ho AM, et al. Spectrum of carpal dislocations and fracture-dislocations: imaging and management. AJR Am J Roentgenol 2014; 203:541–50.
22. Lee RKL, Ng AWH, Tong CSL, et al. Intrinsic ligament and triangular fibrocartilage complex tears of the wrist: comparison of MDCT arthrography, conventional 3-T MRI, and MR arthrography. Skeletal Radiol 2013;42:1277–85.
23. Zhan H, Bai R, Qian Z, et al. Traumatic injury of the triangular fibrocartilage complex (TFCC) – a refinement of the Palmer classification by using high-resolution 3-T MRI. Skeletal Radiol 2020;49:1567–79.
24. Borchers J, Best T. Common finger fractures and dislocations. Am Fam Physician 2012;85(8):805–10.
25. Wieschhoff G, Sheehan S, Wortman J, et al. Traumatic finger injuries: what the orthopedic surgeon wants to know. RadioGraphics 2016;36(4):1106–28.
26. Madan S, Pai D, Kaur A, et al. Injury to ulnar collateral ligament of thumb. Orthop Surg 2014;6(1):1–7.
27. Mahajan M, Tolman C, Wurth B, et al. Clinical evaluation vs magnetic resonance imaging of the skier's thumb: A prospective cohort of 30 patients. Eur J Radiol 2016;85:1750–6.
28. Petchprapa C, Vaswani D. MRI of the fingers: an update. AJR Am J Roentgenol 2019;213(3):534–48.
29. Clavero J, Alomar X, Monill J, et al. MR imaging of ligament and tendon injuries of the fingers. RadioGraphics 2002;22:237–56.
30. Laclere FM, Mathys L, Juon B, et al. The role of dynamic ultrasound in the immediate conservative treatment of volar plate injuries of the PIP joint: a series of 78 patients. Plast Surg 2017;25(3):151–6.
31. Lapegue F, Andre A, Meyrignac O, et al. US-guided percutaneous release of the trigger finger by using a 21-gauge needle: a prospective study of 60 cases. Radiology 2016;280(2):493–9.

MRI of the Meniscus

James Derek Stensby, MD[a],*, Lauren Clough Pringle, MD[b],
Julia Crim, MD[c]

KEYWORDS

- Knee • Meniscus • Meniscal tear • MRI • Anatomy

KEY POINTS

- The normal meniscus is an important fibrocartilage structure in the knee, which is optimally evaluated by MRI.
- Knowledge of normal anatomy, imaging parameters, imaging findings of tear in the native and postoperative meniscus, common anatomic variants, and MRI pitfalls are essential in obtaining the correct imaging diagnosis.
- Postoperative meniscus is a diagnostic challenge that can be improved with details from the operative note and may be optimized by arthrography.

NORMAL ANATOMY AND FUNCTION

The menisci are fibrocartilaginous structures interposed between the articular surface of the femur and tibia. These semilunar-shaped structures function to distribute the force from axial loading of the knee, absorb shock, and act as a secondary stabilizer.[1] The type I collagen fibers that provide structural support to the meniscus are oriented in 3 layers.[1,2] The central, or innermost, layer is composed of thick collagen fibrils that extend circumferentially, paralleling the peripheral rim of the adjacent tibial plateau.[1,2] Peripheral to the circumferential collagen bundles is a lamellar layer with radially oriented collagen fibrils at the periphery. On the surface, the meniscus is covered by a meshwork of thin collagen fibrils.[1,2]

In cross-section, the menisci have a wedge shape—concave on the superior (femoral) surface and flat on the inferior (tibial) surface (**Fig. 1**). The inner margin is tapered to a thin sharp edge, whereas the periphery is thick. As an axial load is applied to the meniscus, the wedge-shaped contour results in the meniscus being pushed outwards. The strong anterior and posterior root attachments anchor the meniscus and the axial loading force is converted to a tensile force, or hoop stress, along the long axis of the meniscus parallel to the thick central collagen fibrils (**Fig. 2**)[1-3].

[a] Diagnostic Radiology, Department of Radiology, DC069.10, University of Missouri, Columbia, MO, USA; [b] Department of Radiology, DC069.10, University of Missouri, Columbia, MO, USA; [c] Musculoskeletal Radiology, Department of Radiology, DC069.10, University of Missouri, Columbia, MO, USA
* Corresponding author.
E-mail address: stensbyj@health.missouri.edu

Clin Sports Med 40 (2021) 641–655
https://doi.org/10.1016/j.csm.2021.05.004
0278-5919/21/© 2021 Elsevier Inc. All rights reserved.

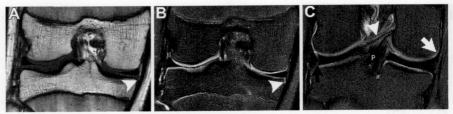

Fig. 1. Normal menisci in the coronal plane. Coronal T1 (*A*) and PD with fat suppression (*B*) images of the normal menisci at the midbody. They are dark (hypointense = low signal intensity) on all MR sequences. The inner margin forms a sharp point. The flat tibial and concave femoral surfaces permit the transmission of axial load as hoop stress to the root attachments. The thin medial meniscotibial ligament (*arrowhead*), an important meniscus stabilizer, should always be well-seen on coronal images. Coronal PD with fat suppression (*C*) through the posterior horns shows that the menisci are block-like, but curved upward at their medial and lateral margins. MM is tightly adherent to the joint capsule (*white arrow*). LM is separated from the popliteus tendon by the narrow popliteus hiatus that contains a small amount of fluid (*black arrow*). The meniscofemoral ligament of Wrisberg (*arrowhead*) is present. Both posterior roots lie immediately adjacent to the posterior cruciate ligament (*P*).

The menisci receive blood flow via a perimeniscal capillary plexus, which in turn is supplied by the genicular arteries.[4] In adult patients, the peripheral 10% to 25% of the meniscus is vascularized and is often referred to as the red-red zone.[4,5] Owing to the decreased blood supply to the inner two-thirds of the meniscus, tears of the middle third, or red-white zone, and inner third, or white-white zone, have decreased ability to heal.[5,6]

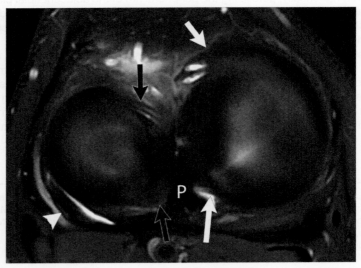

Fig. 2. Meniscal roots. Axial PD with fat suppression image shows the medial (*white arrows*) and lateral (*black arrows*) meniscal roots. The popliteus tendon (*arrowhead*) passes adjacent to the lateral aspect of the posterior horn. *P*, PCL.

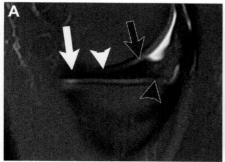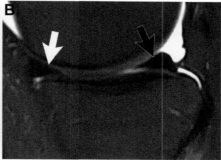

Fig. 3. Normal MM on sagittal images. Note that all sagittal images are shown with the anterior portion of the knee on the left side of the image. Sagittal T2 fat-suppressed image (*A*) through the periphery of the meniscus shows the *"bow tie"* appearance, with the thin meniscal body (*white arrowhead*) connecting the smaller anterior horn (*white arrow*) to the larger posterior horn (*black arrow*). Note the normal appearance of the meniscocapsular junction (*black arrowhead*) at the posteromedial corner; joint fluid (high signal intensity) does not extend between the meniscus and the capsule. Fluid extending the entire height of the meniscocapsular junction indicates a meniscocapsular separation (compared to **Fig. 14**). Sagittal T2 fat-suppressed image (*B*) through the central portion of the meniscus shows the MM anterior horn (*white arrow*) appears similar in size to the posterior horn (*black arrow*). At this point, the meniscal attachment to the posterior capsule is much smaller than it is in the posteromedial corner.

In the axial plane, the medial meniscus (MM) has an uppercase "C" shape. Its anterior and posterior root attachments are farther apart than the lateral meniscus (LM). The posterior horn MM is larger than the anterior horn.[7] The MM covers a smaller portion of the articular surface (50%) when compared with the LM (70%) (**Fig. 3**).[5]

In the axial plane, the anterior and posterior root attachments of the LM are closer together than the MM, and thus has a lowercase "c" shape; it forms a tighter curve than the uppercase 'C' of the MM. The anterior root of the LM has multiple fiber bundles, resulting in a striated appearance on MRI (**Fig. 4**).[8,9] The anterior root attaches lateral to, and blends with, the anterior cruciate ligament (ACL), and is anterior to the lateral tibial tubercle.[8,9] The close proximity of the root attachment results in the LM covering a larger portion of the articular surface, 70%, relative to the MM.[5] Unlike the MM, the LM anterior and posterior horns are equivalent in size (**Fig. 5**).[5]

NORMAL MRI APPEARANCE

Optimal assessment of the menisci requires the use of a high field strength magnet, 1.5 or 3.0 T, and dedicated knee coils, both of which contribute to image acquisition with a high signal-to-noise ratio. The high spatial resolution needed to assess the meniscus is obtained using a slice thickness of less than 4 mm, a field of view of 16 cm or less, and a matrix size of 192 × 256.[10] The magnetic resonance (MR) examination should consist of a combination of T1-weighted images and fluid-sensitive (PD or T2-weighted images) with or without fat suppression.[10]

Normal menisci are homogeneously low in signal intensity, or dark, on both T1-weighted and T2-weighted images because of their fibrocartilaginous composition.[11] In adult patients, linear or globular increased signal in the substance of the meniscus that does not contact the articular surface usually indicates mucinous degeneration (**Fig. 6**).[11,12] In pediatric patients, high signal in the substance of the meniscus that

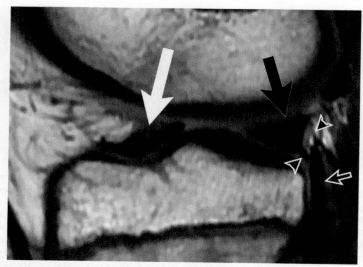

Fig. 4. Normal anterior and posterior horns of the LM. Sagittal PD image shows the normal fibrillar structure of the LM anterior root, shown in long axis in **Fig. 2**, is seen in cross-section on sagittal views as striated (*white arrow*). The posterior horn (*large black arrow*) is triangular, and is attached by thin struts (*arrowheads*) to the sheath of the popliteus tendon (*small black arrow*).

does not contact the articular surface corresponds to the increased vascularity that becomes less prevalent with increasing age.[13]

On sagittal images, the meniscus will have a "bow tie" shape in the midbody and a triangular shape in the anterior and posterior horns, approaching the mid joint line. On coronal images, the body of the meniscus will be triangular, whereas the anterior and posterior horns will be roughly rectangular, but slightly thicker at the medial and lateral corners. The posterior meniscal roots should lie adjacent to the posterior cruciate ligament (PCL). In cross-section, the inner, central margin of the meniscus should form a

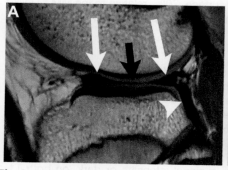
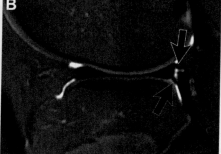

Fig. 5. Normal LM on sagittal images. PD image (*A*) shows the low-signal anterior and posterior horns (*white arrows*), equal in size, and the thin meniscal body near its central portion (*short black arrow*). Arrowhead points to the popliteal tendon. T2 fat-suppressed image (*B*) shows that the meniscus is uniformly hypointense. Normal fluid in the joint outlines the meniscus struts (*arrows*).

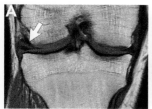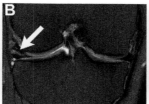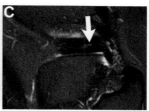

Fig. 6. Mucinous degeneration. Coronal T1 image (*A*) and PD fat-suppressed image (*B*) show that the midbody LM is enlarged relative to the MM. The margins of the meniscus remain low signal intensity, whereas the center (*arrow*) contains globular, mildly increased signal, characteristic of mucinous degeneration. Note that abnormal signal does not extend to an articular surface of the meniscus, distinguishing mucinous degeneration from tear. Sagittal T2 fat-suppressed image (*C*) shows abnormal high signal (*arrow*), which does not extend to the surface.

well-defined point like the apex of the triangle. On sagittal images, the posterior horn of the MM is larger than the anterior horn, whereas on the lateral side, the anterior horn LM is similar in size to the posterior horn.

IMAGING OF MENISCAL TEARS

The International Society of Arthroscopy, Knee Surgery and Orthopedic Sports medicine (ISAKOS) developed a classification to improve reporting standards for arthroscopic evaluation of meniscal tears.[14] Good interobserver reliability of the classification system was subsequently documented.[15] Per the ISAKOS classification, tears are described as partial (involving only one surface) or complete (involving both superior and inferior surfaces or both the free edge and peripheral margin). Tear orientation is divided into longitudinal-vertical (separating central and peripheral meniscus), horizontal (separating superior and inferior meniscus), radial (separating meniscus anterior to posterior in the body or medial to lateral in the anterior and posterior horns), vertical flap, horizontal flap, and complex (a combination of the basic types).[10,14]

Data from a meta-analysis of 27 studies revealed a sensitivity and specificity of 93% and 88%, respectively, for MM tears and 79% and 96% for LM tears.[16] Criteria for diagnosing meniscal tears in patients without a history of knee surgery include identification of intrameniscal signal contacting the meniscal surface and distortion of the normal meniscal shape.[11,17] Many additional imaging signs can be used to increase accuracy in the identification of meniscal tears; these include the two-slice-touch rule, alteration in meniscal shape, ghost meniscus, parameniscal cyst, and meniscal extrusion. Knowledge of specific types of meniscal tear, including Wrisberg rip and ramp lesions, will lead to accurate imaging diagnosis.

The *two-slice-touch* requires abnormal intrameniscal signal contacting the surface on two images—either consecutive sagittal/coronal images or two images in different planes (single coronal image and corresponding single sagittal image) (**Fig. 7**).[18,19] Identification of signal contacting the meniscal surface on a single image should be described as a possible meniscal tear; in a study of 174 patients, the positive predictive value was 43% for an MM tear and 18% for an LM tear as compared to arthroscopy.[19]

A change in the meniscal contour is an important finding in the identification of meniscal tears.[11,17] The change in the meniscal shape depends on the orientation of the tear and the imaging plane. A radial or vertical flap tear may result in truncation

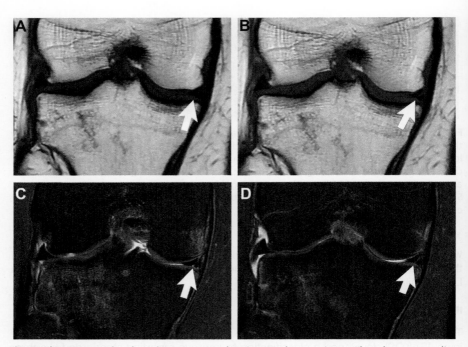

Fig. 7. The *Two-touch rule*. Adjacent coronal T1 images (*A* anterior to *B*) and corresponding PD fat-suppressed images (*C* anterior to *D*) show a thin line of increased signal intensity extending to the inferior surface of the medial meniscus (*arrow*), more easily appreciated on PD images. A meniscus tear can be confidently diagnosed because the abnormal signal extends to the articular surface on 2 slices. Note another sign of tear: the inner contour of the meniscus does not have a sharp, triangular, point.

of the normal triangular appearance of the meniscus when imaged in the same plane as the tear.[20] Widening of the base of the meniscal triangle, particularly when there is meniscal extension above or below the joint line, is indicative of a displaced meniscal flap—common in *horizontal flap* tears (**Fig. 8**).[11,21] Smaller size of a portion of the

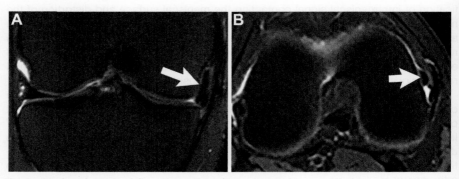

Fig. 8. *Displaced meniscal flap.* Coronal PD fat-suppressed image (*A*) shows that the in-situ meniscus is small, and has a blunted contour. Flap of the torn meniscus (*arrows*) is displaced above the joint line. Axial PD fat-suppressed image (*B*) shows displaced meniscus (*arrow*) between the medial femoral condyle and the medial collateral ligament.

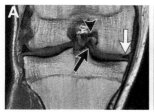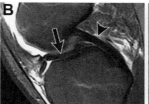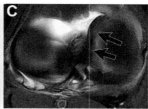

Fig. 9. *Bucket handle* longitudinal tear. Coronal T1 image (*A*) shows a small MM body (*white arrow*), which should prompt search for a displaced flap. In this case, the inner portion of the meniscus is displaced in the intercondylar notch (*black arrow*), immediately inferior to the PCL (*arrowhead*). Sagittal T2 fat-suppressed image (*B*) shows a large portion of the meniscus (*arrow*) displaced into the intercondylar notch. Because it lies anterior and inferior to the PCL (*arrowhead*), this is sometimes called the "double PCL" sign. Axial PD fat-suppressed image (*C*) shows the displaced portion of the MM (*arrows*), which remained attached to the in situ meniscus both anteriorly and posteriorly.

meniscus relative to the remainder of the meniscus or the contralateral meniscus should, in the absence of a history of partial meniscectomy, prompt a search for a displaced meniscal flap. In a longitudinal tear, the central portion of the meniscus may become displaced into the intercondylar notch. When the displaced flap remains attached to the anterior and posterior roots, this is known as a *bucket handle tear* (**Fig. 9**).

A radial tear disrupts the circumferential collagen fibers that distribute hoop stress (**Fig. 10**). The *ghost meniscus* is a sign of a radial tear.[20,22] It occurs when an image is acquired in the same plane and location as a radially oriented tear, for example, sagittal image is obtained through a radial tear in the anterior or posterior horn or a coronal image through a tear in the midbody. If the image is acquired through a tear, bright on T2-weighted images, and the adjacent meniscus, dark on T2-weighted images, the resultant image is an average of the torn and adjacent intact meniscus. The image of the meniscus will be intermediate to bright in signal intensity depending on the size of the tear.

Extrusion of the meniscus is defined as peripheral displacement of the meniscus relative to the margin of the tibial plateau ≥ 3 mm (**Fig. 11**).[23,24] Identification of a meniscal extrusion is an indirect sign of a meniscal tear that should prompt evaluation for a meniscal root or radial tear.[10,25]

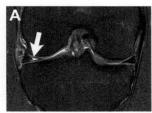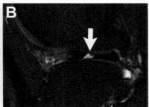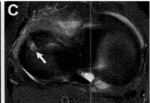

Fig. 10. Radial tear. Coronal PD fat-suppressed image (*A*) through the body of the lateral meniscus shows the meniscus comes to a blunted point, but the central portion of the meniscus is absent (*arrow*), a partial *ghost meniscus*. Sagittal T2 fat-suppressed image (*B*) shows the defect (*arrow*) in the meniscal body. Axial PD fat-suppressed image (*C*) shows the separation of the meniscus (*arrow*) due to the complete radial tear.

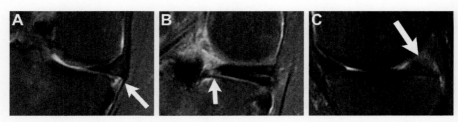

Fig. 11. *Meniscal extrusion* due to meniscal root tear. Coronal PD fat-suppressed image through midbody shows (*A*) the meniscus (*arrow*) is displaced medial to the medial tibial plateau. Coronal PD fat-suppressed image more posteriorly (*B*) shows the radial tear of the meniscal root. The root is displaced medially, with a wide fluid-filled cleft (*arrow*) and irregular margins. Sagittal T2 fat-suppressed image (*C*) through the tear shows the meniscus is small and irregularly shaped (*arrow*).

Parameniscal cysts are very frequently associated with meniscal tears (**Fig. 12**).[26,27] Parameniscal cysts occur more frequently on the medial side.[26–29] Meniscal tears are present with only 64% of cysts adjacent to the anterior horn versus with 100% of cysts adjacent to the midbody and posterior horn.[26]

The meniscofemoral ligaments attach the posterior horn of the LM to the medial femoral condyle. The meniscofemoral ligament of Wrisberg runs posterior to the PCL, and is present in 89% to 94% of patients.[30,31] The ligament of Humphry, identified in up to 27% of patients, runs anterior to the PCL. At the attachment of the meniscofemoral ligament to the LM, a small focus of fluid between the ligament and meniscus may mimic a peripheral meniscal tear (see **Fig. 5**).[32] The rotation and anterior translation that may occur with an ACL tear results in traction at the ligament attachment site, creating a longitudinal tear extending lateral to the normal attachment, known as the *Wrisberg rip* (**Fig. 13**).

Ramp lesions are repairable tears of the peripheral attachment of the posterior horn of the MM less than 2.5 cm in length that occur in the setting of acute ACL tear or chronic ACL insufficiency (**Fig. 14**).[33] Ramp lesions compromise the ability of the posterior horn MM to mechanically stabilize the knee against anterior subluxation. The

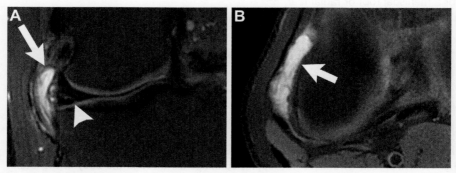

Fig. 12. *Parameniscal cyst.* Coronal PD fat-suppressed image (*A*) shows horizontal tear (*arrowhead*) extending to the inferior surface of the meniscus. There is an adjacent parameniscal cyst (*arrow*). Axial PD fat-suppressed image (*B*) shows the cyst (*arrow*) wraps around the lateral meniscus, compressed between the joint capsule and the tibia.

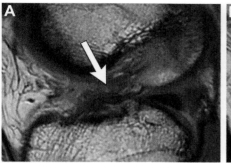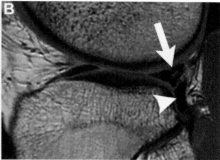

Fig. 13. *Wrisberg rip*, associated with ACL tear. Sagittal PD image through the intercondylar notch (*A*) shows wavy, discontinuous anterior cruciate ligament (*arrow*). Sagittal PD image through the posterior horn LM (*B*) shows the associated vertical tear (*arrow*), which occurs due to traction by the Wrisberg ligament on the posterior horn. Note that the tear is nearly parallel to the normal fluid seen between the meniscus and the popliteal tendon (*arrow*), and can be mistaken for a normal popliteal hiatus.

tear may involve the meniscocapsular ligament or the meniscotibial ligament with or without a tear of peripheral third of the posterior horn MM.[34]

VARIANTS THAT SIMULATE MENISCAL TEARS

Normal structures of the knee can simulate meniscal tears and are important to recognize as potential pitfalls. The *anterior horn of the LM* has a normal striated appearance as it approaches its anterior root attachment and should not be confused with a tear (see **Fig. 4**).[35] The *anterior transverse ligament* connects the anterior horns of the LM

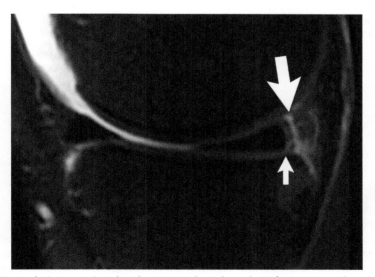

Fig. 14. *Ramp lesion*, associated with ACL tear (not shown). T2 fat-suppressed image shows a meniscocapsular separation (*large arrow*) and a far peripheral, vertically oriented tear of the meniscus (*small arrow*).

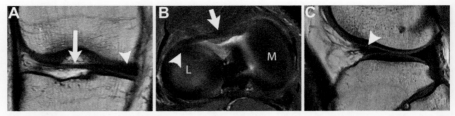

Fig. 15. Anterior intermeniscal ligament. Coronal T1 image (*A*) at the anterior margin of the joint shows the normal anterior intermeniscal ligament (*arrow*) outlined by fat and shows continuity with the anterior horn of the MM (*arrowhead*). Axial PD fat-suppressed image (*B*) shows the anterior intermeniscal ligament (*arrow*) extending between the menisci. Only small portions of the meniscus are visible on this image, but the obliquity of the ligament's attachment to the lateral meniscus is evident (*arrowhead*). Sagittal PD image (*C*) shows the ligament (*arrowhead*), as it approaches the anterior horn of the LM. At this point, the ligament should not be mistaken for a tear. *L, lateral compartment; M, medial compartment.*

and MM and there is often high signal between it and the anterior horn of the LM, which can simulate a tear (**Fig. 15**).[11] The *popliteal hiatus*, or the normal capsular opening through which the popliteus tendon enters the knee joint, is immediately superficial to the posterior horn of the LM (see **Fig. 5**). Along the medial margin of the hiatus, the main anchoring fascicle of the LM is visible in the sagittal plane and can simulate a tear of the posterior horn.[11]

Meniscal flounce is a pitfall that usually occurs when the patient's knee is partially flexed, rather than fully extended, during the MRI examination (**Figs. 16** and **17**).[11,36] In the partially flexed knee, the meniscus may be slightly redundant and appear slightly folded rather than lying flat relative to the tibial plateau. This artifact is more commonly seen during knee arthroscopy with certain positions.[36] Other findings discussed earlier can simulate tear but do not contact an articular surface and include *mucinous degeneration* and *pediatric vascularity*.

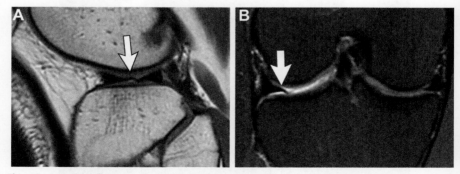

Fig. 16. *Meniscal flounce.* Sagittal T2W fat-suppressed image (*A*) through the body of the meniscus shows the central portion has a crinkled contour (*arrow*), known as the meniscal flounce. This appearance tends to occur when the knee is slightly flexed, as shown here. Coronal PD fat-suppressed image (*B*) shows the normal sharp inner margin in the area of the flounce (*arrow*).

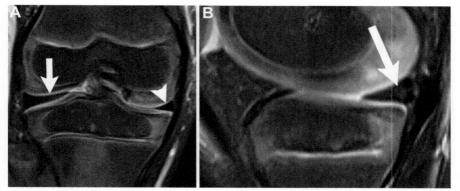

Fig. 17. *Pediatric Meniscal vascularity.* Coronal PD fat-suppressed image (*A*) through the midportion of the knee in a 7 yo scanned for cellulitis shows an incidental discoid LM (*arrow*), which covers nearly the entirety of the tibial plateau. In contrast, the normal body of the MM (*arrowhead*) covers only the periphery of the plateau. Sagittal PD fat-suppressed image (*B*) through the posterior horn of the MM shows high signal due to vascularity (*arrow*), which does not extend to the surface.

POSTOPERATIVE MENISCUS

MR evaluation of the postoperative meniscus remains a diagnostic challenge. After meniscal repair or partial meniscectomy, identification of abnormal signal extending to the articular surface and an abnormal shape of the meniscus are not necessarily indicative of recurrent tear. Diagnosis is aided by comparison to the preoperative MR imaging and operative report. An abnormality seen in an area of the meniscus where a preoperative tear was not present can be reliably diagnosed using the usual criteria. However, an abnormality in a region that has been treated surgically can be difficult to distinguish from normal postoperative findings.

Although noncontrast MRI is the standard to assess for meniscal injury in the native knee joint, a variety of techniques may be used to help assess the postoperative knee. Depending on the clinical question, implants used, patient contraindications, and

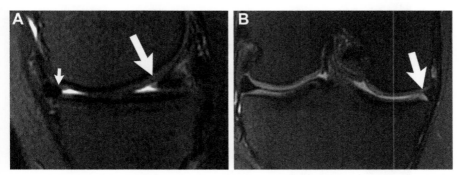

Fig. 18. Partial meniscectomy. Sagittal T2 fat-suppressed (*A*) image through the medial meniscus shows that both the posterior horn (*large arrow*) and anterior horn (*small arrow*) have a blunted contour indicating the free edge of the meniscus has been resected. Coronal PD fat-suppressed image (*B*) shows the MM (*arrow*) tapers to a point, but it is too small, another indication of partial meniscectomy.

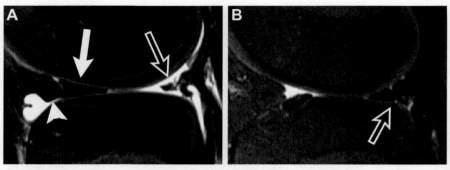

Fig. 19. Meniscal repair. Sagittal T2 fat-suppressed image (*A*) obtained preoperatively shows that the torn posterior meniscus (*black arrow*) is diminutive and irregular in contour. The displaced bucket handle fragment (*white arrow*) lies adjacent to the anterior meniscal horn (*arrowhead*). Sagittal T2 fat-suppressed image (*B*) obtained after meniscal repair shows that the flap has been reduced and sutured. Most of the repair site shows low signal intensity. High signal intensity at the periphery of the suture site (*arrow*) is consistent with granulation tissue.

surgeon preference, noncontrast knee MRI, direct MR arthrography, indirect MR arthrography, or direct CT arthrography may be used.[37]

After partial meniscectomy, the inner margin of the normally sharp meniscal triangle will be blunted and a variable portion of the meniscus will be absent (**Fig. 18**).[38] After meniscal repair, the intensity of abnormal signal in the meniscus on T2-weighted images has been shown to be predictive of recurrent tear. The absence of fluid signal in the meniscus at the site of repair indicates a healed repair (**Fig. 19**).[37] Additional findings of recurrent tear in the postoperative meniscus are irregular contour and displaced meniscal flap.[39] At arthrography, the criteria for recurrent tear are extension of contrast into the substance of the meniscus and displaced meniscal flap (**Fig. 20**).[40] It should be noted that if a postoperative meniscus meets criteria for

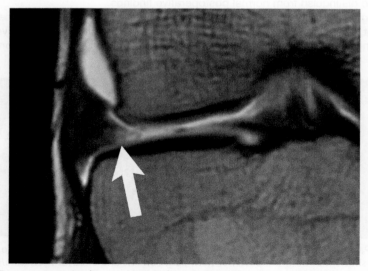

Fig. 20. Recurrent meniscal tear on MR arthrography. Coronal T1-weighted image shows injected contrast extending into a recurrent tear (*arrow*) after partial meniscectomy. Fluid is high signal (*white*) because gadolinium contrast material has been injected into the joint.

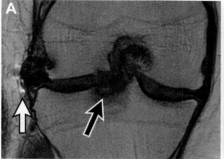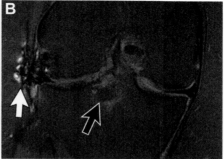

Fig. 21. Meniscal transplant. Coronal T1 (A) and PD fat-suppressed (B) images show bone plug (*black arrow*) transplanted with the meniscus, to better stabilize the meniscal roots. Artifact due to minuscule foci of metal related to repair (*white arrow*) is a normal finding.

tear on conventional MRI but contrast does not extend into the defect at arthrography, a recurrent tear remains likely.[40]

Meniscal allografts may be fixed with suture or bone fixation techniques. Bone fixation for the MM typically involves separate bone plugs for the anterior and posterior root attachments (**Fig. 21**).[41] The proximity of the anterior and posterior roots of the LM allows placement of the graft attached to a continuous bone bridge of varying shapes, which includes attached anterior and posterior roots.[42] Healing of the graft at MR imaging is defined as the absence of contrast extension between the graft and capsule at arthrography.[41] Normal meniscal allografts may have increased signal intensity, not reaching that of fluid, attributed to the graft maturation process. Increased signal in the graft more than 12 months after surgery, fluid signal intensity in the substance of the graph, or change in graft morphology are imaging findings of a torn graft. Shrinkage of the graft and graft extrusion are undesirable imaging outcomes, but are not predictive of a poor clinical outcome.[41]

SUMMARY

The menisci are critical supporting structures of the knee joint. Noninvasive evaluation of these small but important structures requires high-quality MR images, detailed understanding of anatomy and normal variants, and attention to multiple imaging signs of tear. Evaluation of the postoperative meniscus is especially difficult, and accuracy may be improved with arthrography.

DISCLOSURE

The authors have nothing to disclose.

REFERENCES

1. Fithian DC, Kelly MA, Mow VC. Material properties and structure-function relationships in the menisci. Clin Orthop Relat Res 1990;(252):19–31.

2. Petersen W, Tillmann B. Collagenous fibril texture of the human knee joint menisci. Anat Embryol (Berl) 1998;197:317–24.

3. Seedhom BB, Hargreaves DJ. Transmission of the Load in the Knee Joint with Special Reference to the Role of the Menisci. Eng Med 1979;8:220–8.

4. Arnoczky SP, Warren RF. Microvasculature of the human meniscus. Am J Sports Med 1982;10:90–5.
5. Rath E, Richmond JC. The menisci: Basic science and advances in treatment. Br J Sports Med 2000;34:252–7.
6. Cooper DE, Arnoczky SP, Warren RF. Arthroscopic meniscal repair. Clin Sports Med 1990;9:589–607.
7. Rosas HG, De Smet AA. Magnetic Resonance Imaging of the Meniscus. Top Magn Reson Imaging 2009;20:151–73.
8. Brody JM, Hulstyn MJ, Fleming BC, et al. The Meniscal Roots: Gross Anatomic Correlation with 3-T MRI Findings. Am J Roentgenol 2007;188:W446–50.
9. Sharif B, Ashraf T, Saifuddin A. Magnetic resonance imaging of the meniscal roots. Skeletal Radiol Skeletal Radiol 2020;49:661–76.
10. Nguyen JC, De Smet AA, Graf BK, et al. MR imaging-based diagnosis and classification of meniscal tears. Radiographics 2014;34:981–99.
11. De Smet AA. How I diagnose meniscal tears on knee MRI. Am J Roentgenol 2012;199:181–499.
12. Stoller DW, Martin C, Crues JV, et al. Meniscal tears: Pathologic correlation with MR imaging. Radiology 1987;163:731–5.
13. Francavilla ML, Restrepo R, Zamora KW, et al. Meniscal pathology in children: Differences and similarities with the adult meniscus. Pediatr Radiol 2014;44:910–25.
14. Anderson A. The ISAKOS Classification of Meniscal Tears. ISAKOS Newsl 2010;1–3.
15. Anderson AF, Irrgang JJ, Dunn W, et al. Interobserver reliability of the International Society of Arthroscopy, Knee Surgery and Orthopaedic Sports Medicine (ISAKOS) classification of meniscal tears. Am J Sports Med 2011;39:926–32.
16. Oei EHG, Nikken JJ, Verstijnen ACM, et al. MR imaging of the menisci and cruciate ligaments: A systematic review. Radiology 2003;226:837–48.
17. Manaster BJ. Magnetic resonance imaging of the knee. Semin Ultrasound CT MRI 1990;11:307–26.
18. De Smet AA, Norris MA, Yandow DR, et al. MR diagnosis of meniscal tears of the knee: importance of high signal in the meniscus that extends to the surface. AJR Am J Roentgenol 1993;161:101–7.
19. De Smet AA, Tuite MJ. Use of the "two-slice-touch" rule for the MRI diagnosis of meniscal tears. Am J Roentgenol 2006;187:911–4.
20. Harper KW, Helms CA, Lambert HS, et al. Radial meniscal tears: Significance, incidence, and MR appearance. Am J Roentgenol 2005;185:1429–34.
21. McKnight A, Southgate J, Price A, et al. Meniscal tears with displaced fragments: Common patterns on magnetic resonance imaging. Skeletal Radiol 2010;39:279–83.
22. Tuckman GA, Miller WJ, Remo JW, et al. Radial tears of the menisci: MR findings. AJR Am J Roentgenol 1994;163:395–400.
23. Costa CR, Morrison WB, Carrino JA. Medial meniscus extrusion on knee MRI: Is extent associated with severity of degeneration or type of tear? Am J Roentgenol 2004;183:17–23.
24. Lerer DB, Umans HR, Xu MX, et al. The role of meniscal root pathology and radial meniscal tear in medial meniscal extrusion. Skeletal Radiol 2004;33:569–74.
25. Choi C-J, Choi Y-J, Lee J-J, et al. Magnetic Resonance Imaging Evidence of Meniscal Extrusion in Medial Meniscus Posterior Root Tear. Arthrosc J Arthrosc Relat Surg 2010;26:1602–6.

26. De Smet AA, Graf BK, Del Rio AM. Association of parameniscal cysts with underlying meniscal tears as identified on MRI and arthroscopy. Am J Roentgenol 2011;196:180–6.

27. Anderson JJ, Connor GF, Helms CA. New observations on meniscal cysts. Skeletal Radiol 2010;39:1187–91.

28. Tasker AD, Ostlere SJ. Relative incidence and morphology of lateral and medial meniscal cysts detected by magnetic resonance imaging. Clin Radiol 1995;50: 778–81.

29. De Maeseneer M, Shahabpour M, Vanderdood K, et al. MR imaging of meniscal cysts: evaluation of location and extension using a three-layer approach. Eur J Radiol 2001;39:117–24.

30. Cho JM, Suh JS, Na JB, et al. Variations in meniscofemoral ligaments at anatomical study and MR imaging. Skeletal Radiol 1999;28:189–95.

31. Abreu MR, Chung CB, Trudell D, et al. Meniscofemoral ligaments: Patterns of tears and pseudotears of the menisci using cadaveric and clinical material. Skeletal Radiol 2007;36:729–35.

32. Vahey TN, Bennett HT, Arrington LE, et al. MR imaging of the knee: Pseudotear of the lateral meniscus caused by the meniscofemoral ligament. Am J Roentgenol 1990;154:1237–9.

33. Liu X, Feng H, Zhang H, et al. Arthroscopic prevalence of ramp lesion in 868 patients with anterior cruciate ligament injury. Am J Sports Med 2011;39:832–7.

34. Greif DN, Baraga MG, Rizzo MG, et al. MRI appearance of the different meniscal ramp lesion types, with clinical and arthroscopic correlation. Skeletal Radiol 2020;49:677–89.

35. Shankman S, Beltran J, Melamed E, et al. Anterior horn of the lateral meniscus: another potential pitfall in MR imaging of the knee. Radiology 1997;204:181–4.

36. Park JS, Ryu KN, Yoon KH. Meniscal flounce on knee MRI: Correlation with meniscal locations after positional changes. Am J Roentgenol 2006;187:364–70.

37. Boutin RD, Fritz RC, Marder RA. Magnetic Resonance Imaging of the Postoperative Meniscus. Magn Reson Imaging Clin N Am 2014;22:517–55.

38. Recht MP, Kramer J. MR Imaging of the Postoperative Knee: A Pictorial Essay. RadioGraphics 2002;22:765–74.

39. Kijowski R, Rosas H, Williams A, et al. MRI characteristics of torn and untorn postoperative menisci. Skeletal Radiol 2017;46:1353–60.

40. Magee T. Accuracy of 3-Tesla MR and MR arthrography in diagnosis of meniscal retear in the post-operative knee. Skeletal Radiol 2014;43:1057–64.

41. Dianat S, Small KM, Shah N, et al. Imaging of meniscal allograft transplantation: what the radiologist needs to know. Skeletal Radiol 2020;50(4):615–27.

42. Farr J, Gersoff W. Current meniscal allograft transplantation. Sports Med Arthrosc 2004;12:69–82.

Knee Ligament Imaging
Preoperative and Postoperative Evaluation

Andrew G. Geeslin, MD[a], Diego F. Lemos, MD[b,c],
Matthew G. Geeslin, MD, MEng[d,*]

KEYWORDS

- Ligament imaging • MRI • Stress radiography • Postoperative
- Anterolateral complex • Knee

KEY POINTS

- Awareness of knee ligament disruption patterns improves injury detection and supports timely and appropriate surgical planning.
- Stress radiography is a useful tool for quantifying ligamentous laxity, particularly in chronic settings and when MRI findings and clinical presentation are discordant.
- Postoperative imaging evaluation hinges on the appropriate utilization of available modalities and requires familiarity with the normal and abnormal postoperative appearance of ligament repair and reconstruction.

INTRODUCTION

Knee ligament injuries are very common and imaging diagnosis is a vital first step in the treatment pathway. This article will review basic and advanced topics in knee ligament imaging, with the goal of highlighting challenging aspects of imaging throughout the course of injury management.

Comprehensive management of knee ligament injury hinges on thorough preoperative imaging review such that all injuries may be detected at initial imaging to allow for appropriate surgical planning. Familiarity with the surgical significance of image findings across modalities supports efficient and appropriate patient management, particularly when urgent referral to an orthopedic subspecialist is required for more complex treatment. MRI is often considered the gold standard for the assessment of ligamentous injury although standard radiography, stress radiography, and computed tomography (CT) also have important roles. In the forthcoming discussion,

[a] Department of Orthopedic Surgery, University of Vermont Medical Center, 192 Tilley Drive, South Burlington, VT 05403, USA; [b] Radiology and Orthopedic Surgery, University of Vermont Medical Center, Burlington, VT, USA; [c] Department of Radiology, 111 Colchester Avenue, Burlington, VT 05401, USA; [d] Department of Radiology, University of Vermont Medical Center, 111 Colchester Avenue, Burlington, VT 05401, USA
* Corresponding author.
E-mail address: Matthew.geeslin@uvmhealth.org

Clin Sports Med 40 (2021) 657–675
https://doi.org/10.1016/j.csm.2021.05.005
0278-5919/21/© 2021 Elsevier Inc. All rights reserved.

sportsmed.theclinics.com

we will begin by reviewing the utility of each imaging modality as it is optimally deployed for ligamentous evaluation in the preoperative setting.

Evaluation of knee ligament injury does not conclude at the initial diagnosis of native ligament disruption. Frequently, postoperative imaging assessment presents the greatest diagnostic challenge. Appropriate utilization of available imaging modalities for postoperative ligament assessment and familiarity with the normal and abnormal postoperative appearance of ligament reconstruction is required.

DISCUSSION
Preoperative Evaluation

Image modality utilization

Standard radiographs are a first-line modality for the assessment of knee injury. Relative to cross-sectional imaging, they are efficient and low-cost. However, their sensitivity for ligamentous injury is largely limited to the secondary osseous findings associated with ligamentous injury.

The lower extremity mechanical axis strongly influences the surgical approach for ligamentous injuries. Weight-bearing mechanical axis radiographs to assess coronal plane malalignment (ie, varus or valgus) are critical when considering surgical reconstruction of chronic injuries. Sagittal plane malalignment secondary to abnormal tibial slope has been implicated in anterior cruciate ligament (ACL) reconstruction graft failure; true lateral knee radiographs allow assessment of tibial slope and should be obtained in all patients undergoing ACL reconstruction as well as in those with residual laxity postoperatively.

Stress radiography has been shown to provide objective and reproducible quantification of knee ligament injury. This method is particularly useful in patients with multiligament injury, chronic injuries, previous reconstruction procedures, as well as those with equivocal MRI findings but persistent laxity on examination. Stress radiography requires acquisition of bilateral knee radiographs with force applied at a defined location and side-to-side comparison of compartment gapping or tibial translation. The results of stress radiography may be incorporated for surgical decision-making with consideration of patient activity level, the presence of multiligament injury, and the severity of additionally injured ligaments.

Prior biomechanical studies have established a relationship between injury grade and measurements obtained by stress radiography (**Table 1**). Varus[1,2] and valgus[3] stress radiographs are obtained with each knee imaged in the anterior-posterior dimension with knee flexion set at 20°. Varus stress radiography is used to assess lateral compartment gapping and thereby the lateral and posterolateral supporting structures, principally the fibular collateral ligament (FCL) and posterolateral corner (PLC) (**Fig. 1**). Valgus stress radiography is performed to assess medial compartment gapping and injury to the medial and posteromedial supporting structures, chiefly the medial collateral ligament (MCL) and posterior oblique ligament (POL) (**Fig. 2**). Kneeling (posterior) stress radiography is obtained with the knee flexed at 90°, and each knee imaged separately with a comparison of the side-to-side difference in posterior tibial translation[4] (**Fig. 3**). The primary structure evaluated with this mechanism is the PCL, however, depending on the severity of posterior tibial translation, injury to the posterolateral and or posteromedial corner can also be inferred.

MRI provides the greatest soft tissue contrast and thereby the most sensitive evaluation for ligament integrity. It is this soft tissue contrast that allows MRI to detect fiber disruption as well as intraligamentous and periligamentous edema, a secondary finding of injury. As noted earlier, an intact ligament does not necessarily imply a

Table 1
Summary of stress radiographic findings and corresponding ligamentous injury grading[1-4]

Stress View	Structures Evaluated	Side-to-Side Difference	Significance
Varus (lateral compartment gapping)	FCL and PLC	0–2.1 mm	Partial FCL tear
		2.2–4.0 mm	Complete FCL tear
		>4.0 mm	Complete PLC tear
Valgus (medial compartment gapping)	MCL and PMC	0–3.1 mm	Partial MCL tear
		3.2–9.7 mm	Complete MCL tear
		>9.8 mm	Complete PMC tear
Kneeling (posterior tibial translation)	PCL and PLC/PMC	0–8.0 mm	Partial PCL tear
		8.1–12.0 mm	Complete PCL tear
		>12.0 mm	Combined PCL tear and PLC or PMC injury

Abbreviation: PMC, posteromedial corner.

functional ligament. In cases of MRI discordance with clinical presentation, stress radiography may be required for a "functional" evaluation of suspected ligament insufficiency.

Systematic preoperative imaging evaluation of knee ligament injury

Cruciate ligaments—The ACL is the most commonly reconstructed ligament.[5] Key secondary signs of ACL disruption can be detected radiographically and include depression of the lateral femoral notch (deep lateral femoral notch sign),[6] avulsion fracture from the anterolateral tibia (Segond fracture)[7] (**Fig. 4**), and anterior tibial translation. As the most common ligamentous reconstruction, efficient and accurate diagnosis of ACL disruption on MRI is well established. MRI for ACL disruption requires careful examination of both its anteromedial and posterolateral fiber bundles in the coronal, axial, and sagittal planes for the greatest sensitivity. Tears should be described as partial or complete and tear location should be described as repair of proximal (femoral) avulsions is increasing.[8] Avulsion fractures of the tibial spine should include measurement of the osseous fragment size and a description of the position

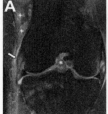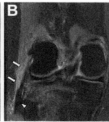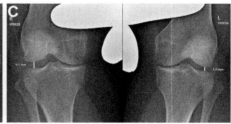

Fig. 1. Coronal PD fat sat images at the midanterior (*A*) and more posterior (*B*) aspects of the right knee show a grade 2 injury of the FCL with intrasubstance partial tear proximally (*white straight arrow*) as well as periligamentous edema along the entire length of the ligament (*white arrowheads*). The distal FCL and biceps femoris are intact at their insertion on the fibular head (*white*). Soft tissue edema along the course of the Kaplan fibers (*white stars*) and a high-grade ACL tear (*white asterisk*) are also noted. Varus stress radiographs (*C*) demonstrate increased right knee lateral compartment gapping by 3.4 mm (side-to-side difference) consistent with an insufficient FCL.

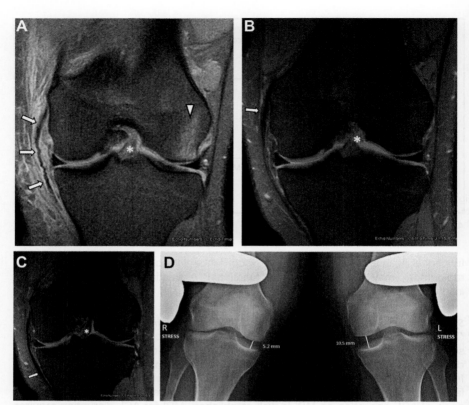

Fig. 2. Coronal PD MR image (*A*) of the left knee obtained in an 18-year-old male shows a grade 3 tear of the MCL at its distal insertion on the tibia. The torn MCL is wavy and proximally retracted (*white straight arrows*). There is a bone marrow contusion on the lateral femoral condyle (*white arrowhead*) as well as a grade 2 partial tear of the ACL (*white asterisk*). Two consecutive coronal PD fat sat images obtained 3 years later due to persistent instability (*B, C*) demonstrate mild thickening and irregularity of the superficial MCL (*straight white arrows*), although the study was interpreted as "normal." The ACL shows interval healing (*white asterisks*). Bilateral comparison valgus stress radiographs (*D*) were obtained and demonstrate a 5.3 mm side-to-side difference in the gapping of the medial femorotibial compartments, clinically and radiographically consistent with an insufficient superficial MCL on the left knee.

relative to the anterior meniscal attachments as well as the amount of displacement (angulation and translation). An established secondary sign of ACL disruption on MRI is lateral compartment bone bruising.[9]

There are several associated injuries that are recognized in the setting of ACL disruption, including the MCL, PLC,[5] medial and lateral menisci,[10] and anterolateral complex (ALC).[11] Awareness of the presence of such injury associations helps increase the index of suspicion for the radiologist and surgeon and promote careful scrutiny of particular anatomic structures.

The PCL consists of two bundles (anterolateral and posteromedial) and is the primary restraint to posterior tibial translation. Injury to the PCL is far more common in the setting of multiligament injury than in isolation.[12] PCL tear location and grade as well as the presence of associated injury has been shown to direct management

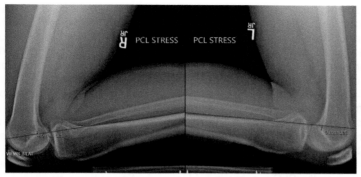

Fig. 3. Kneeling (posterior) stress radiographs are shown in a patient with a grade 3 chronic left knee PCL and PLC injury demonstrating 13.5 mm increased posterior tibial translation of the left knee compared with the intact right knee.

with regard to conservative versus surgical treatment, and such findings should be carefully documented during MRI evaluation.[13] Additional findings including posterior tibial subluxation on MRI should be noted when abnormality of the PCL is identified.[14]

Medial and Posteromedial Knee—The MCL is the most commonly injured ligament in the knee.[15] Acute injuries are usually clinically evident because of localized pain and swelling and injury location may be predicted based on the region of tenderness. Chronic injuries may be evident because of increased medial joint opening during valgus stress testing and this can be quantified with stress radiographs. MRI provides a qualitative assessment of medial ligamentous structure integrity and is most useful in the acute setting. The superficial MCL (ie, tibial collateral ligament) has a proximal femoral attachment as well as proximal and distal tibial attachments (1.2 cm and 6 cm below the joint line, respectively)[16] and to avoid missing distal MCL injuries, the imaging protocol must include a field of view 6 cm below the joint line on coronal sequences.

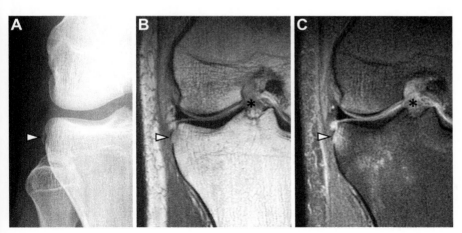

Fig. 4. AP radiograph (*A*) and coronal PD and PD fat sat MRI (*B, C*) demonstrating a minimally displaced Segond fracture (*white arrowhead*) and complete ACL tear (*black asterisk*) (*B,C*).

Most isolated proximal and midsubstance MCL injuries heal adequately with nonsurgical treatment, whereas acute surgical treatment is often indicated for tibial-based grade 3 injuries (especially when the torn MCL fibers are displaced superficial to the pes anserinus (**Fig. 5**) or if they are intra-articularly entrapped (**Fig. 6**) and in multi-ligamentous injuries). MCL reporting should therefore include location (tibial, femoral, or midsubstance) as well as grade (partial vs complete).[17,18] A secondary finding of acute MCL tears is lateral compartment bone bruising, which must be distinguished from that seen with ACL tears.[19]

Posterolateral Knee — The three primary static stabilizers of the PLC include the FCL, popliteus tendon, and popliteofibular ligament (PFL).[20] These three structures, along with the biceps femoris tendon, are readily identifiable components of the PLC on MRI and their injured appearance has been well documented.[21] Image-based diagnosis of injury to the PLC requires individual evaluation of these structures. As in the case of the MCL, reporting of ligamentous injury should include severity (partial vs complete) as well as location (femoral or fibular avulsions, as well as midsubstance injuries). An important secondary sign of grade 3 PLC injuries is medial compartment bone bruising.[22] A useful secondary sign of popliteus injury is the presence of muscle belly edema, and such a finding should prompt careful evaluation of the tendon and myotendinous region. Varus stress radiographs may be used in acute and chronic settings and are especially useful in evaluating injuries to this region of the knee due to frequently identified physiologic laxity on physical examination.

Injury to the PLC most commonly occurs in the setting of other knee ligament disruption. In fact, only approximately 28% of PLC injuries occur in isolation.[22–24] These data highlight the importance of careful MRI review of the PLC on knee examinations obtained with a history of recent trauma, particularly when cruciate ligament injury has been identified. The radiologist should understand that detection of grade 3 tearing of the LCL, popliteus, or PFL has surgical consequences and requires orthopedic evaluation (**Fig. 7**). Additional indications for PLC repair or reconstruction

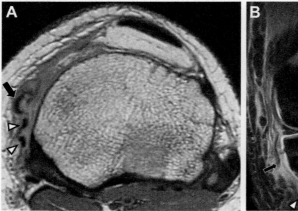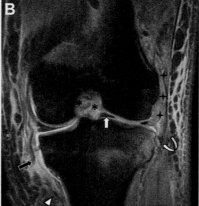

Fig. 5. Axial PD (*A*) and coronal T2W fat sat (*B*) MR images show a Stener-like lesion of the knee. There is a complete distal tear of the superficial MCL at its insertion in the tibia. The torn MCL is proximally retracted (*black straight arrow*) and superficial to the plane of the interposed pes anserinus tendons (*white arrowheads*). There are high-grade tears of the ACL and PCL (*black asterisks*) as well as tearing of the Kaplan fibers and ALL (*black stars*). A Segond fracture (*curved white arrow*) and bucket handle tear of the lateral meniscus are present as well (*white straight arrow*).

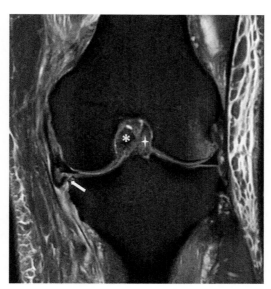

Fig. 6. Coronal T2W fat sat MR image shows a complete tear of the superficial MCL at its distal insertion on the tibia. The torn MCL is proximally retracted and partially entrapped along the periphery of the medial femorotibial compartment (*white straight arrow*). There are low-grade partial tears of the ACL (*white star*) and the PCL (*white asterisk*).

include displaced osseous avulsions and soft tissue avulsions of the biceps femoris.[24] Further underscoring the importance of prompt diagnosis of PLC injury is the association of improved outcomes when injury is surgically addressed within 3 weeks.[24]

Anterolateral Knee—Increasing attention has been paid to the ALC of the knee because of the relationship between injury to this region in combination with ACL tears. The anatomic composition of the ALC of the knee includes the superficial and deep aspects of the iliotibial band (ITB) with its Kaplan fiber attachments on the distal femur, the capsuloosseous layer of the ITB, and the anterolateral ligament (ALL).[11]

The ALL originates posterior and slightly proximal to the FCL and courses anteroinferiorly to its insertion on the anterolateral tibia, midway between the center of Gerdy's tubercle and the anterior aspect of the fibular head.[25] A combination of axial and coronal MRI planes is best suited to visualize this band of fibers. The Kaplan fibers arise from the deep aspect of the IT band at the level of the distal femur and consist of two distinct fiber bundles attaching on the distal femur to two osseous ridges.[26]

Biomechanical and outcomes-based studies have evaluated the ALC with regard to its role in anterolateral stability, particularly in the setting of ACL disruption, laxity, and reconstruction. The increased incidence of ALL injury in the setting of ACL disruption provides further evidence for its role in stability, and investigations report a range of ALL injury between 10% and 62%, in patients with a complete ACL tear.[27,28] The Kaplan fibers are readily identified on MRI and studies have shown up to 30% injury rate in the setting of ACL tear[29,30] (**Fig. 8**). The superficial ITB band inserts onto Gerdy's tubercle and has also demonstrated a high incidence of injury (albeit low grade) in the setting of ACL disruption.

Anteromedial Knee—The static stabilizers of the anteromedial knee include the medial patellofemoral ligament, medial patellotibial ligament, and medial patellomeniscal ligament.[31] The reader is referred to an article in the present issue on the supporting structures of the anteromedial knee, as they relate to patellofemoral stability.

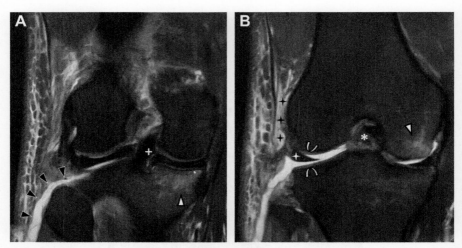

Fig. 7. Two coronal fluid-sensitive MR images (*A, B*) show complete detachment of the lateral and posterolateral supporting structures of the knee inserting in the fibular head, denoted by a fluid-filled gap highlighting the naked insertional footprints on the fibula (*black arrowheads*) including those for the biceps femoris and fibular collateral ligament as well as the popliteofibular ligament. Supporting structures of the anterolateral complex are also injured, including the anterolateral ligament and iliotibial band, the latter with extensive soft tissue edema along the proximal and distal Kaplan fibers (*black stars*). There is a moderate- to high-grade partial tear of the ACL (*white asterisk*) as well as a "floating" lateral meniscus due to loss of its tibial attachments (*white star*) with gapping of the lateral femorotibial compartment (*white curved arrows*). The PCL was intact (*white cross*). There are bone marrow contusions in the medial femoral condyle and medial tibial plateau (*white arrowheads*).

Postoperative Imaging of Ligament Repair and Reconstruction

Image modality utilization

Imaging modalities most commonly used for postoperative assessment of ligamentous repair and reconstruction include standard radiography, stress radiography, CT, and MRI.

Standard Radiographs—Standard radiographs are routinely obtained at 1 to 2 weeks for postoperative assessment of ligament reconstruction with anteroposterior (AP) and lateral views. Radiographic image review should be completed with the assessment of screw and anchor position for prominence, subsidence, or migration. Radiography is also used to assess tunnel position to ensure anatomic reconstruction. The consequences of tunnel malposition, such as graft impingement, are better demonstrated on MRI. Peri-hardware osteolysis manifesting as lucency is another postsurgical complication that can be detected radiographically, but is not expected on early postoperative imaging.

Stress Radiographs—Stress radiography can be conducted with varus, valgus, and kneeling (posterior) stress views to assess lateral and medial supporting structures as well as the PCL, respectively. Stress radiographs can be obtained in the postoperative setting to quantify ligamentous laxity and are routinely performed at 6 months after surgery. As emphasized in **Fig. 2**, an "intact" ligament as defined by the absence of frank fiber disruption on MRI, is not always clinically stable. Stress radiography is ideally suited to provide quantifiable results for such discordant scenarios.

Computed Tomography—CT is used in the postoperative setting for the evaluation of osseous details relative to ligament reconstruction. Tunnel diameter measurement

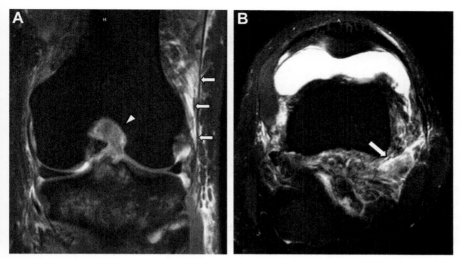

Fig. 8. Left knee coronal (A) and axial (B) PD fat sat MR images demonstrate edema along the course of the distal Kaplan fibers (straight white arrows) compatible with partial tearing. The empty notch sign on the coronal PD FS MRI demonstrates a high-grade ACL tear (A) (white arrowhead).

(to evaluate for osteolysis) and tunnel position are two key aspects of postoperative CT for ligament reconstruction. CT is also used to evaluate bone stock and osseous graft incorporation for 2-stage revision cruciate ligament reconstruction (**Fig. 9**).[32]

MRI—MRI is generally considered the imaging modality of choice to evaluate ligament and graft integrity in both the preoperative and postoperative setting (**Fig. 10**).

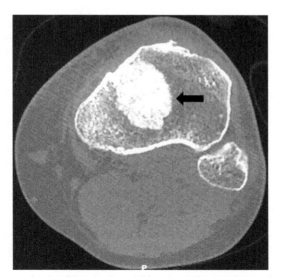

Fig. 9. Axial CT image obtained in a patient with prior ACL tunnel osteolysis after first-stage bone grafting before a second-stage revision ACL reconstruction. There is evidence of excellent osseous incorporation of the bone graft (black arrow).

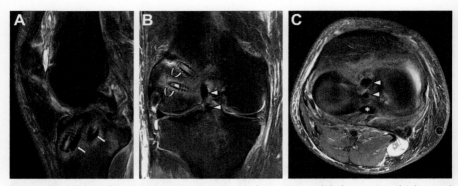

Fig. 10. Double bundle ACL reconstruction. Sagittal T2W image (*A*) shows two tibial tunnels for the anteromedial and posterolateral bundles (*white straight arrows*). Coronal T2W image (*B*) shows the two corresponding femoral tunnels for both bundles of the ACL graft (*white curved arrows*). Axial T2W image (*C*) at the level of the joint line shows the two intact anteromedial and posterolateral bundles of the ACL graft (*white arrowheads*), the intact native PCL (*white asterisk*) is noted posterior to the ACL graft bundles. The posterolateral bundle tunnel in the tibia may have destabilized the lateral meniscal posterior root because of the posterior position of this tunnel. (Case courtesy of Dr Atul Taneja from São Paulo, Brazil.)

Compared with standard and stress radiography, MRI is not ordered in the postoperative period for routine follow-up, but rather to assess suspicion for failure of the repair/reconstruction.

Systematic postoperative imaging evaluation of knee ligament repair and reconstruction

Assessment of postoperative imaging is more complex than preoperative imaging as the reviewer must understand the normal anatomic appearance and attachment locations as well as the basic surgical principles, fixation devices, and procedures performed, and incorporate these findings to interpret the normal and abnormal appearance. Tunnel/socket size, reconstruction position (including tunnel, graft, and fixation device), security of fixation device, and graft structural integrity must be assessed.

Procedure performed—Postoperative imaging evaluation should begin with confirmation of the surgical procedure that was performed. This step helps set expectations for tunnel placement (**Fig. 11**), hardware usage, and potential complications. The surgery performed is often visually evident in cases of single ligament repair or reconstruction. However, owing to technical differences between surgeons and evolving surgical techniques, imaging evaluation of multiligament reconstructions (**Fig. 12**) should be preceded by review of the operative note if possible. In cases of multiligament imaging, review of preoperative imaging also helps the reviewer set expectations for postoperative image review.

Hardware type and position—The most commonly used fixation devices for ligament surgery include anchors, screws, suture washers, screw-washer combinations, and staples. Anchors are most frequently used in repairs but may also be used in reconstruction procedures for only fixation. Interference and tenodesis screws are placed within a tunnel or socket and secure the graft, compressing it against the adjacent bone. Suture washers are placed adjacent to cortical bone to secure a graft within a tunnel and are common in intra-articular (ie, cruciate ligament) reconstruction but

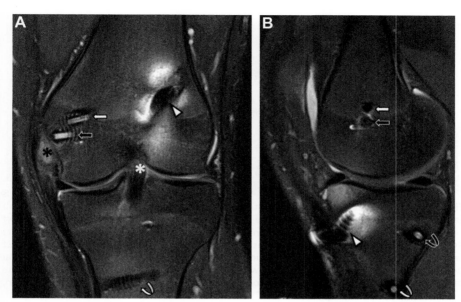

Fig. 11. Coronal (*A*) and sagittal (*B*) T2W fat sat images show postsurgical changes from an MCL and POL reconstruction with 2 grafts, 2 femoral tunnels, and 2 tibial tunnels in a patient with additional postsurgical changes from a single bundle ACL reconstruction. Note the proximal screw (*straight white arrow*) and distal screw (*curved white arrow*) for the POL graft, as well as the proximal screw (*straight black arrow*) and distal screw (*curved black arrow*) for the MCL graft, which is partially torn proximally (*black asterisk*). Note the metallic screws in the tibial and femoral tunnels (*white arrowheads*) for the ACL graft, which is intact (*white asterisk*).

may also be used in extra-articular ligament reconstruction. Screw-washer devices may be used in both cruciate and collateral ligament reconstruction when intratunnel fixation is not selected. Staples may be used in certain cruciate ligament reconstruction techniques as well as with lateral extra-articular tenodesis (LET).

Owing to material differences in components used for ligament repair and reconstruction, hardware may be isodense or hyperdense to the adjacent bone surface or osseous tunnel. In some instances, hardware migration is pronounced and easily detected because of its metallic hyperdensity (**Fig. 13**). Detection of subtle, isodense hardware migration is improved through attention to hardware position relative to osseous tunnels and use of cross-sectional imaging or acquisition of two orthogonal radiographic views.

Tunnel Position—Procedures to restore the anatomy are most commonly used when considering knee ligament reconstruction. Some procedures such as LET (**Fig. 14**) and certain PLC reconstructions are felt to be nonanatomic but serve to accomplish a biomechanical aim. It should be recognized that surgical and patient factors, as well as differences in interpretation of anatomic principles, may influence surgical technique for reconstruction procedures. However, accepted anatomic principles should be observed. Tunnels placed in nonanatomic position (eg, malpositioned ACL reconstruction) may lead to postoperative complications such as loss of knee extension, graft failure, or failure to achieve a biomechanical aim (**Fig. 15**). The orthopedic surgeon reviewing postoperative imaging must carefully observe tunnel location; the radiologist also has a role in noting tunnel position although emphasis

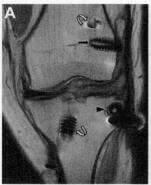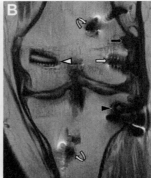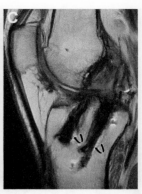

Fig. 12. Three MR images depicting multiligament reconstruction, illustrating the importance of tunnel position planning because of the limited bone volume in the knee. Two coronal PD images (*A, B*) and a sagittal PD image (*C*) show postsurgical changes from ACL and PCL reconstructions as well as a PLC reconstruction. Note the two interference screws in the lateral femoral condyle for proximal fixation of the FCL graft (*black straight arrow*) and the popliteus graft (*white straight arrow*), as well as the interference screw in the lateral aspect of the proximal tibia for distal graft fixation (*black arrowhead*). The tunnel and screw in the proximal fibula, which are part of the PLC reconstruction, are not included in these images, only the susceptibility artifact from the adjacent metallic fibular screw is noted. There is an additional interference screw in the medial aspect of the distal femur for fixation of the PCL graft (*white arrowhead*) in addition to screws in the femur and tibia near the midline for fixation of the ACL graft on both sides (*white curved arrows*). The tibial tunnels for the ACL and PCL grafts are both well seen in the sagittal image (*black curved arrows*). The femoral tunnel for the PCL graft is approximately one tunnel width anterior to its anatomic position. Intra-articular course of ACL and PCL grafts is not shown.

should be placed on presenting the information in an objective fashion and allowing the treating surgeon to make appropriate conclusions based on the objective information. Given the limited bone volume in the knee, tunnel position requires precise planning in cases where more than one osseous tunnel is required. The radiologist should carefully observe tunnel position and report tunnel convergence or collision if present, as multiligament reconstructions are at increased risk for this.[33]

Osteolysis—Evaluation of the osseous tunnels for peri-hardware osteolysis is required. Tunnel osteolysis, which may compromise bony integrity and complicates tunnel placement in revision setting, manifests on radiographs and CT as peri-screw lucency, and on MRI as a combination of tunnel widening and often T2 hyperintensity replacing bone-screw apposition (**Fig. 16**). The challenge of tunnel osteolysis is most commonly associated with ACL reconstruction although it can be seen with any intra-articular tunnel such as PCL reconstruction. True osteolysis is not commonly seen with collateral ligament reconstruction (unless there is convergence with an intra-articular tunnel) although bony integrity around a collateral ligament tunnel should be assessed.

Femoral-Tibial Subluxation—Close attention to femoral tibial alignment and course of the graft fibers is recommended and abnormalities merit reporting. Tibial subluxation serves as a supplemental "stress" view on MRI and evaluation of femorotibial alignment is required, as an "intact" graft does not always correspond to a functional graft. The oblique course of the cruciate ligaments sets up a corresponding subluxation pattern for graft laxity. An insufficient ACL may result in anterior subluxation of the

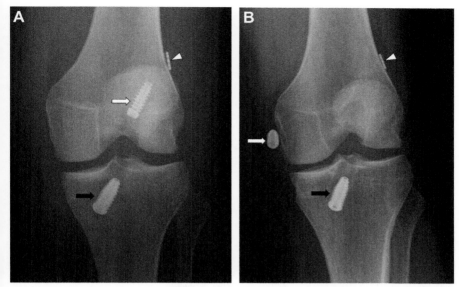

Fig. 13. AP radiograph of the knee (*A*) in a patient with a single bundle ACL reconstruction shows single interference screws in the tibial tunnel (*black arrow*) and the femoral tunnel (*white arrow*) for fixation of the ACL graft as well as a cortical button for suspensory fixation. Follow-up AP radiograph (*B*) obtained approximately a year later shows complete migration of the femoral screw, which now is located in the medial soft tissues adjacent to the medial femoral condyle (*white arrow*).

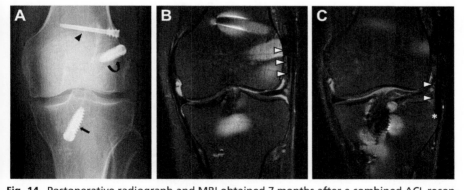

Fig. 14. Postoperative radiograph and MRI obtained 7 months after a combined ACL reconstruction with a LET using a strip harvested from the ITB. The frontal knee radiograph (*A*) shows a metallic interference screw in the tibial tunnel (*black straight arrow*) for fixation of the ACL graft, as well as a femoral cortical cross pin (*black arrowhead*) for suspensory fixation of the ACL graft on the femoral tunnel. An additional, more laterally located, metallic screw in the lateral femoral epicondyle (*black curved arrow*) is for proximal fixation of the ITB strip for the LET. Note that there is no fixation device for the ITB strip distally as its normal distal insertional footprint at Gerdy's tubercle (*white asterisk*) is preserved during this type of surgery. The two coronal PD fat sat images (*B, C*) show an intact LET (*white arrowheads*) as it passes proximally deep to the lateral collateral ligament and from there courses deep to the plane of the ITB. (Case courtesy of Dr. Marcelo Bordalo-Rodrigues from São Paulo, Brazil.)

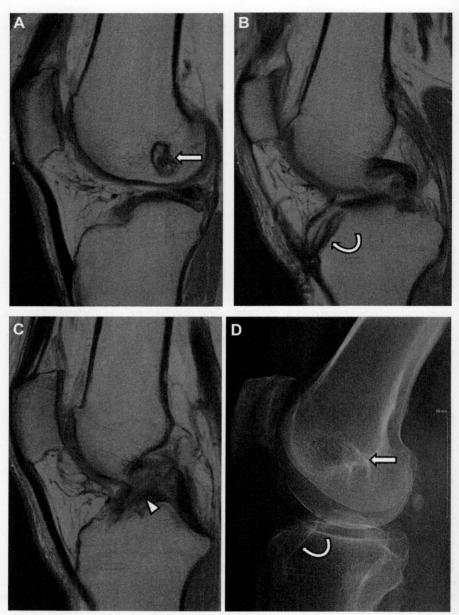

Fig. 15. Three sagittal PD images (*A–C*) as well as a lateral knee radiograph (*D*) show post-surgical changes from a single bundle ACL reconstruction. Note the malposition of the tibial tunnel (*curved arrow*) as well as the femoral tunnel (*straight arrow*), which are both too anterior, predisposing to impingement of the ACL graft, which itself appears indistinct and degenerated with high-grade tearing (*arrowhead*).

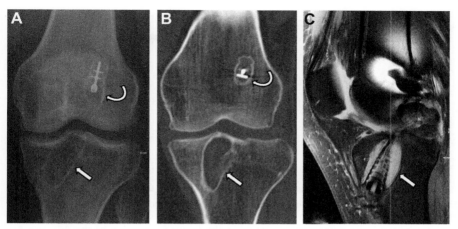

Fig. 16. Frontal knee radiograph (*A*), coronal CT (*B*), and sagittal PD fat sat MR image (*C*) show postsurgical changes from a single bundle ACL reconstruction. There is significant osteolysis in the tibial tunnel (*straight white arrow*) and to a lesser extent in the femoral tunnel (*curved white arrow*). Note the presence of fluid within the tibial tunnel likely related to ganglion cyst formation.

lateral tibial plateau and an insufficient PCL may result in posteromedial tibial subluxation.[14]

Soft tissue complications—Arthrofibrosis can occur after open or arthroscopic surgery and can be focal or diffuse. It is typically described in the setting of ACL

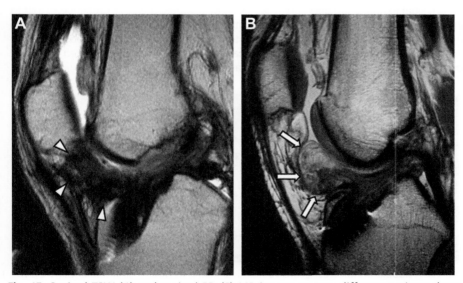

Fig. 17. Sagittal T2W (*A*) and sagittal PD (*B*) MR images on two different patients show diffuse and focal forms of arthrofibrosis in the setting of ACL reconstructions. Diffuse arthrofibrosis (*A*) is depicted with diffuse low signal infiltrating the infrapatellar fat pad (*arrowheads*) as well as the anterior aspect of the ACL graft, and to a lesser extent the suprapatellar recess. Focal arthrofibrosis (*B*) is shown with a large cyclops lesion (*straight arrows*), which is intimate with the ACL graft, and in this case, results in mass effect and displacement of the infrapatellar fat pad.

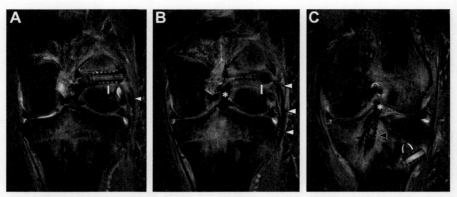

Fig. 18. Postoperative MRI obtained 1 month after a combined ALL and ACL reconstruction. The first and second coronal PD fat sat images (*A, B*) show a single bioabsorbable interference screw within a single common tunnel in the femur for fixation of the ACL and ALL grafts (*white straight arrow*). The last coronal PD fat sat image (*C*) shows a single bioabsorbable screw for distal fixation of the ALL graft to the tibia (*white curved arrow*), as well as a separate screw for fixation of the ACL graft within the tibial tunnel (*black arrowhead*). The ALL graft is intact (*white arrowheads*). The ACL graft is also intact (*white asterisks*). There is residual bone marrow edema surrounding the single femoral tunnel as well as the two tibial tunnels, an expected finding on this MR obtained 1 month after surgery. (Case courtesy of Dr. Marcelo Bordalo-Rodrigues from São Paulo, Brazil.)

reconstruction (**Fig. 17**). Suspicion for arthrofibrosis is linked to limited knee extension on physical examination and confirmation on MRI is based on the presence of low to intermediate signal intensity soft tissue with heterogeneous morphology, sometimes more focal and nodular located anterior to the ACL graft, the so-called "Cyclops" lesion. In severe cases, arthrofibrosis can be diffuse, with generalized capsular contraction, necessitating more widespread debridement.

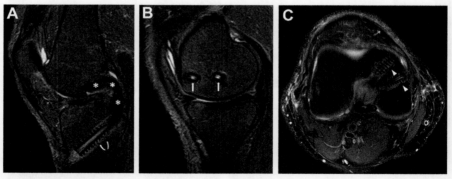

Fig. 19. A double-bundle PCL reconstruction is showing in three STIR MR images (*A–C*). The first sagittal STIR image (*A*) shows a single tibial tunnel for both bundles of the PCL graft secured with a single interference screw (*curved white arrow*), the PCL graft is intact (*white asterisk*). The second sagittal STIR image (*B*) shows the two corresponding femoral tunnels (*straight white arrows*), one for the anterolateral bundle and one for the posteromedial bundle. The axial STIR image (*C*) reveals the two interference screws for fixation of the two PCL bundles in the femur (*white arrowheads*). (Case courtesy of Dr Atul Taneja from São Paulo, Brazil.)

Graft integrity—MRI is the modality of choice for the postoperative assessment of ligament and graft integrity (**Fig. 18**). Grafts should be continuous throughout their course (**Fig. 19**). Linearity and caliber should also be assessed as nonlinearity (PCL excluded) and areas of attenuation or caliber change can be signs of partial tearing. Signal properties should also be assessed in the context of time elapsed since reconstruction.

SUMMARY

Knee ligament evaluation is a challenging area of musculoskeletal imaging. The imager must be familiar with patterns of injury to support timely preoperative detection and surgical planning. Image modality selection based on the strengths and weaknesses of each modality is a key component of care optimization. Postoperative ligament evaluation is often the greatest challenge and requires awareness of the normal and abnormal postoperative appearance as well as understanding of the surgical procedure performed.

CLINICS CARE POINTS

- Stress radiography serves as a "functional" imaging modality for quantifying ligamentous laxity and assists surgical planning in cases of multiligament injury.
- Stress radiography supports surgical decision-making in scenarios where MRI findings and clinical presentation are discordant.
- Knowledge of ligament injury patterns promotes detection of subtle associated injuries and supports timely orthopedic subspecialty referral and appropriate surgical planning.
- Postoperative imaging evaluation requires knowledge of the operation performed and familiarity with the normal and abnormal appearance of repaired or reconstructed ligaments.

DISCLOSURE

A.G. Geeslin: Arthrex, Inc: Paid presenter or speaker, Arthroscopy: Editorial or governing board Ossur: Paid presenter or speaker, Smith & Nephew: Paid consultant; Paid presenter or speaker.

REFERENCES

1. Kane PW, Cinque ME, Moatshe G, et al. Fibular Collateral Ligament: Varus Stress Radiographic Analysis Using 3 Different Clinical Techniques. Orthop J Sports Med 2018;6(5). 2325967118770170.
2. LaPrade RF, Heikes C, Bakker AJ, et al. The reproducibility and repeatability of varus stress radiographs in the assessment of isolated fibular collateral ligament and grade-III posterolateral knee injuries. An in vitro biomechanical study. J Bone Joint Surg Am 2008;90(10):2069–76.
3. LaPrade RF, Bernhardson AS, Griffith CJ, et al. Correlation of valgus stress radiographs with medial knee ligament injuries: an in vitro biomechanical study. Am J Sports Med 2010;38(2):330–8.
4. Jackman T, LaPrade RF, Pontinen T, et al. Intraobserver and interobserver reliability of the kneeling technique of stress radiography for the evaluation of posterior knee laxity. Am J Sports Med 2008;36(8):1571–6.

5. Dean RS, LaPrade RF. ACL and Posterolateral Corner Injuries. Curr Rev Musculoskelet Med 2020;13(1):123–32.
6. Pao DG. The lateral femoral notch sign. Radiology 2001;219(3):800–1.
7. Gottsegen CJ, Eyer BA, White EA, et al. Avulsion fractures of the knee: imaging findings and clinical significance. Radiographics 2008;28(6):1755–70.
8. Vermeijden HD, van der List JP, O'Brien R, et al. Return to sports following arthroscopic primary repair of the anterior cruciate ligament in the adult population. Knee 2020;27(3):906–14.
9. Graf BK, Cook DA, De Smet AA, et al. Bone bruises" on magnetic resonance imaging evaluation of anterior cruciate ligament injuries. Am J Sports Med 1993; 21(2):220–3.
10. Duchman KR, Westermann RW, Spindler KP, et al. The Fate of Meniscus Tears Left In Situ at the Time of Anterior Cruciate Ligament Reconstruction: A 6-Year Follow-up Study From the MOON Cohort. Am J Sports Med 2015;43(11):2688–95.
11. Getgood A, Brown C, Lording T, et al. The anterolateral complex of the knee: results from the International ALC Consensus Group Meeting. Knee Surg Sports Traumatol Arthrosc 2019;27(1):166–76.
12. Anderson MA, Simeone FJ, Palmer WE, et al. Acute posterior cruciate ligament injuries: effect of location, severity, and associated injuries on surgical management. Skeletal Radiol 2018;47(11):1523–32.
13. Pache S, Aman ZS, Kennedy M, et al. Posterior Cruciate Ligament: Current Concepts Review. Arch Bone Joint Surg 2018;6(1):8–18.
14. DePhillipo NN, Cinque ME, Godin JA, et al. Posterior Tibial Translation Measurements on Magnetic Resonance Imaging Improve Diagnostic Sensitivity for Chronic Posterior Cruciate Ligament Injuries and Graft Tears. Am J Sports Med 2018;46(2):341–7.
15. Varelas AN, Erickson BJ, Cvetanovich GL, et al. Medial Collateral Ligament Reconstruction in Patients With Medial Knee Instability: A Systematic Review. Orthop J Sports Med 2017;5(5). 2325967117703920.
16. LaPrade RF, Engebretsen AH, Ly TV, et al. The anatomy of the medial part of the knee. J Bone Joint Surg Am 2007;89(9):2000–10.
17. Geeslin AG, Geeslin MG, LaPrade RF. Ligamentous Reconstruction of the Knee: What Orthopaedic Surgeons Want Radiologists to Know. Semin Musculoskelet Radiol 2017;21(2):75–88.
18. LaPrade RF, Wijdicks CA. The management of injuries to the medial side of the knee. J Orthop Sports Phys Ther 2012;42(3):221–33.
19. Miller MD, Osborne JR, Gordon WT, et al. The natural history of bone bruises. A prospective study of magnetic resonance imaging-detected trabecular microfractures in patients with isolated medial collateral ligament injuries. Am J Sports Med 1998;26(1):15–9.
20. LaPrade RF, Ly TV, Wentorf FA, et al. The posterolateral attachments of the knee: a qualitative and quantitative morphologic analysis of the fibular collateral ligament, popliteus tendon, popliteofibular ligament, and lateral gastrocnemius tendon. Am J Sports Med 2003;31(6):854–60.
21. LaPrade RF, Gilbert TJ, Bollom TS, et al. The magnetic resonance imaging appearance of individual structures of the posterolateral knee. A prospective study of normal knees and knees with surgically verified grade III injuries. Am J Sports Med 2000;28(2):191–9.
22. Geeslin AG, LaPrade RF. Location of bone bruises and other osseous injuries associated with acute grade III isolated and combined posterolateral knee injuries. Am J Sports Med 2010;38(12):2502–8.

23. LaPrade RF, Johansen S, Agel J, et al. Outcomes of an anatomic posterolateral knee reconstruction. J Bone Joint Surg Am 2010;92(1):16–22.

24. Geeslin AG, LaPrade RF. Outcomes of treatment of acute grade-III isolated and combined posterolateral knee injuries: a prospective case series and surgical technique. J Bone Joint Surg Am 2011;93(18):1672–83.

25. Kennedy MI, Claes S, Fuso FA, et al. The Anterolateral Ligament: An Anatomic, Radiographic, and Biomechanical Analysis. Am J Sports Med 2015;43(7): 1606–15.

26. Godin JA, Chahla J, Moatshe G, et al. A Comprehensive Reanalysis of the Distal Iliotibial Band: Quantitative Anatomy, Radiographic Markers, and Biomechanical Properties. Am J Sports Med 2017;45(11):2595–603.

27. Gaunder C, Campbell S, Sciortino M, et al. Incidence of Anterolateral Ligament Tears in the Anterior Cruciate Ligament-Deficient Knee: A Magnetic Resonance Imaging Analysis. Arthroscopy 2018;34(7):2170–6.

28. Helito CP, Helito PV, Costa HP, et al. Assessment of the Anterolateral Ligament of the Knee by Magnetic Resonance Imaging in Acute Injuries of the Anterior Cruciate Ligament. Arthroscopy 2017;33(1):140–6.

29. Van Dyck P, De Smet E, Roelant E, et al. Assessment of Anterolateral Complex Injuries by Magnetic Resonance Imaging in Patients With Acute Rupture of the Anterior Cruciate Ligament. Arthroscopy 2019;35(2):521–7.

30. Marom N, Greditzer HGt, Roux M, et al. The Incidence of Kaplan Fiber Injury Associated With Acute Anterior Cruciate Ligament Tear Based on Magnetic Resonance Imaging. Am J Sports Med 2020;48(13):3194–9.

31. LaPrade MD, Kallenbach SL, Aman ZS, et al. Biomechanical Evaluation of the Medial Stabilizers of the Patella. Am J Sports Med 2018;46(7):1575–82.

32. Salem HS, Axibal DP, Wolcott ML, et al. Two-Stage Revision Anterior Cruciate Ligament Reconstruction: A Systematic Review of Bone Graft Options for Tunnel Augmentation. Am J Sports Med 2020;48(3):767–77.

33. Moatshe G, Slette EL, Engebretsen L, et al. Intertunnel Relationships in the Tibia During Reconstruction of Multiple Knee Ligaments: How to Avoid Tunnel Convergence. Am J Sports Med 2016;44(11):2864–9.

Knee Cartilage Imaging

Karen Y. Cheng, MD[a], Alecio F. Lombardi, MD[a,b], Eric Y. Chang, MD[a,b],
Christine B. Chung, MD[a,b,*]

KEYWORDS

- MRI • Cartilage • Knee • Histologic structure • Compositional imaging

KEY POINTS

- Understanding the histologic structure of cartilage is important to appreciate the normal appearance of cartilage on MRI, which in turn allows for better recognition of abnormal appearances of cartilage.
- Standard MRI sequences allow for evaluation of cartilage morphology and signal changes, providing comparable information to arthroscopic evaluation.
- Translational MRI sequences allow for evaluation of cartilage biochemical composition and structural integrity, and the identification of changes that may precede morphologic changes visible on either MRI or arthroscopy.
- Identification of cartilage abnormalities on MRI may determine the appropriate course of treatment or help explain the clinical symptoms experienced by the patient.

INTRODUCTION

Articular cartilage is a highly specialized connective tissue overlying the adjoining bone surfaces in diarthrodial joints, which enables frictionless movement and repetitive weight-bearing. Cartilage injury and degeneration represent common causes of joint pain, particularly at the knee. There is growing recognition of symptomatic chondral lesions and a corresponding increase in the surgical management of focal cartilage lesions, with an estimated 5% growth in the annual incidence of cartilage procedures in the United States.[1] Moreover, some studies demonstrate that the presence of a cartilage lesion on MRI in patients with osteoarthritis correlates more strongly with pain and poor function than conventional radiographic grading of osteoarthritis severity.[2] MRI provides an effective and noninvasive means of evaluating the structure of cartilage and predicting injuries amenable to surgical intervention. This review begins with a description of the structure of cartilage focusing on its histologic appearance to emphasize that structure will dictate patterns of tissue failure as well as magnetic resonance (MR) appearance.

[a] Department of Radiology, UC San Diego Health, 200 W. Arbor Drive MC 8226, San Diego, CA 92103, USA; [b] VA San Diego Healthcare System, Radiology Service, 3350 La Jolla Village Drive, MC 114, San Diego, CA 92161, USA
* Corresponding author. Department of Radiology - 9114, Center for Translational Imaging and Precision Medicine, 9427 Health Sciences Drive, La Jolla, CA 92093.
E-mail address: cbchung@health.ucsd.edu

Clin Sports Med 40 (2021) 677–692
https://doi.org/10.1016/j.csm.2021.05.006
0278-5919/21/© 2021 Elsevier Inc. All rights reserved.
sportsmed.theclinics.com

CARTILAGE COMPOSITION: HISTOLOGIC AND BIOCHEMICAL

Normal articular cartilage is composed of a relatively small number of specialized cells called chondrocytes, which function primarily to produce the collagen fibers and proteoglycans comprising the abundant extracellular matrix in which they reside.[3,4] The distribution of collagen bundles in cartilage contributes to their function in resisting the tension produced by deformation of the cartilage that occurs with weightbearing.[5] Proteoglycans are large negatively charged macromolecules composed of a protein core and polysaccharide chains called glycosaminoglycans that provide the osmotic force to maintain a high water content within cartilage, with water accounting for 67% to 74% of the chemical composition of cartilage.[6] No blood vessels, nerves, or lymphatics course through cartilage.[7] As a result of this avascularity, articular cartilage must receive nutrients from adjacent structures. Deeper portions of the cartilage are supplied by the subchondral bone, whereas more superficial layers are nourished via diffusion of substances from the synovial fluid.[4]

Articular cartilage has a layered architecture, with the zonal variation in each of its components allowing it to be uniquely adapted to the function of evenly transmitting load to the underlying subchondral bone. Collagen fibrils, which provide the scaffolding for cartilage structure, have been described as arcades anchored in the subchondral bone. They are oriented vertically in the layers closest to the subchondral bone: the zone of calcified cartilage (zone IV) and the radial zone (zone III),[8] which are separated by a line of transition demarcating the upper limit of calcification called the "tidemark."[9] The collagen fibers become more disorganized in the overlying transitional zone (zone II) as they change to a parallel orientation in the superficial zone (zone I) (**Fig. 1**).[3,9] Proteoglycan concentration also varies by cartilage depth, with concentrations highest in the deepest zone and decreasing more superficially.[6,9,10]

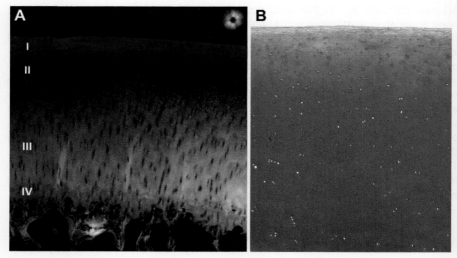

Fig. 1. Normal histologic appearance of cartilage. (*A*) Quantitative polarization image with color representing collagen fiber orientation (color wheel in the upper right) and brightness representing retardance. Collagen fiber orientation varies between 60° to 90° when compared between zones I and III. Zone II shows lower intensity, reflecting relative fiber disorganization. Note that chondrocyte density decreases with increasing depth. (*B*) Photomicrograph of Safranin-O-stained slide shows normal proteoglycan distribution, with the strongest concentration at the deepest zone and lowest concentration more superficially.

Chondrocytes, on the other hand, demonstrate an inverse pattern of density, with large numbers of thin, ellipsoid cells superficially, and fewer larger-sized, rounded chondrocytes in the deeper transitional and radial zones.[3,11] The chondrocytes also differ in function by depth, with the deeper cells demonstrating greater capacity for synthetic function and the superficial cells in a relatively quiescent state.[3]

Histologic analysis of articular cartilage focuses on the preservation of tissue architecture, cellularity, collagen integrity, and proteoglycan content.[10,12–14] On gross examination, in contrast to the bluish-white, smooth, and glistening appearance of healthy articular cartilage, damaged cartilage has been described as dull or yellowish and swollen in appearance.[15] Aging, osteoarthritic cartilage has been associated with increased chondrocyte activity with increased sulfate uptake and utilization,[10] increased DNA synthesis and cell replication,[12] as well as increased water content due to damaged collagen structure resulting in loss of normal restraint to osmotic pressure despite decreasing proteoglycan content.[6,12,16]

MR APPEARANCE OF NORMAL CARTILAGE
Normal Cartilage Morphology

Two-dimensional (2D) spin echo and gradient echo sequences in multiple planes are the workhorses of standard clinical evaluation of cartilage. On T1-weighted images, normal cartilage has a relatively homogeneous appearance, with intermediate signal intensity compared with the higher signal of fat and marrow and lower signal of calcified cartilage and compact bone. Although there is a contrast between noncalcified cartilage and calcified cartilage/subchondral bone on these sequences and good delineation of anatomic detail,[17] a major limitation of T1-weighted imaging is the inability to distinguish cartilage from joint fluid, either physiologic or pathologic. The low signal of joint fluid, real or simulated, on these sequences is often indistinguishable from the cartilage surface.[4,17–19] The distinction between joint fluid and cartilage is much better appreciated on T2-weighted images, on which bright joint fluid is starkly contrasted to dark-appearing cartilage, producing a pseudo-"arthrogram" effect.[4,20] Intermediate (IM)-weighted images (also referred to as proton density [PD]-weighted images) combine some of the advantages of both T1-weighted and T2-weighted images, providing contrast between the intermediate signal of normal noncalcified articular cartilage with the high signal of joint fluid and synovium and the low signal of calcified cartilage and subchondral bone.[21] IM-weighted sequences allow for better characterization of noncartilage structures in the knee, improving evaluation for possible associated meniscal or ligamentous injuries.[22,23] In addition, IM-weighted sequences also allow for visualization of a laminar appearance of the intrinsic cartilage signal called "gray-scale stratification," with a lower signal radial zone and higher signal in the transitional zone that reflects the differences in T2 relaxation time resulting from the anisotropic interaction of water molecules with the varying collagen structure between these two histologic layers (**Fig. 2**A).[24–26] At higher resolution, an additional low signal superficial zone may also be visible, producing a trilaminar appearance.[27–30]

A major disadvantage of 2D techniques is partial volume averaging, which is resolved with three dimensional (3D) gradient-echo-based sequences such as 3D spoiled gradient-recalled echo (SPGR).[31–34] However, these sequences are limited by long acquisition time, lower intrinsic cartilage contrast, and relatively poor definition of noncartilage structures.[32] More recently, T2-weighted and IM-weighted 3D fast spin echo sequences have been applied to the imaging of cartilage, allowing for improved assessment of other knee joint structures and concurrent high-resolution cartilage assessment, but are not yet widely used in routine imaging.[35–37]

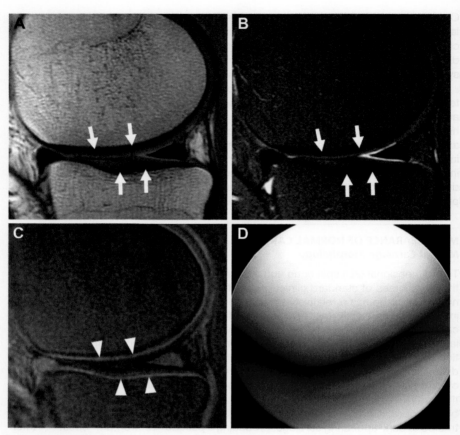

Fig. 2. Normal appearance of articular cartilage in vivo. Sagittal (*A*) IM-weighted and (*B*) T2-weighted fat-suppressed MR images show the laminar appearance of healthy cartilage with hypointense deep radial zone (*arrows*). (*C*) Inversion recovery UTE MR image highlights the intact osteochondral junction (*arrowheads*). (*D*) Arthroscopic image shows the smooth, healthy cartilage in the medial femorotibial compartment.

For any given sequence selected, magnetic field strength is another variable that may be considered in the selection of optimal cartilage imaging parameters. The image quality and spatial resolution achievable with the higher signal-to-noise ratio (SNR) of a higher magnetic field strength may improve diagnostic performance for the detection of cartilage lesions at 3.0 T as compared with 1.5 T.[38,39] However, other studies have failed to find a significant difference between 1.5 and 3.0 T imaging in routine clinical practice.[40]

Normal Cartilage Biochemical Composition

Collagen

Quantitative T2 maps can be created by fitting signal intensities from multiple T2-weighted acquisitions at different echo times (TE) to an exponential decay curve to estimate the T2 relaxation time for any given region of interest. Normal cartilage has low T2 relaxation values, ranging from 32 ms in the radial zone to a maximum of 67 ms in the superficial zone.[41,42] These low values are thought to reflect the restriction of water mobility within the constraint of intact collagen structure, resulting in increased spin-spin interactions and rapid dephasing. The interlaminar variation in T2 values of normal cartilage thus reflects the different collagen organization in each histologic layer. In the setting of collagen damage and loss of this architecture, T2 values increase.[39,43,44] Of note, the radial and calcified zones of cartilage and subchondral bone have very short T2 values with resultant low SNR on images with longer TEs (see **Fig. 2**B), such as those used for conventional T2 maps. Dedicated ultrashort TE techniques can capture signal from these tissues before decay (see **Fig. 2**C).[45]

Similarly, the T2* relaxation time of cartilage reflects changes in collagen organization, possibly with greater sensitivity and shorter scan times than T2 mapping because of its reflection of local field inhomogeneity, particularly for short T2 tissues when used in combination with ultrashort TE techniques.[46–48] Like T2, T2* values demonstrate zonal variation, with increasing values moving from the radial to superficial zone.[49] Cartilage degeneration typically results in lower T2* values, especially in the superficial zone, as compared with normal cartilage.[46,49,50] T2*-weighted imaging is primarily limited by its sensitivity to susceptibility and chemical shift artifact.[47,51]

Diffusion-weighted imaging (DWI) and diffusion tensor imaging (DTI) are alternative methods for evaluating the cartilage architecture based on information about how the collagen structure restricts the movement of water. With the loss of collagen integrity as seen in degeneration, there is an increase in water mobility that manifests as an increase in the apparent diffusion coefficient.[52] DTI adds additional information about directionality/anisotropy of the collagen structure.[53,54] However, diffusion imaging of cartilage is technically challenging as standard diffusion sequences yield low SNR, rendering it difficult to achieve adequate resolution, and prolonged imaging times increase the sensitivity to patient motion artifacts.[55]

Magnetization transfer contrast (MTC) has also been demonstrated to be sensitive to collagen content.[56] This technique generates contrast based on the interactions of protons in bulk water and protons bound to macromolecules and is, therefore, of particular interest in the evaluation of cartilage where there is a strong interaction of collagen-bound protons and cartilage water protons.[57] In cartilage degeneration, there is a diminished magnetization transfer signal corresponding to focally increased collagen concentration.[58,59]

Proteoglycan content

As proteoglycans are negatively charged, they attract positively charged sodium ions. In the setting of cartilage degeneration, the loss of proteoglycans leads to a corresponding decrease in sodium content, which can be quantified by sodium MRI.[60–63] A major limitation of this technique is the low quantity of sodium present in articular cartilage (compared with the abundance of protons), resulting in a requirement for higher magnetic field strength than most clinically available MR scanners or long acquisition times to produce images of adequate SNR to quantify proteoglycan loss.[64]

Delayed gadolinium-enhanced MRI of cartilage (dGEMRIC) also quantifies proteoglycan concentration based on the negative charge of the glycosaminoglycan chains. Gadolinium chelate is also negatively charged and is repelled by the negative charge present in proteoglycan-rich normal cartilage. When proteoglycans are lost, as in cartilage degeneration, the decreased negative charge allows more contrast agent to distribute into the less negative cartilage matrix and shorten the T1 relaxation time. Thus, proteoglycan loss results in a corresponding decrease in T1 relaxation time.[65,66] The major limitations of this imaging technique are the requirement for intravenous contrast, and the logistical challenges of requiring a 40 to 45 minute delay after contrast injection as the patient exercises the knee to allow contrast to equilibrate.

The T1 (spin-lattice) relaxation time in the rotating frame (T1ρ), which reflects the interactions between water molecules with local macromolecules, has also been shown to correlate to proteoglycan levels. With proteoglycan loss, T1ρ relaxation time increases (**Fig. 3**).[67–70] Unfortunately, with more advanced cartilage degeneration, T1ρ begins to reflect a combination of collagen abnormality and proteoglycan loss, although it remains specific to proteoglycan quantities at earlier stages of degeneration.[71]

Chemical exchange saturation transfer (gagCEST) is an imaging technique which draws upon some of the same principles as MTC and has emerged as a means of determining the proteoglycan content of cartilage. In this technique, the exchangeable protons of glycosaminoglycans ($-NH$, $-OH$, $-NH_2$) are saturated with a selective pulse. Chemical exchange between these protons and bulk water protons results in transfer of saturation, which produces image contrast based on the glycosaminoglycan content.[66,72] However, although reflective of glycosaminoglycan content at 7T, some authors have suggested that gagCEST values are negligible at 3T, which may limit the potential for routine clinical use.[73]

MR APPEARANCE OF ABNORMAL CARTILAGE
Cartilage Loss

Cartilage may be morphologically abnormal in the setting of a single acute traumatic event, multiple repetitive injuries, osteonecrosis, chronic degenerative change, or inflammatory joint disease. Irrespective of etiology, the historical gold standard for evaluation of cartilage has been arthroscopy. As a result, MR classification of cartilage has relied heavily on modified versions of arthroscopic grading systems, which include the Noyes and Stabler,[38,39,74] Outerbridge,[22,23,40,75] and Shahriaree[4,17,21,31,76,77] grading systems, and more recently an arthroscopic system based on the International Cartilage Repair Society (ICRS) histologic grading system.[78] The ICRS system is now the

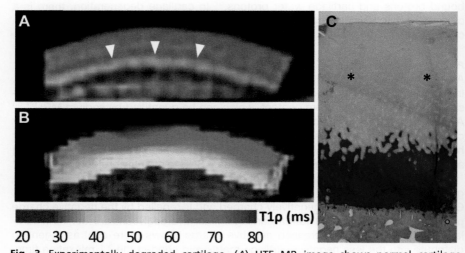

Fig. 3. Experimentally degraded cartilage. (*A*) UTE MR image shows normal cartilage appearance with intact osteochondral junction (*arrowheads*). (*B*) Despite normal cartilage thickness, T1ρ map shows abnormally increased values in the superficial and transitional zones (*red regions*). (*C*) Photomicrograph of Safranin-O-stained slide confirms marked decrease of proteoglycan in areas with elevated T1ρ value (*asterisks*).

most commonly used by orthopedic surgeons to identify isolated high-grade cartilage defects that are amenable to surgical repair.

In the ICRS system, cartilage defects are distinguished by depth of involvement (**Fig. 4**). Grade 0 represents normal or near-normal cartilage. Grade 1 represents surface or superficial irregularity. Grade 2 abnormalities extend deeper in the cartilage but involve less than 50% of the total cartilage depth. Grade 3 abnormalities represent deep defects that extend for more than 50% of the cartilage depth but do not expose subchondral bone. Finally, grade 4 defects extend to and involve the subchondral bone. The grade 3 and 4 chondral lesions are often candidates for surgical management with procedures such as microfracture, reconstruction with autograft or allograft, autologous chondrocyte implantation, and local application of growth factors and mesenchymal stem cells, whereas lower grade defects are typically treated conservatively. Defect size is also an important feature that can be determined by MRI and factors into treatment decisions, with many surgeons limiting microfracture to lesions less than 2 cm^2 in area.[79]

The surface morphology visualized on arthroscopy may be translated in a straightforward fashion to the morphology of cartilage visualized on MRI. On fluid-sensitive sequences, high signal intensity joint fluid can be visualized outlining superficial fibrillations, filling cartilage defects in continuity with the cartilage surface, and undercutting loose osteochondral fragments.[4,19] Bredella and colleagues reported overall sensitivity and specificity of 93% and 99%, respectively, for the detection of 86 arthroscopically proven cartilage abnormalities in 36 patients using the combination of axial and coronal T2-weighted fast-spin echo sequences with fat saturation.[77] High degree of agreement was also found between arthroscopic lesion grade and MR grade of chondral lesions on IM-weighted images in multiple studies,[21,23,80] as well as on 3D SPGR images.[31]

In addition to focal cartilage loss, MRI can demonstrate diffuse cartilage thinning, which may be seen in the setting of osteoarthritis. Although the earliest detectable change of osteoarthritis is actually an increase in cartilage thickness that likely reflects increased water content due to loss of collagen integrity,[81] more advanced stages of degeneration show cartilage thinning or absence, with longitudinal studies of osteoarthritis demonstrating progressive cartilage loss.[82] As such, there has been significant interest in quantifying cartilage volume. Although some have argued that MR has limited clinical utility for grading cartilage in osteoarthritis[83] or that there are no associations between cartilage loss and symptoms,[2] others have reported associations between tibial cartilage volume and the symptoms of osteoarthritis,[84] as well as between patellar cartilage volume and knee pain.[85]

Abnormal Signal in Morphologically Normal Cartilage

Although on arthroscopic evaluation the surgeon focuses primarily on areas of cartilage loss, MRI is able to detect signal changes in cartilage even when the surface morphology is completely normal. This is, of course, a primary goal of techniques focused on imaging the biochemical composition of cartilage described above but can also be appreciated on conventional sequences designed to evaluate cartilage morphology. This feature of MRI enables the radiologist to identify cartilage at risk for more extensive injury in the future on routine clinical MRI. As MRI may have surpassed management in sensitivity, the availability of treatments for these early stages of cartilage injury may be limited at present. The ability to identify this cartilage at risk, however, could lay the groundwork for the development of future treatments to prevent progression to cartilage loss.

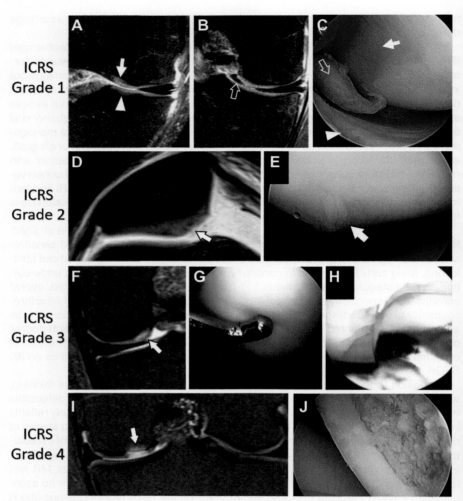

Fig. 4. ICRS Grading System. Grade 1: (*A* and *B*) Coronal T2-weighted FS MR images show hyperintense femoral (*arrow*) and tibial (*arrowhead*) cartilage with displaced medial meniscal flap (open *arrow*) in a 39-year-old man. (*C*) The corresponding arthroscopic image confirmed the discolored, superficial cartilage lesions which were soft on probing and meniscal flap. Grade 2: (*D* and *E*) Axial IM-weighted fat-suppressed MR and arthroscopic images in a 41-year-old woman show fissuring at the patellar median ridge extending less than 50% of cartilage depth (*arrows*). Grade 3: (*F*) Coronal IM-weighted fat-suppressed MR image shows a chondral blister at the medial femoral condyle in a 24-year-old woman. (*G*) Arthroscopic image shows chondral softening with marked bogginess on palpation. (*H*) Surface was debrided and lesion extending approximately 80% of the cartilage depth was unveiled. Grade 4: (*I*) Coronal IM-weighted fat-suppressed MR image shows a chondral defect at the medial femoral condyle extending down to subchondral bone with bone marrow edema (*arrow*). (*J*) Arthroscopic image confirms the detection with exposed subchondral bone.

Loss of gray-scale stratification/laminar appearance

As the laminar appearance of normal cartilage is a reflection of the ultrastructural properties of cartilage, it is not surprising that loss of that stratification reflects damage to the normal tissue architecture. Loss of the laminar appearance has been reported in association with chondral lesions of the retropatellar cartilage[86] and cartilage elsewhere in the knee,[31] and may also reflect early degeneration[87] or predict future delamination.[88]

Intrinsic high signal on fluid-sensitive sequences

Intrinsic high signal intensity on T2-weighted images has been described to correspond to an arthroscopic grade 1 (cartilage softening) chondral lesion.[77] Intrinsic cartilage signal change without abnormal morphology may also appear as focal hyperintensity on IM-weighted images.[23] Interestingly, Potter and colleagues noted that they tended to overdiagnose grade 1 (softening or blistering) cartilage

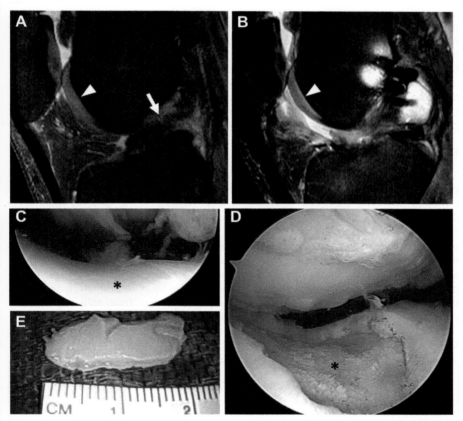

Fig. 5. A 22-year-old man with ACL tear and subsequent chondral delamination. (A) Sagittal IM-weighted MR image shows a complete ACL rupture (*arrow*). Note the normal chondral signal at the trochlea (*arrowhead*). (B) Sagittal IM-weighted MR image obtained 9 months later shows interval ACL reconstruction with abnormal high signal at the osteochondral junction, consistent with delamination. (C) Arthroscopic image shows an intact trochlear surface (*asterisk*), but abnormal ballotability was noted on palpation confirming extensive osteochondral delamination. (D and E) The bony surface (*asterisk*) is revealed postexcision of the 2 cm long chondral flap. ACL, anterior cruciate ligament.

abnormalities on IM-weighted MRI when compared to arthroscopy, speculating that while this could reflect artifactual signal alteration, an alternative explanation is that arthroscopy is less sensitive for early cartilage softening than MRI.

In addition, fluid-sensitive sequences may demonstrate high signal at the interface of noncalcified and calcified cartilage—a point of mechanical vulnerability because of changing structural properties—suggesting a delamination injury in the setting of shear stress.[89] This type of injury would likely be associated with normal surface morphology on both MRI and arthroscopy, and could easily go unnoticed by a surgeon who failed to specifically probe the area of delamination for ballotability or bogginess (**Fig. 5**). This would result in significant morbidity as untreated delamination injuries often progress to large full-thickness chondral defects and early osteoarthritis.[90]

Intrinsic low signal

Thin linear low signal in the central femoral trochlea on T2-weighted images has been found to correspond to the arthroscopic finding of cartilage fissuring, which may herald progression to full-thickness chondral defects.[91,92] Although most frequently found at the patellofemoral joint,[93] focal low signal can be found on other cartilage surfaces in correlation to findings of chondromalacia or degeneration on either arthroscopy[76,80] or histologic analysis from biopsy specimens.[94] In a study by Markhardt and colleagues, 64.1% of dark cartilage lesions corresponded to arthroscopic findings of degeneration (cartilage softening, fibrillation, partial-thickness flaps and defects), with a higher proportion of positive arthroscopic findings noted with increasing patient age. These signal abnormalities likely reflect early alterations in normal internal tissue architecture that precede morphologic changes visible on MRI, and perhaps even on arthroscopy.

SUMMARY

MRI is an accurate, noninvasive means to evaluate articular cartilage. The appearance of cartilage is variable depending on the chosen MR sequence, with each set of parameters providing particular advantages and disadvantages. Beyond routine 2D (and 3D) sequences, there are many translational techniques that allow for the assessment of cartilage composition and structure. Although arthroscopy remains the gold standard for cartilage evaluation, MRI has been shown to be comparable in its sensitivity for chondral lesions. In addition to identifying cartilage loss, MRI can demonstrate signal changes that correspond to intrinsic structural abnormalities, which place the cartilage at risk for subsequent more serious injury or premature degeneration, some of which may be poorly evaluated by arthroscopy. Thus, MRI may allow for earlier intervention and treatment of important causes of pain and morbidity.

CLINICS CARE POINTS

- Understanding the histologic structure of cartilage is important to appreciate the normal appearance of cartilage on MRI, which in turn allows for better recognition of abnormal appearances of cartilage.

- Standard MRI sequences allow for evaluation of cartilage morphology and signal changes, providing comparable information to arthroscopic evaluation.

- Translational MRI sequences allow for evaluation of cartilage biochemical composition and structural integrity, and the identification of changes that may precede morphologic changes visible on either MRI or arthroscopy.

- Identification of cartilage abnormalities on MRI may determine the appropriate course of treatment or help explain the clinical symptoms experienced by the patient.

DISCLOSURE

The authors acknowledge grant support from VA Merit Awards (I01RX002604 and I01CX001388).

REFERENCES

1. McCormick F, Harris JD, Abrams GD, et al. Trends in the surgical treatment of articular cartilage lesions in the United States: an analysis of a large private-payer database over a period of 8 years. Arthrosc J Arthrosc Relat Surg 2014; 30(2):222–6.
2. Link TM, Steinbach LS, Ghosh S, et al. Osteoarthritis: MR imaging findings in different stages of disease and correlation with clinical findings. Radiology 2003;226(2):373–81.
3. Weiss C, Rosenberg L, Helfet A. An ultrastructural study of normal young adult human articular cartilage. J Bone Joint Surg Am 1968;50(4):663–74.
4. Yulish BS, Montanez J, Goodfellow DB, et al. Chondromalacia patellae: assessment with MR imaging. Radiology 1987;164(3):763–6.
5. MacConaill MA. The movements of bones and joints. J Bone Joint Surg Br 1951; 33-B(2):251–7.
6. Venn M, Maroudas A. Chemical composition and swelling of normal and osteoarthrotic femoral head cartilage. I. Chemical composition. Ann Rheum Dis 1977; 36(2):121–9.
7. Foster JE, Maciewicz RA, Taberner J, et al. Structural periodicity in human articular cartilage: comparison between magnetic resonance imaging and histological findings. Osteoarthritis Cartilage 1999;7(5):480–5.
8. Jeffery A, Blunn G, Archer C, et al. Three-dimensional collagen architecture in bovine articular cartilage. J Bone Joint Surg Br 1991;73-B(5):795–801.
9. Fawns HT, Landells JW. Histochemical studies of rheumatic conditions. Ann Rheum Dis 1953;12(2):105–13.
10. Collins DH, McElligott TF. Sulphate (35SO4) uptake by chondrocytes in relation to histological changes in osteo-arthritic human articular cartilage. Ann Rheum Dis 1960;19(4):318–30.
11. Klein TJ, Malda J, Sah RL, et al. Tissue engineering of articular cartilage with biomimetic zones. Tissue Eng Part B Rev 2009;15(2):143–57.
12. Mankin HJ, Dorfman H, Lippiello L, et al. Biochemical and metabolic abnormalities in articular cartilage from osteo-arthritic human hips: II. Correlation of morphology with biochemical and metabolic data. J Bone Joint Surg Am 1971; 53(3):523–37.
13. Pauli C, Whiteside R, Heras FL, et al. Comparison of cartilage histopathology assessment on human knee joints at all stages of osteoarthritis development. Osteoarthritis Cartilage 2012;20(6):476–85.
14. Pritzker KPH, Gay S, Jimenez SA, et al. Osteoarthritis cartilage histopathology: grading and staging. Osteoarthritis Cartilage 2006;14(1):13–29.
15. Outerbridge RE. The etiology of chondromalacia patellae. J Bone Joint Surg Br 1961;43-B(4):752–7.
16. Maroudas A, Venn M. Chemical composition and swelling of normal and osteoarthrotic femoral head cartilage. II. Swelling. Ann Rheum Dis 1977;36(5):399–406.
17. Hayes CW, Sawyer RW, Conway WF. Patellar cartilage lesions: in vitro detection and staging with MR imaging and pathologic correlation. Radiology 1990; 176(2):479–83.

18. Burk D, Kanal E, Brunberg J, et al. 1.5-T surface-coil MRI of the knee. Am J Roentgenol 1986;147(2):293–300.

19. Gylys-Morin V, Hajek P, Sartoris D, et al. Articular cartilage defects: detectability in cadaver knees with MR. Am J Roentgenol 1987;148(6):1153–7.

20. Vallotton JA, Meuli RA, Leyvraz PF, et al. Comparison between magnetic resonance imaging and arthroscopy in the diagnosis of patellar cartilage lesions. Knee Surg Sports Traumatol Arthrosc 1995;3(3):157–62.

21. Sonin AH, Pensy RA, Mulligan ME, et al. Grading articular cartilage of the knee using fast spin-echo proton density-weighted MR imaging without fat suppression. Am J Roentgenol 2002;179(5):1159–66.

22. Oeppen RS, Connolly SA, Bencardino JT, et al. Acute injury of the articular cartilage and subchondral bone: a common but unrecognized lesion in the immature knee. Am J Roentgenol 2004;182(1):111–7.

23. Potter HG, Linklater JM, Allen AA, et al. Magnetic resonance imaging of articular cartilage in the knee. An evaluation with use of fast-spin-echo imaging*. J Bone Joint Surg Am 1998;80(9):1276–84.

24. Dardzinski BJ, Mosher TJ, Li S, et al. Spatial variation of T2 in human articular cartilage. Radiology 1997;205(2):546–50.

25. Xia Y, Farquhar T, Burton-Wurster N, et al. Origin of cartilage laminae in MRI. J Magn Reson Imaging 1997;7(5):887–94.

26. Mlynárik V, Degrassi A, Toffanin R, et al. Investigation of laminar appearance of articular cartilage by means of magnetic resonance microscopy. Magn Reson Imaging 1996;14(4):435–42.

27. Goodwin DW, Wadghiri YZ, Zhu H, et al. Macroscopic structure of articular cartilage of the tibial plateau: influence of a characteristic matrix architecture on MRI appearance. Am J Roentgenol 2004;182(2):311–8.

28. Chalkias SM, Pozzi-Mucelli RS, Pozzi-Mucelli M, et al. Hyaline articular cartilage: relaxation times, pulse-sequence parameters and MR appearance at 1.5 T. Eur Radiol 1994;4(4):353–9.

29. Modl JM, Sether LA, Haughton VM, et al. Articular cartilage: correlation of histologic zones with signal intensity at MR imaging. Radiology 1991;181(3):853–5.

30. Cova M, Toffanin R, Frezza F, et al. Magnetic resonance imaging of articular cartilage: ex vivo study on normal cartilage correlated with magnetic resonance microscopy. Eur Radiol 1998;8(7):1130–6.

31. Disler DG, McCauley TR, Wirth CR, et al. Detection of knee hyaline cartilage defects using fat-suppressed three-dimensional spoiled gradient-echo MR imaging: comparison with standard MR imaging and correlation with arthroscopy. Am J Roentgenol 1995;165(2):377–82.

32. Disler DG, Peters TL, Muscoreil SJ, et al. Fat-suppressed spoiled GRASS imaging of knee hyaline cartilage: technique optimization and comparison with conventional MR imaging. Am J Roentgenol 1994;163(4):887–92.

33. Yoshioka H, Stevens K, Hargreaves BA, et al. Magnetic resonance imaging of articular cartilage of the knee: Comparison between fat-suppressed three-dimensional SPGR imaging, fat-suppressed FSE imaging, and fat-suppressed three-dimensional DEFT imaging, and correlation with arthroscopy. J Magn Reson Imaging 2004;20(5):857–64.

34. Siepmann DB, McGovern J, Brittain JH, et al. High-resolution 3D cartilage imaging with IDEAL–SPGR at 3 T. Am J Roentgenol 2007;189(6):1510–5.

35. Jung JY, Yoon YC, Kim HR, et al. Knee derangements: comparison of isotropic 3D fast spin-echo, isotropic 3D balanced fast field-echo, and conventional 2D fast spin-echo MR imaging. Radiology 2013;268(3):802–13.

36. Chen CA, Kijowski R, Shapiro LM, et al. Cartilage morphology at 3.0T: assessment of three-dimensional MR imaging techniques. J Magn Reson Imaging 2010;32(1):173–83.
37. Crema MD, Nogueira-Barbosa MH, Roemer FW, et al. Three-dimensional turbo spin-echo magnetic resonance imaging (MRI) and semiquantitative assessment of knee osteoarthritis: comparison with two-dimensional routine MRI. Osteoarthritis Cartilage 2013;21(3):428–33.
38. Van Dyck P, Kenis C, Vanhoenacker FM, et al. Comparison of 1.5- and 3-T MR imaging for evaluating the articular cartilage of the knee. Knee Surg Sports Traumatol Arthrosc 2014;22(6):1376–84.
39. Kijowski R, Blankenbaker DG, Davis KW, et al. Comparison of 1.5- and 3.0-T MR imaging for evaluating the articular cartilage of the knee joint. Radiology 2009; 250(3):839–48.
40. Mandell JC, Rhodes JA, Shah N, et al. Routine clinical knee MR reports: comparison of diagnostic performance at 1.5 T and 3.0 T for assessment of the articular cartilage. Skeletal Radiol 2017;46(11):1487–98.
41. Dardzinski BJ, Laor T, Schmithorst VJ, et al. Mapping T2 relaxation time in the pediatric knee: feasibility with a clinical 1.5-T MR imaging system. Radiology 2002; 225(1):233–9.
42. Smith HE, Mosher TJ, Dardzinski BJ, et al. Spatial variation in cartilage T2 of the knee. J Magn Reson Imaging 2001;14(1):50–5.
43. Pan J, Pialat J-B, Joseph T, et al. Knee cartilage T2 characteristics and evolution in relation to morphologic abnormalities detected at 3-T MR imaging: a longitudinal study of the normal control cohort from the osteoarthritis initiative. Radiology 2011;261(2):507–15.
44. Subburaj K, Souza RB, Stehling C, et al. Association of MR relaxation and cartilage deformation in knee osteoarthritis. J Orthop Res 2012;30(6):919–26.
45. Bae WC, Biswas R, Chen K, et al. UTE MRI of the osteochondral junction. Curr Radiol Rep 2014;2(2):35.
46. Williams A, Qian Y, Bear D, et al. Assessing degeneration of human articular cartilage with ultra-short echo time (UTE) T2* mapping. Osteoarthritis Cartilage 2010; 18(4):539–46.
47. Newbould RD, Miller SR, Toms LD, et al. T2* measurement of the knee articular cartilage in osteoarthritis at 3T. J Magn Reson Imaging 2012;35(6):1422–9.
48. Murphy BJ. Evaluation of grades 3 and 4 chondromalacia of the knee using T2*-weighted 3D gradient-echo articular cartilage imaging. Skeletal Radiol 2001; 30(6):305–11.
49. Mamisch TC, Hughes T, Mosher TJ, et al. T2 star relaxation times for assessment of articular cartilage at 3 T: a feasibility study. Skeletal Radiol 2012;41(3):287–92.
50. Bittersohl B, Hosalkar HS, Miese FR, et al. Zonal T2* and T1Gd assessment of knee joint cartilage in various histological grades of cartilage degeneration: an observational in vitro study. BMJ Open 2015;5(2):e006895.
51. Kirsch S, Kreinest M, Reisig G, et al. In vitro mapping of 1H ultrashort T2* and T2 of porcine menisci. NMR Biomed 2013;26(9):1167–75.
52. Mlynárik V, Sulzbacher I, Bittšanský M, et al. Investigation of apparent diffusion constant as an indicator of early degenerative disease in articular cartilage. J Magn Reson Imaging 2003;17(4):440–4.
53. Filidoro L, Dietrich O, Weber J, et al. High-resolution diffusion tensor imaging of human patellar cartilage: feasibility and preliminary findings. Magn Reson Med 2005;53(5):993–8.

54. Raya JG, Melkus G, Adam-Neumair S, et al. Diffusion-tensor imaging of human articular cartilage specimens with early signs of cartilage damage. Radiology 2013;266(3):831–41.

55. Miller KL, Hargreaves BA, Gold GE, et al. Steady-state diffusion-weighted imaging of in vivo knee cartilage. Magn Reson Med 2004;51(2):394–8.

56. Seo GS, Aoki J, Moriya H, et al. Hyaline cartilage: in vivo and in vitro assessment with magnetization transfer imaging. Radiology 1996;201(2):525–30.

57. Wolff SD, Chesnick S, Frank JA, et al. Magnetization transfer contrast: MR imaging of the knee. Radiology 1991;179(3):623–8.

58. Vahlensieck M, Dombrowski F, Leutner C, et al. Magnetization transfer contrast (MTC) and MTC-subtraction: enhancement of cartilage lesions and intracartilaginous degeneration in vitro. Skeletal Radiol 1994;23(7):535–9.

59. Koskinen SK, Ylä-Outinen H, Aho HJ, et al. Magnetization transfer and spin lock MR imaging of patellar cartilage degeneration at 0.1 T. Acta Radiol 1997;38(6): 1071–5.

60. Borthakur A, Shapiro EM, Beers J, et al. Sensitivity of MRI to proteoglycan depletion in cartilage: comparison of sodium and proton MRI. Osteoarthritis Cartilage 2000;8(4):288–93.

61. Madelin G, Babb J, Xia D, et al. Articular cartilage: evaluation with fluid-suppressed 7.0-T sodium MR Imaging in subjects with and subjects without osteoarthritis. Radiology 2013;268(2):481–91.

62. Madelin G, Xia D, Brown R, et al. Longitudinal Study of sodium MRI of articular cartilage in patients with knee osteoarthritis: initial experience with 16-month follow-up. Eur Radiol 2018;28(1):133–42.

63. Reddy R, Insko EK, Noyszewski EA, et al. Sodium MRI of human articular cartilagein vivo. Magn Reson Med 1998;39(5):697–701.

64. Reproducibility and repeatability of quantitative sodium magnetic resonance imaging in vivo in articular cartilage at 3 T and 7 T - Madelin - 2012 - Magnetic Resonance in Medicine - Wiley Online Library. Available at: https://onlinelibrary.wiley.com/doi/full/10.1002/mrm.23307. [Accessed 2 November 2020].

65. Tiderius CJ, Olsson LE, Leander P, et al. Delayed gadolinium-enhanced MRI of cartilage (dGEMRIC) in early knee osteoarthritis. Magn Reson Med 2003;49(3): 488–92.

66. Wei W, Lambach B, Jia G, et al. A Phase I clinical trial of the knee to assess the correlation of gagCEST MRI, delayed gadolinium-enhanced MRI of cartilage and T2 mapping. Eur J Radiol 2017;90:220–4.

67. Akella SVS, Regatte RR, Gougoutas AJ, et al. Proteoglycan-induced changes in T1ρ-relaxation of articular cartilage at 4T. Magn Reson Med 2001;46(3):419–23.

68. Borthakur A, Mellon E, Niyogi S, et al. Sodium and T1ρ MRI for molecular and diagnostic imaging of articular cartilage. NMR Biomed 2006;19(7):781–821.

69. Pakin SK, Xu J, Schweitzer ME, et al. Rapid 3D-T1ρ mapping of the knee joint at 3.0T with parallel imaging. Magn Reson Med 2006;56(3):563–71.

70. Wang L, Chang G, Xu J, et al. T1rho MRI of menisci and cartilage in patients with osteoarthritis at 3T. Eur J Radiol 2012;81(9):2329–36.

71. Menezes NM, Gray ML, Hartke JR, et al. T2 and T1ρ MRI in articular cartilage systems. Magn Reson Med 2004;51(3):503–9.

72. Brinkhof S, Nizak R, Khlebnikov V, et al. Detection of early cartilage damage: feasibility and potential of gagCEST imaging at 7T. Eur Radiol 2018;28(7): 2874–81.

73. Singh A, Haris M, Cai K, et al. Chemical exchange saturation transfer magnetic resonance imaging of human knee cartilage at 3 T and 7 T. Magn Reson Med 2012;68(2):588–94.

74. Cha JG, Yoo JH, Rhee SJ, et al. MR imaging of articular cartilage at 1.5T and 3.0T: comparison of IDEAL 2D FSE and 3D SPGR with fat-saturated 2D FSE and 3D SPGR in a porcine model. Acta Radiol 2014;55(4):462–9.

75. Recht MP, Kramer J, Marcelis S, et al. Abnormalities of articular cartilage in the knee: analysis of available MR techniques. Radiology 1993;187(2):473–8.

76. McCauley TR, Kier R, Lynch KJ, et al. Chondromalacia patellae: diagnosis with MR imaging. Am J Roentgenol 1992;158(1):101–5.

77. Bredella MA, Tirman PF, Peterfy CG, et al. Accuracy of T2-weighted fast spin-echo MR imaging with fat saturation in detecting cartilage defects in the knee: comparison with arthroscopy in 130 patients. Am J Roentgenol 1999;172(4): 1073–80.

78. Dwyer T, Martin CR, Kendra R, et al. Reliability and validity of the arthroscopic international cartilage repair society classification system: correlation with histological assessment of depth. Arthrosc J Arthrosc Relat Surg 2017;33(6):1219–24.

79. Medina J, Garcia-Mansilla I, Fabricant PD, et al. Microfracture for the treatment of symptomatic cartilage lesions of the knee: a survey of international cartilage regeneration & joint preservation society. Cartilage 2020. https://doi.org/10.1177/1947603520954503. 1947603520954503.

80. Broderick LS, Turner DA, Renfrew DL, et al. Severity of articular cartilage abnormality in patients with osteoarthritis: evaluation with fast spin-echo MR vs arthroscopy. Am J Roentgenol 1994;162(1):99–103.

81. Calvo E, Palacios I, Delgado E, et al. Histopathological correlation of cartilage swelling detected by magnetic resonance imaging in early experimental osteoarthritis. Osteoarthritis Cartilage 2004;12(11):878–86.

82. Phan CM, Link TM, Blumenkrantz G, et al. MR imaging findings in the follow-up of patients with different stages of knee osteoarthritis and the correlation with clinical symptoms. Eur Radiol 2006;16(3):608–18.

83. von Engelhardt LV, Lahner M, Klussmann A, et al. Arthroscopy vs. MRI for a detailed assessment of cartilage disease in osteoarthritis: diagnostic value of MRI in clinical practice. BMC Musculoskelet Disord 2010;11(1):75.

84. Wluka A, Wolfe R, Stuckey S, et al. How does tibial cartilage volume relate to symptoms in subjects with knee osteoarthritis? Ann Rheum Dis 2004;63(3):264–8.

85. Hunter DJ, March L, Sambrook PN. The association of cartilage volume with knee pain. Osteoarthritis Cartilage 2003;11(10):725–9.

86. Uhl M, Ihling C, Allmann KH, et al. Human articular cartilage: in vitro correlation of MRI and histologic findings. Eur Radiol 1998;8(7):1123–9.

87. Gold SL, Burge AJ, Potter HG. MRI of hip cartilage: joint morphology, structure, and composition. Clin Orthop 2012;470(12):3321–31.

88. Potter HG, Koff MF. MR imaging tools to assess cartilage and joint structures. HSS J 2012;8(1):29–32.

89. Kendell SD, Helms CA, Rampton JW, et al. MRI appearance of chondral delamination injuries of the knee. Am J Roentgenol 2005;184(5):1486–9.

90. White CL, Chauvin NA, Waryasz GR, et al. MRI of native knee cartilage delamination injuries. Am J Roentgenol 2017;209(5):W317–21.

91. Wissman RD, Ingalls J, Nepute J, et al. The trochlear cleft: the "black line" of the trochlear trough. Skeletal Radiol 2012;41(9):1121–6.

92. Stephens T, Diduch DR, Balin JI, et al. The cartilage black line sign: an unexpected MRI appearance of deep cartilage fissuring in three patients. Skeletal Radiol 2011;40(1):113–6.
93. Markhardt BK, Kijowski R. The clinical significance of dark cartilage lesions identified on MRI. Am J Roentgenol 2015;205(6):1251–9.
94. König H, Sauter R, Deimling M, et al. Cartilage disorders: comparison of spin-echo, CHESS, and FLASH sequence MR images. Radiology 1987;164(3):753–8.

Imaging of Patellofemoral Instability

Erin McCrum, MD[a],*, Kyle Cooper, MD[a], Jocelyn Wittstein, MD[b],
Robert J. French, MD[a]

KEYWORDS

- Patellofemoral instability • Patellar dislocation • MPFL reconstruction

KEY POINTS

- Patellar instability is a broad term that encompasses patellar dislocation, patellar subluxation, and patellar instability.
- Patella alta, trochlear dysplasia, and lateralization of the tibial tubercle are important anatomic causes of patellofemoral instability.
- Radiographs and MRI demonstrate characteristic findings of patellofemoral instability.
- Surgical methods to address the sequalae and underlying etiologies of patellar instability vary.

INTRODUCTION

Patellar instability is a broad term that encompasses patellar dislocation, patellar subluxation, and patellar instability.

Acute traumatic patellar dislocation has an estimated prevalence that ranges from 6 to 77 per 100,000 and is typically due to injury that occurs during physical activity in a flexed knee with a twisting or valgus stress applied to a planted foot with or without direct contact to the patella.[1,2] While most primary dislocations occur in adolescents with the highest incidence in the 10- to 17-year-old age group, a primary dislocation event in a patient younger than 12 years is suggestive of underlying abnormal morphology.[3,4] The most important of the structural abnormalities are thought to be patella alta, trochlear dysplasia, and lateralization of the tibial tubercle.[1] Second dislocation events in skeletally mature patients have been reported in 15% to 44% of patients and are more common in female patients or in patients with a history of dislocation in the contralateral knee.[5–7] Although fewer than half of the patients

[a] Division of Musculoskeletal Imaging, Department of Radiology, Duke University Medical Center, Duke University Hospital, Box 3808, Durham, NC 27710, USA; [b] Department of Orthopaedic Surgery, Duke Health Heritage, Duke University School of Medicine, 3000 Rogers Road, Wake Forest, Durham, NC 27587, USA
* Corresponding author.
E-mail address: erin.mccrum@duke.edu

Clin Sports Med 40 (2021) 693–712
https://doi.org/10.1016/j.csm.2021.05.007
0278-5919/21/© 2021 Elsevier Inc. All rights reserved.
sportsmed.theclinics.com

experience a second dislocation event, 58% of patients reported significant functional limitations with strenuous physical activity.[8]

Patients with symptoms of patellofemoral instability often present with a history of knee "giving way," and in the setting of acute dislocation, they may have hemarthrosis and pain along the course of the medial patellofemoral ligament (MPFL). Although the physical examination can be indeterminate in the acute setting because of pain and guarding, positive patellar apprehension and increased patellar lateral translation are highly suggestive of patellar instability. A positive patellar grind test is suggestive of patellofemoral chondral degeneration which, among other etiologies, can be seen in the setting of chronic instability.[9]

Radiologists can aid their clinical colleagues not only in the assessment of abnormal patellofemoral morphology and alignment but also by assessing the integrity of the stabilizing ligamentous structures, concomitant injury to the collateral ligaments or menisci, and the presence of osteochondral lesions or loose bodies which necessitate surgical intervention.

Although surgical practices vary, the goals of surgery are to stabilize the patellofemoral joint by correcting underlying anatomic contributions to instability and to address any osteochondral and soft-tissue injuries that result from patellar dislocation.

NORMAL PATELLOFEMORAL ANATOMY

The patellofemoral joint refers to the articulation between the triangular patella sesamoid bone and the femoral trochlea. The patella sits within a concave trochlear groove with patellar and trochlear medial and lateral articulating facets. The lateral trochlear facet typically has a larger and steeper morphology.[10] The articular surfaces are lined by a thick layer of hyaline cartilage with the patellar cartilage among the thickest in the body.[11] Joint stability is dependent on a proper fit between the femoral trochlea and patella as well as a complex combination of ligaments, tendons, and aponeuroses providing stabilization in both transverse and longitudinal dimensions.

Superiorly the trilaminar quadriceps tendon inserts onto the patella.[12] Inferiorly, the rectus femoris component of the quadriceps tendon continues as the patellar tendon, which inserts proximally at the patellar apex and distally onto the tibial tubercle. In the transverse dimension, the patella is stabilized by medial and lateral retinacula. The lateral retinaculum receives contributions from the deep muscular fascia, iliotibial band, quadriceps aponeurosis, and joint capsule.[12–15] These lateral stabilizers exert a lateral force on the patella. Opposing force is provided by the medial retinacular structures, which contribute to the second of the three anatomic layers of the knee and are positioned between the superficial investing fascia and joint capsule.[16] The medial retinacular structures consist primarily of three ligaments. The MPFL has been shown to be the most important resistance to lateral patellar translation with a smaller contribution provided by the medial patellomeniscal ligament (MPML) and associated capsular fibers. In contrast, the medial patellotibial ligament (MPTL) is thought to be functionally unimportant in preventing lateral patellar subluxation.[17,18]

ASSESSMENT OF ABNORMAL PATELLOFEMORAL ANATOMY

Malalignment produced by poor fit between the patella and trochlear and/or unequal pull from its complex of support structures can produce patellofemoral pain and result in patellar instability.[13,17–19] The most important of the structural abnormalities are thought to be patella alta, trochlear dysplasia, and lateralization of the tibial tubercle. Abnormal tibiofemoral version may be an important secondary cause of patellofemoral instability.[1]

Trochlear Dysplasia

Trochlear dysplasia refers to a dysplastic alteration in the normal morphology of the femoral trochlea, primarily affecting the superior portion of the trochlea, and is an important factor contributing to patellar instability.[20] Quantitative and qualitative methods for assessing trochlear morphology on radiographs and cross-sectional imaging have been adopted for use in clinical practice.

Dejour Classification

The most used qualitative classification schema for trochlear dysplasia is the Dejour classification system. Working primarily with lateral radiographs, Henri Dejour and colleagues identified several radiographic concepts for assessment of the dysplastic trochlea.[21] These were subsequently refined through the work of his son, David Dejour, resulting in three primary radiographic criteria: crossing sign, trochlear spur, and double contour sign.[22] In conjunction with cross-sectional imaging findings, these radiographic signs form the basis of the modern Dejour classification of trochlear morphology (**Fig. 1**).

Type A: Crossing sign present. Shallow trochlea on cross-sectional imaging.

Type B: Crossing sign and trochlear spur present. Flat trochlea on cross-sectional imaging.

Type C: Crossing and double contour signs present. Convex trochlea and lateral facet with hypoplastic medial facet on cross-sectional imaging.

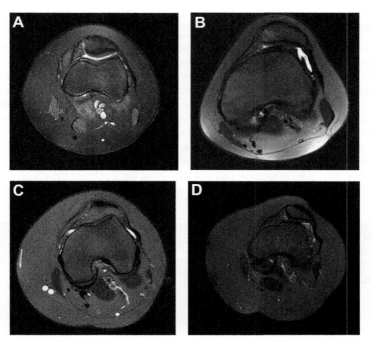

Fig. 1. Dejour classification on axial T2-weighted fat-saturated MRI images of the knee. (*A*) Type A demonstrates a shallow trochlea. (*B*) Type B demonstrates a flat trochlea on cross-sectional imaging. (*C*) Type C demonstrates a hypoplastic medial facet. (*D*) Type D demonstrates a cliff-like appearance separating the medial and lateral facets. (*Courtesy of* Gaetke-Udager K. Used with permission.)

Type D: Crossing sign, trochlear spur, and double contour signs present. Cliff-like appearance separating the medial and lateral facets on cross-sectional imaging.

The use of the Dejour system is somewhat problematic. Interreader agreement in classifying lateral radiographs with the initial Henry Dejour system was poor but improved with the use of the revised David Dejour classification system.[23] Studies have also shown that radiographic and MRI Dejour morphology categorization are frequently discordant, with MR evaluation typically suggesting a higher degree of dysplasia.[24–27] Furthermore, studies have shown poor correlation between three of the most used quantitative methods for assessing trochlear dysplasia: lateral trochlear inclination (LTI), trochlear facet asymmetry, and trochlear depth and the corresponding Dejour grade. Correlation improves when distinguishing between low- and high-grade trochlear dysplasia.[27]

Sulcus Angle

The trochlear sulcus angle was historically measured on the radiographic Merchant view of the knee and considered suggestive of dysplasia if the angle between the medial and lateral trochlear facets is greater than 145° to 150°. Subsequent studies with cross-sectional imaging have demonstrated that radiography significantly underestimates the degree of dysplasia of the proximal trochlea.[26] Furthermore, cross-sectional studies have confirmed that bony trochlear dysplasia is exacerbated by overlying trochlear cartilage resulting in a significant "cartilage-bone mismatch" (**Fig. 2**) with decreased reproducibility of measured angles at higher degrees of dysplasia.[28]

Lateral Trochlear Inclination

LTI is one of the most commonly used quantitative measurements with a reported sensitivity and specificity of 93% and 87%, respectively, with high interreader and intrareader reliability.[1,29,30] The LTI is obtained by measuring the angle between the subchondral bone of the lateral trochlear facet and posterior femoral condyle tangential line at the most cranial axial MR image showing cartilage (**Fig. 3**). An inclination angle of less than 11° is suggestive of trochlear dysplasia.[1] Although not as widely adopted in clinical practice, an alternative measurement method has been reported in which the posterior femoral condylar tangential line is obtained more distally at the level where the femoral condyles are well formed. Using this method, an inclination angle of less than 8.9° is reported as the threshold for trochlear dysplasia. Although sensitivity and specificity are reported as 68% and 90%, respectively, Cheng and

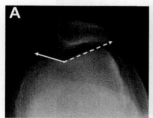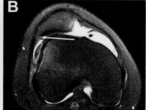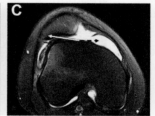

Fig. 2. Sulcus angle. (*A*) Measurement of the sulcus angle on the Merchant view radiograph which demonstrates a sulcus angle of 142° as measured between the medial (*solid arrow*) and lateral (*dashed arrow*) trochlear facets. The sulcus angle increases to 159° (*B*) and 162° (*C*) when measured between the medial trochlear facet (*solid arrow*) and lateral trochlear facet (*black dashed arrow*) along the subchondral bone (*B*) and chondral surface (*C*).

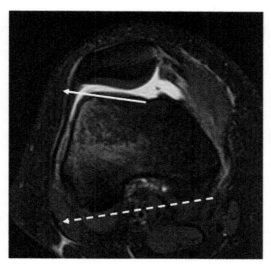

Fig. 3. Lateral trochlear inclination of 8° as measured between a line along the lateral trochlear facet (*solid arrow*) and a posterior condylar tangential line (*dashed line*) suggestive of trochlear dysplasia.

colleagues suggest that this may be a more accurate measurement because the traditional method may underestimate the true rotational axis of the femur.[29–31]

TROCHLEAR FACET ASYMMETRY

Trochlear facet asymmetry is calculated as the ratio of the length of the medial to lateral trochlear facets 3 cm above the tibiofemoral joint with values less than 40% suggesting trochlear dysplasia. The ratio has high sensitivity and specificities of 100% and 96%, respectively, as reported by Pfirrman and colleagues who used a lateral radiograph of the knee as a standard of reference.[32] However, in practice, the level 3 cm above the tibiofemoral joint may represent different topographic portions of the trochlear groove in knees of a different size. As an alternative, numerous intrinsic landmarks have been variably used, such as the level in which chondral cartilage is first evident[33] or the level in which trochlear chondral coverage is complete,[34] but it is unclear if these yield more accurate measurements (**Fig. 4**).

TROCHLEAR DEPTH

Trochlear depth measurements are obtained at the level of facet asymmetry measurement.[1] In the most common method for this calculation, the perpendicular anteroposterior (AP) lengths of the most anterior aspect of the medial and lateral trochlear chondral facets to a posterior femoral condylar tangential line are averaged, and the perpendicular AP length of the spanning the chondral surface of the trochlear sulcus to the posterior femoral condylar line is subtracted (**Fig. 5**). Values of less than 3 mm are suggestive of trochlear dysplasia with a sensitivity and specificity of 100% and 96%, respectively, as reported by Pfirrman and colleagues.[1,32] As with other measurements of trochlear dysplasia, numerous alternative methods have been proposed to measure trochlear depth which are not mathematically equivalent to the method reported by Pfirmann. Because of the numerous methodologies in use, trochlear

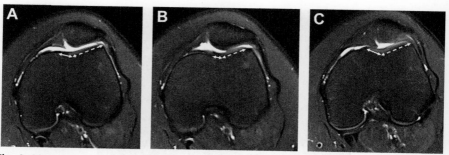

Fig. 4. Measurement of facet asymmetry. A ratio of the medial trochlear facet (*solid arrow* in *A*, *B*, and *C*) to the lateral trochlear facet (*dashed arrows* in *A*, *B*, and *C*). Measurements were acquired at 3 cm above the level of the joint (*A*), at the level of the first axial MR slice demonstrating cartilage (*B*), and at the level of complete trochlear chondral coverage (*C*). Ratios were found to be 39%, 24%, and 50% in *A*, *B*, and *C*, respectively, suggesting variability in the measurement based on the level of the axial image used for measurement. (*Courtesy of* Gaetke-Udager K. Used with permission.)

depth–reported values should include a description of the technique used to reduce miscommunication between radiologists and clinical colleagues.

PATELLAR TILT

Assessment of patellar tilt is also useful in the evaluation of extensor alignment. Numerous methods have been developed to assess for patellar alignment; however, the most frequently used ones are the Laurin lateral patellofemoral angle (PFA) and the patellar tilt angle. The PFA is evaluated on the Merchant radiograph and is formed

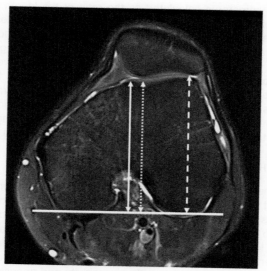

Fig. 5. Perpendicular AP lengths of the most anterior aspect of the medial (*solid arrow*) and lateral trochlear chondral facets (*dashed arrow*) to a posterior femoral condylar tangential line (*solid line*) are averaged and the perpendicular AP length of the spanning the chondral surface to the trochlear sulcus (*dotted arrow*) to the posterior femoral condylar line is subtracted. In this case, the trochlear depth measured 1.6 mm, suggestive of dysplasia.

between the lateral patellar facet and a line along the anterior medial and lateral femoral condyles measured at the level of the mid-patella. In a normally aligned patella, the PFA angle opens laterally, whereas with abnormal patellar tilt, the PFA is flat or opens medially.[35–37] Patellar tilt can also be quantitatively assessed with the patellar tilt angle. The patellar tilt angle refers to the angle between the longest transverse diameter of the patella and a tangential line to the posterior femoral condyles (**Fig. 6**) measured on an axial MR image. Abnormal patellar alignment is suggested if the patellar tilt angle is greater than 5°.[38]

TIBIAL TUBERCLE LATERALIZATION

The tibial tubercle to trochlear groove distance (TT-TG) provides a quantitative evaluation of the degree of tibial tubercle lateralization. A line is drawn along the posterior margin of the femoral condyles followed by perpendicular lines bisecting the tibial tuberosity and the deepest point of the trochlea on axial MR imaging. A distance is then measured between the tibial tubercle and trochlear groove (**Fig. 7**). Measurements less than 15 mm are considered normal with 15 to 20 mm borderline and greater than 20 mm positive for significant tibial tubercle lateralization.[39] Abnormal TT-TG values are predictive of patellofemoral instability,[40] and identification of patients with patellar instability and abnormal TT-TG intervals allows selection of patients who may benefit from surgical tibial tubercle transfer.[41–44] CT can also be used to obtain the TT-TG interval; however, the measurements are slightly greater than those on MRI.[45]

PATELLA ALTA

Patella alta refers to an abnormal vertical or high-riding position of the patella with respect to the femoral trochlea. The patella normally resides vertical to the femoral trochlea during passive extension with patellofemoral engagement occurring at progressively higher degrees of flexion. However, the high-riding patella alters this process with the patella engaging later during flexion resulting in increased compressive forces across the patellofemoral joint with consequent chondral

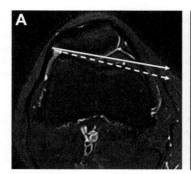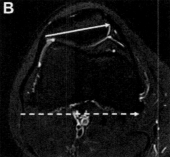

Fig. 6. (A) Qualitative assessment of patellar tilt with PFA obtained between the lateral patellar facet (*solid arrow*) and a line connecting the anterior medial and lateral femoral condyles (*dashed arrow*) opening medially, suggestive of trochlear dysplasia. In (B), the patellar tilt angle is measured between longest transverse diameter of the patella (*solid arrows*) and a posterior condylar tangential line (*dashed arrow*). The value of this angle was found to be 20° suggestive of trochlear dysplasia.

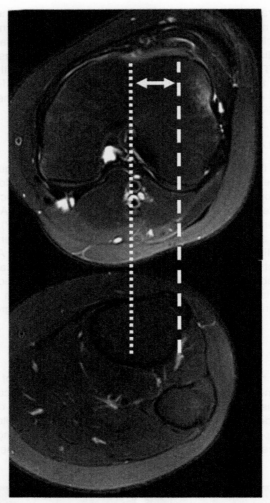

Fig. 7. The TT-TG interval is measured on axial fat-saturated T2-weighted imaging by measuring the interval between a line perpendicular to the femoral condyles through the deepest part of the trochlear groove (*dotted line* in the top slice of the knee) and a line bisecting the tibial tubercle (*dashed line* in the bottom slice of the knee). This patient had a borderline TT-TG interval of 18 mm.

stresses.[46] Although patella alta can be a normal finding, it can also lead to abnormal lateral patellar displacement and tilt with a resultant predisposition to dislocation.[47,48]

Numerous radiographic and MR techniques for quantification of patellar height have been described. The most common radiographic measurements are the Insall-Salvati index (ISI), the modified Insall Salvati index (MISI), and the Caton-Deschamps index (CDI) which are measured on the lateral radiograph with the knee in 30° of flexion.[49–53] The ISI is a simple ratio of the patellar tendon length to the maximum length of the patella with normal values ranging from 0.8 to 1.2 and values greater than 1.2 indicative of patella alta. The MISI was developed to address error introduced in the Insall-Salvati measurement of patella alta in the setting of an elongated or truncated nonarticular inferior patellar pole. The MISI ratio is the length from the inferior articular surface of the patella to the patellar tendon insertion divided by the length of the patellar articular surface. Values greater than 2.0 are suggestive of patella alta. The CDI was developed to address cases in which measurement of the patellar tendon length is challenging such as in patients with Osgood-Schlatter disease and is helpful in preoperative and postoperative assessments as the ratio improves with distalization procedures, whereas the ISI does not. The index is considered suggestive of patella alta if a ratio of a line spanning the tip of the patellar articular surface to the most anterior tibial plateau to the length of the patellar articular surface is greater than 1.2 (**Fig. 8**). This method can be problematic if there is alteration of the normal tibial plateau margins, such as by degenerative change.[53,54]

Femoral Version

Femoral version refers to the twisting of the femur along its course. This is commonly assessed with a line drawn through the long axis of the femoral neck and along the posterior margin of the femoral condyles with the resultant angle measured.[55] Some amount of anteversion is expected with 30 to 40° normal at birth and a subsequent decrease to slightly less than 15° as adults. Abnormal degrees of femoral anteversion have been shown to cause increased pressure on the lateral patellar facets by the lateral trochlea, in effect pushing the patella laterally.[56]

STRUCTURAL CHANGES DUE TO PATELLAR DISLOCATION AND MALTRACKING
Radiographic Findings

In the setting of traumatic injury to the knee, the initial imaging examination of choice is a radiographic knee series. The presence of a small osseous avulsion fracture adjacent to the peripheral margin of the medial patellar facet, dubbed the "sliver sign", may suggest a patellar dislocation as the underlying mechanism of injury.[57] Inclusion of a dedicated patellar view, such as a sunrise view, is of paramount importance as it

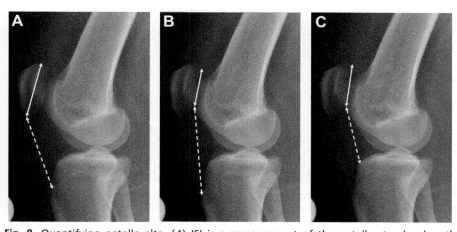

Fig. 8. Quantifying patella alta. (*A*) ISI is a measurement of the patellar tendon length (*dashed arrow*) divided by the longest patellar length (*solid arrow*). (*B*) The MISI measurement measures the length of a line spanning from the inferior articular surface (*dashed arrow*) to the length of the patellar articular surface (*solid arrow*). (*C*) CDI is a ratio of the line spanning the tip of the patellar articular surface to the most anterior tibial plateau (*dashed arrow*) and to the length of the patellar articular surface (*solid arrow*).

has been reported that 30% of medial patellar avulsion fractures could only be identified on the dedicated patellar view.[58] The slivered osseous avulsion fracture originates from the patellar attachment of at least one component of the medial patellar retinaculum (MPR), either the MPFL attachment, the more inferiorly located MPTL/MPML attachment, or a combination of the components (**Fig. 9**).[59] When the avulsion fracture fragment is identified on the radiograph, an MRI should be considered for further evaluation of additional stigmata of prior patellar dislocation.

Magnetic Resonance Findings

Contusion patterns

The patellofemoral contusion pattern after an episode of transient lateral patellar dislocation manifests as edema-like signal at the inferomedial margin of the patella and the peripheral aspect of the weight-bearing lateral femoral condyle.

Injury to the Medial Patellar Stabilizers

Both the MPR and the MPFL are important medial stabilizers of the patella. In practice, it can be difficult to differentiate the two structures near the patellar attachment on

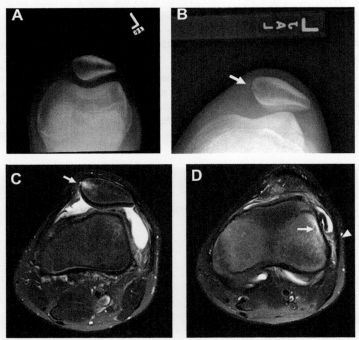

Fig. 9. A 20-year-old patient who presented with a recent patellar dislocation. (*A*) Radiographs made 2 years before initial presentation. (*B*) A small avulsion fracture from the medial patellar facet (*arrow*) which is highly characteristic of a patellar dislocation event. The patella appears laterally subluxed which is also suggestive of injury to the MPFL. (*C*) An axial fat saturated T2-weighted image demonstrates the avulsion fracture from the medial patellar facet with associated tearing at the patellar insertion of the MPFL. (*D*) Axial fat-saturated T2-weighted image demonstrates the characteristic contusion on the lateral femoral condyle (*arrow*) with the suggestion of injury to the femoral attachment of the MPFL (*arrow head*).

MRI. MRI examinations of patients with lateral patellar dislocations reveal injuries to the MPR and/or MPFL in 70% to 100% of cases.[1,60,61] Medial retinacular injuries are best evaluated on T2-weighted imaging in the axial plane and often categorized as being complete, referring to a region of substance loss, or partial when some fibers remain intact. One study also described the location of the injury along its ligamentous course, from the femoral attachment (76%), its midsubstance (30%), or its patellar attachment (49%) (**Fig. 10**).[60] When the MPFL is completely torn, particularly from its patellar attachment, there is an association with chondral/osteochondral abnormalities at the lateral femoral condyle.[62] Alternatively, complete MPFL tears from the femoral attachment on initial lateral patellar dislocation have a higher incidence of persistent patellar instability and second lateral patellar dislocation injury.[63,64] The location of MPFL rupture appears to be related to patient age: Young patients often rupture from the patellar attachment, and older patients rupture from the femoral attachment.[65,66] A more recent study suggests that 84% of the patellar avulsion fractures were located in the inferomedial patellar border suggesting that injury occurred at the MPTL/MPML attachments as opposed to the more classically thought MPFL attachment at the superomedial patellar border[59] or, alternatively, due to impaction injury.

Osteochondral Defect/Loose Bodies

The identification of osteochondral defects and loose bodies on MRI is critical because their presence can prompt more urgent surgical management. Osteochondral fractures are present in up to 70% of acute of recurrent lateral patellar dislocation cases.[37] In fact, a concave osteochondral impaction deformity at the inferomedial patella secondary to the impaction-type injury has been described as a highly specific sign for lateral patellar dislocation.[60] Patellar predominant cartilage lesions have been described on MRI in patients with acute dislocations (71%), recurrent dislocations (82%), and chronic dislocations (97%).[67] Patients with chronic patellar instability have a higher incidence and severity of trochlear cartilage abnormalities.[68] It has been suggested that lateral femoral condylar cartilage defects occur in approximately 40% of lateral patellar dislocations (**Fig. 11**) and that the anterior to posterior location of the defect on the lateral femoral condyle is based on the degree of flexion at time of injury.[69]

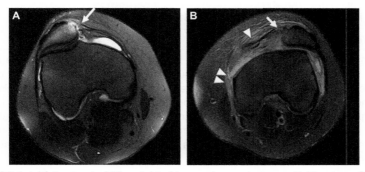

Fig. 10. (*A*) Axial fat-saturated T2-weighted image demonstrates partial tearing of the MPFL at the patellar attachment (*arrow*). (*B*) Axial fat-saturated T2-weighted image demonstrates multiple sites of injury to the MPFL including the patellar attachment (*arrow*), midsubstance (*arrow head*), and femoral attachment (*double arrowhead*).

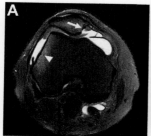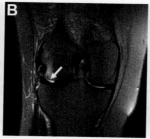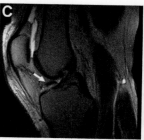

Fig. 11. A 25-year-old patient with a history of recurrent patellar dislocation. (*A*) Axial fat-saturated T2-weighted image of the knee demonstrates characteristic appearance of a recent patellar dislocation event with an osteochondral fracture of the medial patellar facet with associated MPFL injury and contusion of the lateral femoral condyle (*arrow head*). (*B*) Coronal fat-saturated T2-weighted image demonstrates a large cartilage defect in the peripheral lateral femoral condyle (*arrow*). (*C*) Sagittal fat-saturated T2-weighted image demonstrates the corresponding loose body anterior to the ACL (*arrow*). (*Courtesy of* Gaetke-Udager K. Used with permission.)

Other

Additional soft-tissue injuries have been described in lateral patellar dislocation injuries. One study reports that 25% of medial collateral ligament (MCL) injuries in injured adolescent athletes occurred in conjunction with manifestations of patellar instability injuries.[70] Also, soft-tissue edema or hemorrhage, and less commonly muscle elevation, can be present along the inferior margin of the vastus medialis obliquus muscle after acute lateral patellar dislocations.[60]

PATELLAR LATERAL FEMORAL FRICTION SYNDROME

Patients with MRI findings of patellar lateral femoral friction syndrome (PLFFS) are associated with morphologic predisposition to patellofemoral instability, as well as patellar chondral lesions (35%) and patella-trochlear osteochondral lesions (48%).[71] Characteristic findings on MRI in the setting of PLFFS includes an abnormal edema-like signal in the lateral margin of the infrapatellar fat pad (**Fig. 12**). Anatomically, this region of abnormal signal is present within the fat interposed between the lateral margin of the proximal patellar tendon and the peripheral aspect of the lateral femoral trochlea. Further quantitative analysis on MRI not only confirms the association between PLFFS and subtle patellofemoral instability but may also help elucidate the biomechanics of PLFFS.[72]

Surgical Techniques

Unless an osteochondral fracture, femoral MPFL avulsion fracture, or loose body is identified which requires arthroscopic or surgical fixation, studies have not demonstrated a clear long-term benefit to operative intervention after a primary patellar dislocation, and the preferred treatment is nonoperative.[3,73,74]

Although surgical management and practices are variable, MPFL reconstruction and tibial tubercle realignment are the primary surgical techniques used to address patellofemoral instability. Trochleoplasty is an additional surgical consideration but is less commonly performed.

MPFL Reconstruction

In the past, MPFL repair or medial capsular plication was the preferred surgical approach for medial soft-tissue deficiency. However, these surgeries had a high

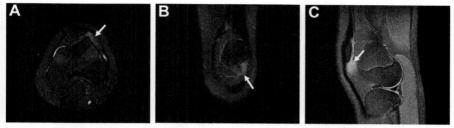

Fig. 12. A 14-year-old runner with patellofemoral pain. Axial (*A*), coronal (*B*), and sagittal (*C*) fat-saturated T2- weighted images demonstrate edema (*arrows*) in the lateral margin of the infrapatellar fat pad which is characteristic of patellar lateral femoral friction syndrome.

rate of failure (**Fig. 13**).[75] Studies showed that not only was it difficult to determine the location of injury of the MPFL during arthroscopy or imaging but also the MPFL was often injured at multiple locations which ultimately led to failed repair or recurrent dislocation if not appropriately addressed.[76]

In surgical candidates with a TT-TG of 20 mm or less, MPFL reconstruction has been shown to offer a drastic improvement over MPFL repair or medial capsular plication techniques[77] with only a reported 4.5% recurrent dislocation rate. While studies have not demonstrated a clear benefit to reconstruction with an allograft versus autograft, multiple studies have demonstrated that femoral placement of the graft and appropriate graft tensioning are critical to success. Femoral tunnel positioning is determined intraoperatively on a laterally positioned fluoroscopic image. Schöttle's point[78] is the most frequently used location in clinical practice as it can reproducibly place the femoral tunnel within 5 mm of the MPFL anatomic insertion (**Fig. 14**).[76]

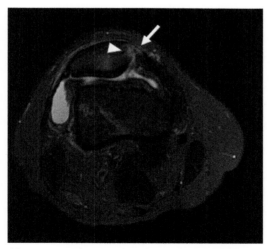

Fig. 13. A 38-year-old patient with a history of prior MPFL repair. Axial fat-saturated T2-weighted images demonstrate findings suggestive of failed MPFL repair including fluid undercutting the graft with increased signal within the graft fibers at the patellar attachment (*arrow*). Contusion of the medial patellar facet (*arrowhead*) and lateral femoral condyle (not shown) is suggestive or recurrent dislocation.

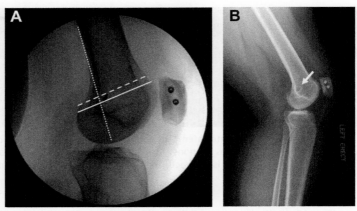

Fig. 14. (*A*) Intraoperative radiograph demonstrating Schöttle's point which is denoted by the black surgical instrument. Schöttle's is slightly anterior (1–2 mm) to the posterior cortex extension line (*dotted line*), 2.5 mm distal to a line drawn through the posterior medial femoral condyle (*dashed line*), and just proximal to the posterior aspect of Blumensaat's line (*solid line*). (*B*) Normal postoperative appearance of a lateral knee radiograph status after MPFL reconstruction (*arrow* denotes femoral tunnel at Schöttle's point).

On MRI, the MPFL graft may appear single- or double-bundled or have a two-tailed configuration and should appear taut and low in signal intensity on both T1- and T2-weighted imaging (**Fig. 15**).[76,79] The graft should originate on the femur just distal to the adductor magnus and insert on the proximal half to one-third of the patella.[79] Patellar tunnels should have a diameter of less than 4.5 mm and are often placed in a parallel oblique orientation which helps reduce patellar fracture. Patellar tunnels may not be evident if a quadriceps turndown autograft was used, a technique which

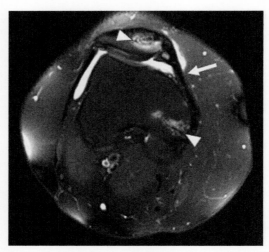

Fig. 15. Axial T2 fat-saturated image of a normal appearance of an MPFL reconstruction. The MPFL graft (*arrow*) appears taut and hypointense. A small avulsion fracture fragment adjacent to the graft was the stigmata of prior patellar dislocation and present on prior studies. Foci of susceptibility (*arrowheads*) in the patella and femoral condyles from patellar and femoral hardware.

is typically reserved for pediatric patients with open physes.[76,79] In addition, small implants may have a diameter as small as just under 2 mm in techniques using anchor fixation without graft placed in tunnels in the patella.

Regardless of graft selection, the MPFL graft strength should exceed that of the native MPFL. However, overtensioning the graft or small variations in graft placement can result in abnormally increased contact pressure to the medial patellofemoral articular surfaces resulting in accelerated chondral degeneration.[9,76,79] Continued symptoms of patellar instability have been reported at 3% to 5% despite surgical intervention.

Trochleoplasty

Trochlear dysplasia is also an important cause of patellofemoral instability. In skeletally mature patients without preexisting arthritis with high-grade trochlear dysplasia (Dejour types B-D) or a lateral elevation, a trochleoplasty can be performed to reduce patellar instability. Although there are various techniques, the aim is to reshape the groove to improve patellar engagement. Reported surgical outcomes are heterogenous because of the variable procedures that are concurrently performed, but Hiemstra and colleagues reported improvement in functional scores at 50 months after surgery with a low rate of redislocation.[80]

The most common complication of trochleoplasty is arthrofibrosis, with reported prevalence ranging from 0% to 46%. Additional complications include fracturing at the site of groove deepening or subchondral collapse at the margins of the reshaped trochlea. And while this technique improves patellar instability, the alteration of the articular surface can accelerate chondral degeneration and hasten patellofemoral osteoarthritis.[76]

TIBIAL TUBEROSITY REALIGNMENT

Although there are many surgical approaches to medialization of the tibial tuberosity, the most commonly performed one is the anteromedialization tibial tuberosity

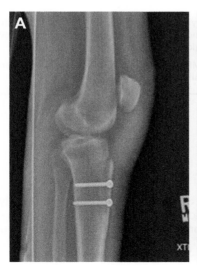
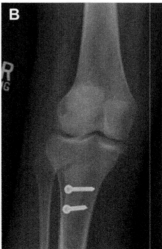

Fig. 16. Lateral (A) and AP (B) radiographs of the knee demonstrates a normal appearance of a recent Fulkerson osteotomy. Two screws are oriented in the AP direction, and the osteotomy margins have not yet healed.

osteotomy, or Fulkerson osteotomy. In patients with a TT-TG interval of 15 to 20 mm or greater, or those with patella alta and CDI greater than 1.2, a Fulkerson osteotomy can help recenter the patella within the groove, with the goal of correcting the TT-TG interval to approximately 10 mm and improving patella alta. Although this surgery is generally successful in reducing patellar instability and improving functional scores, it increases the time required for surgical recovery and may decrease overall return to athletics rate.[76] A straight medialization procedure can be performed in patients without significant chondromalacia.

The overall complication rate for a Fulkerson osteotomy rate is reported at 4.6% with painful hardware requiring removal in 36.7% of cases.[76] Radiographs will show a tibial tubercle osteotomy with two parallel screws oriented in the anterior to posterior direction (**Fig. 16**).[79] Osteotomy margins should become less distinct over time. Although the incidence is low, nonunion and tibial fractures are known complications with rates of 0.8% and 1%, respectively.[76]

SUMMARY

Both functional and structural factors can contribute to patellofemoral pain and result in patellar instability. When evaluating preoperative imaging, the radiologist can aid their surgical colleagues by identifying the stigmata of patellar instability and accurately describing underlying abnormal osseous morphology to help guide surgical management. Familiarity with the normal and abnormal postoperative appearance of common surgical techniques used to address patellofemoral instability can help radiologists identify common imaged postoperative complications.

CLINICS CARE POINTS

- Although the physical exam can be indeterminate in the acute setting, positive patellar apprehension and increased patellar lateral translation are highly suggestive of patellar instability. Additionally, patients may report a history of their knee "giving out."

- Radiographs and MRI can not only identify the stigmata of patellofemoral instability, but also allow for evaluation of underlying abnormal morphology which predisposes towards patellar instability and can help guide surgical management.

- Unless an osteochondral fracture, femoral MPFL avulsion fracture, or loose body is identified, treatment in a first time dislocator is typically non-operative.

DISCLOSURE

The authors have nothing to disclose.

REFERENCES

1. Diederichs G, Issever AS, Scheffler S. MR imaging of patellar instability: injury patterns and assessment of risk factors. RadioGraphics 2010;30(4):961–81.
2. Duthon VB. Acute traumatic patellar dislocation. Orthop Traumatol Surg Res 2015;101(1, Supplement):S59–67.
3. Jain NP, Khan N, Fithian DC. A treatment algorithm for primary patellar dislocations. Sports Health 2011;3(2):170–4.
4. Thompson P, Metcalfe AJ. Current concepts in the surgical management of patellar instability. Knee 2019;26(6):1171–81.

5. Hawkins RJ, Bell RH, Anisette G. Acute patellar dislocations. Am J Sports Med 1986;14(2):117–20.

6. Fithian DC, Paxton EW, Stone ML, et al. Epidemiology and natural history of acute patellar dislocation. Am J Sports Med 2004;32(5):1114–21.

7. Cofield RH, Bryan RS. Acute dislocation of the patella: results of conservative treatment. J Trauma Acute Care Surg 1977;17(7):526–31.

8. Atkin DM, Fithian DC, Marangi KS, et al. Characteristics of patients with primary acute lateral patellar dislocation and their recovery within the first 6 months of injury. Am J Sports Med 2000;28(4):472–9.

9. Redziniak DE, Diduch DR, Mihalko WM, et al. Patellar instability. J Bone Joint Surg Am 2009;91(9):2264–75.

10. Amis AA. Current concepts on anatomy and biomechanics of patellar stability. Sports Med Arthrosc Rev 2007;15(2):48–56.

11. Grelsamer RP, Klein JR. The biomechanics of the patellofemoral joint. J Orthop Sports Phys Ther 1998;28(5):286–98.

12. Reider B, Marshall JL, Koslin B, et al. The anterior aspect of the knee joint. J Bone Joint Surg Am 1981;63(3):351–6.

13. Merican AM, Amis AA. Anatomy of the lateral retinaculum of the knee. J Bone Joint Surg Br 2008;90(4):527–34.

14. Fulkerson JP, Gossling HR. Anatomy of the knee joint lateral retinaculum. Clin Orthop 1980;153:183–8.

15. Kaplan EB. Some aspects of functional anatomy of the human knee joint. Clin Orthop 1962;23:18–29.

16. Warren L, Marshall J. The supporting structures and layers on the medial side of the knee: an anatomical analysis. J Bone Joint Surg Am 1979;61(1):56–62.

17. Conlan T, Garth WP, Lemons JE. Evaluation of the medial soft-tissue restraints of the extensor mechanism of the knee. J Bone Joint Surg Am 1993;75(5):682–93.

18. Desio SM, Burks RT, Bachus KN. Soft tissue restraints to lateral patellar translation in the human knee. Am J Sports Med 1998;26(1):59–65.

19. Wittstein JR, O'Brien SD, Vinson EN, et al. MRI evaluation of anterior knee pain: predicting response to nonoperative treatment. Skeletal Radiol 2009;38(9): 895–901.

20. Amis AA, Oguz C, Bull AMJ, et al. The effect of trochleoplasty on patellar stability and kinematics: a biomechanical study in vitro. J Bone Joint Surg Br 2008;90(7): 864–9.

21. Dejour H, Walch G, Nove-Josserand L, et al. Factors of patellar instability: an anatomic radiographic study. Knee Surg Sports Traumatol Arthrosc 1994;2(1): 19–26.

22. DeJour D, Saggin P. The sulcus deepening trochleoplasty—the Lyon's procedure. Int Orthop 2010;34(2):311–6.

23. Remy F, Besson A, Migaud H, et al. Reproducibility of the radiographic analysis of dysplasia of the femoral trochlea. Intra- and interobserver analysis of 68 knees. Rev Chir Orthop Reparatrice Appar Mot 1998;84(8):728–33.

24. Trochlear Dysplasia. Radsource. 2015. Available at: https://radsource.us/trochlear-dysplasia/. [Accessed 6 April 2021].

25. Lippacher S, Dejour D, Elsharkawi M, et al. Observer agreement on the Dejour trochlear dysplasia classification: a comparison of true lateral radiographs and axial magnetic resonance images. Am J Sports Med 2012;40(4):837–43.

26. Salzmann GM, Weber TS, Spang JT, et al. Comparison of native axial radiographs with axial MR imaging for determination of the trochlear morphology in patients with trochlear dysplasia. Arch Orthop Trauma Surg 2010;130(3):335–40.

27. Nelitz M, Lippacher S, Reichel H, et al. Evaluation of trochlear dysplasia using MRI: correlation between the classification system of Dejour and objective parameters of trochlear dysplasia. Knee Surg Sports Traumatol Arthrosc 2014; 22(1):120–7.

28. van Huyssteen AL, Hendrix MRG, Barnett AJ, et al. Cartilage-bone mismatch in the dysplastic trochlea. An MRI study. J Bone Joint Surg Br 2006;88(5):688–91.

29. Cheng C, Hedgecock J, Solomito M, et al. Defining trochlear dysplasia via the lateral trochlear inclination angle. Orthop J Sports Med 2020;8(4_suppl3). 2325967120S00179.

30. Joseph SM, Cheng C, Solomito MJ, et al. Lateral trochlear inclination in children and adolescents: modified measurement technique to characterize patellar instability. Orthop J Sports Med 2019;7(3_suppl). 2325967119S00146.

31. Cheng C, Joseph SM, Solomito MJ, et al. The effect of trochlear dysplasia on commonly used radiographic parameters to assess patellar instability. Orthop J Sports Med 2019;7(3_suppl). 2325967119S00048.

32. Pfirrmann CW, Zanetti M, Romero J, et al. Femoral trochlear dysplasia: MR findings. Radiology 2000;216(3):858–64.

33. Carrillon Y, Abidi H, Dejour D, et al. Patellar instability: assessment on MR images by measuring the lateral trochlear inclination-initial experience. Radiology 2000; 216(2):582–5.

34. Escala JS, Mellado JM, Olona M, et al. Objective patellar instability: MR-based quantitative assessment of potentially associated anatomical features. Knee Surg Sports Traumatol Arthrosc 2006;14(3):264–72.

35. Ye Q, Yu T, Wu Y, et al. Patellar instability: the reliability of magnetic resonance imaging measurement parameters. BMC Musculoskelet Disord 2019;20(1):317.

36. Endo Y, Stein BES, Potter HG. Radiologic assessment of patellofemoral pain in the athlete. Sports Health 2011;3(2):195–210.

37. Jibri Z, Jamieson P, Rakhra KS, et al. Patellar maltracking: an update on the diagnosis and treatment strategies. Insights Imaging 2019;10(1):65.

38. Grelsamer R, Bazos A, Proctor C. Radiographic analysis of patellar tilt. J Bone Joint Surg Br 1993;75-B(5):822–4.

39. Colvin AC, West RV. Patellar instability. J Bone Joint Surg Am 2008;90(12): 2751–62.

40. Vairo GL, Moya-Angeler J, Siorta MA, et al. Tibial tubercle-trochlear groove distance is a reliable and accurate indicator of patellofemoral instability. Clin Orthop 2019;477(6):1450–8.

41. Diks M, Wymenga A, Anderson P. Patients with lateral tracking patella have better pain relief following CT-guided tuberosity transfer than patients with unstable patella. Knee Surg Sports Traumatol Arthrosc 2003;11(6):384–8.

42. Palmer SH, Servant CTJ, Maguire J, et al. Surgical reconstruction of severe patellofemoral maltracking. Clin Orthop 2004;419:144–8.

43. Pritsch T, Haim A, Arbel R, et al. Tailored tibial tubercle transfer for patellofemoral malalignment: analysis of clinical outcomes. Knee Surg Sports Traumatol Arthrosc 2007;15(8):994–1002.

44. Koëter S, Diks MJF, Anderson PG, et al. A modified tibial tubercle osteotomy for patellar maltracking: results at two years. J Bone Joint Surg Br 2007;89(2):180–5.

45. Hinckel BB, Gobbi RG, Filho ENK, et al. Are the osseous and tendinous-cartilaginous tibial tuberosity-trochlear groove distances the same on CT and MRI? Skeletal Radiol 2015;44(8):1085–93.

46. Singerman R, Davy DT, Goldberg VM. Effects of patella alta and patella infera on patellofemoral contact forces. J Biomech 1994;27(8):1059–65.

47. Ward SR, Terk MR, Powers CM. Patella alta: association with patellofemoral alignment and changes in contact area during weight-bearing. J Bone Joint Surg Am 2007;89(8):1749–55.

48. Magnussen RA, De Simone V, Lustig S, et al. Treatment of patella alta in patients with episodic patellar dislocation: a systematic review. Knee Surg Sports Traumatol Arthrosc 2014;22(10):2545–50.

49. Insall J, Salvati E. Patella position in the normal knee joint. Radiology 1971;101(1): 101–4.

50. Grelsamer RP, Proctor CS, Bazos AN. Evaluation of patellar shape in the sagittal plane. A clinical analysis. Am J Sports Med 1994;22(1):61–6.

51. Grelsamer RP, Meadows S. The modified Insall-Salvati ratio for assessment of patellar height. Clin Orthop 1992;(282):170–6.

52. Caton J, Deschamps G, Chambat P, et al. Patella infera. Apropos of 128 cases. Rev Chir Orthop Reparatrice Appar Mot 1982;68(5):317–25.

53. Patella Alta and Baja. Radsource. 2010. Available at: https://radsource.us/patella-alta-and-baja/. [Accessed 6 April 2021].

54. Gracitelli GC, Pierami R, Tonelli TA, et al. Assessment of patellar height measurement methods from digital radiography. Rev Bras Ortop 2012;47(2):210–3.

55. Souza RB, Powers CM. Concurrent criterion-related validity and reliability of a clinical test to measure femoral anteversion. J Orthop Sports Phys Ther 2009; 39(8):586–92.

56. Lee TQ, Anzel SH, Bennett KA, et al. The influence of fixed rotational deformities of the femur on the patellofemoral contact pressures in human cadaver knees. Clin Orthop 1994;(302):69–74.

57. Pierce JL, McCrum EC, Rozas AK, et al. Tip-of-the-iceberg fractures: small fractures that mean big trouble. Am J Roentgenol 2015;205(3):524–32.

58. Haas JP, Collins MS, Stuart MJ. The "sliver sign": a specific radiographic sign of acute lateral patellar dislocation. Skeletal Radiol 2012;41(5):595–601.

59. Mochizuki T, Tanifuji O, Watanabe S, et al. The majority of patellar avulsion fractures in first-time acute patellar dislocations included the inferomedial patellar border that was different from the medial patellofemoral ligament attachment. Knee Surg Sports Traumatol Arthrosc 2020;28(12):3942–8.

60. Elias DA, White LM, Fithian DC. Acute lateral patellar dislocation at MR imaging: injury patterns of medial patellar soft-tissue restraints and osteochondral injuries of the inferomedial patella. Radiology 2002;225(3):736–43.

61. Zhang G-Y, Zheng L, Ding H-Y, et al. Evaluation of medial patellofemoral ligament tears after acute lateral patellar dislocation: comparison of high-frequency ultrasound and MR. Eur Radiol 2015;25(1):274–81.

62. Zheng L, Shi H, Feng Y, et al. Injury patterns of medial patellofemoral ligament and correlation analysis with articular cartilage lesions of the lateral femoral condyle after acute lateral patellar dislocation in children and adolescents: an MRI evaluation. Injury 2015;46(6):1137–44.

63. Zhang G, Zhu H, Li E, et al. The correlation between the injury patterns of the medial patellofemoral ligament in an acute first-time lateral patellar dislocation on MR imaging and the incidence of a second-time lateral patellar dislocation. Korean J Radiol 2018;19(2):292–300.

64. Sillanpää PJ, Peltola E, Mattila VM, et al. Femoral avulsion of the medial patellofemoral ligament after primary traumatic patellar dislocation predicts subsequent instability in men: a mean 7-year nonoperative follow-up study. Am J Sports Med 2009;37(8):1513–21.

65. Petri M, von Falck C, Broese M, et al. Influence of rupture patterns of the medial patellofemoral ligament (MPFL) on the outcome after operative treatment of traumatic patellar dislocation. Knee Surg Sports Traumatol Arthrosc 2013;21(3): 683–9.

66. Askenberger M, Arendt EA, Ekström W, et al. Medial patellofemoral ligament injuries in children with first-time lateral patellar dislocations: a magnetic resonance imaging and arthroscopic study. Am J Sports Med 2016;44(1):152–8.

67. Vollnberg B, Koehlitz T, Jung T, et al. Prevalence of cartilage lesions and early osteoarthritis in patients with patellar dislocation. Eur Radiol 2012;22(11): 2347–56.

68. Franzone JM, Vitale MA, Shubin Stein BE, et al. Is there an association between chronicity of patellar instability and patellofemoral cartilage lesions? An arthroscopic assessment of chondral injury. J Knee Surg 2012;25(5):411–6.

69. Sanders TG, Paruchuri NB, Zlatkin MB. MRI of osteochondral defects of the lateral femoral condyle: incidence and pattern of injury after transient lateral dislocation of the patella. AJR Am J Roentgenol 2006;187(5):1332–7.

70. Kramer DE, Miller PE, Berrahou IK, et al. Collateral Ligament Knee Injuries in Pediatric and Adolescent Athletes. J Pediatr Orthop 2020;40(2):71–7.

71. Barbier-Brion B, Lerais J-M, Aubry S, et al. Magnetic resonance imaging in patellar lateral femoral friction syndrome (PLFFS): prospective case-control study. Diagn Interv Imaging 2012;93(3):e171–82.

72. Li J, Sheng B, Yu F, et al. Quantitative magnetic resonance imaging in patellar tendon-lateral femoral condyle friction syndrome: relationship with subtle patellofemoral instability. Skeletal Radiol 2019;48(8):1251–9.

73. Zhang K, Jiang H, Li J, et al. Comparison between surgical and nonsurgical treatment for primary patellar dislocations in adolescents: a systematic review and meta-analysis of comparative studies. Orthop J Sports Med 2020;8(9).

74. Smith TO, Donell S, Song F, et al. Surgical versus non-surgical interventions for treating patellar dislocation. Cochrane Database Syst Rev 2015;2:CD008106.

75. Gravesen KS, Kallemose T, Blønd L, et al. High failure rate after medial patellofemoral ligament reconstructions. a nationwide epidemiological study investigating 2.572 medial patellofemoral ligament reconstructions and 24.154 primary dislocations. Arthroscopy 2017;33(10):e70–1.

76. Laidlaw MS, Diduch DR. Current concepts in the management of patellar instability. Indian J Orthop 2017;51(5):493–504.

77. Erickson BJ, Nguyen J, Gasik K, et al. Isolated medial patellofemoral ligament reconstruction for patellar instability regardless of tibial tubercle-trochlear groove distance and patellar height: outcomes at 1 and 2 years. Am J Sports Med 2019; 47(6):1331–7.

78. Schöttle PB, Schmeling A, Rosenstiel N, et al. Radiographic landmarks for femoral tunnel placement in medial patellofemoral ligament reconstruction. Am J Sports Med 2007;35(5):801–4.

79. Purohit N, Hancock N, Saifuddin A. Surgical management of patellofemoral instability part 2: post-operative imaging. Skeletal Radiol 2019;48(7):1001–9.

80. Hiemstra LA, Peterson D, Youssef M, et al. Trochleoplasty provides good clinical outcomes and an acceptable complication profile in both short and long-term follow-up. Knee Surg Sports Traumatol Arthrosc 2019;27(9):2967–83.

Hip Pain
Imaging of Intra-articular and Extra-articular Causes

Katherine M. Bojicic, MD[a], Nathaniel B. Meyer, MD[b],
Corrie M. Yablon, MD[b], Monica Kalume Brigido, MD[b],
Kara Gaetke-Udager, MD[b],*

KEYWORDS

- Hip imaging • FAI imaging • Athletic pubalgia • Snapping hip • Hip ultrasound

KEY POINTS

- MR arthrography allows detailed evaluation of hip intra-articular processes in athletes, including pathologies such as labral tears, cartilage abnormalities, and ligamentum teres injuries.
- Imaging of femoroacetabular impingement includes radiographs, CT, and MRI to assess for morphology, long-term complications such as osteoarthrosis and labral tears, and for preoperative planning.
- Ultrasound is a useful modality when evaluating athletic injuries of the hip, as it allows dynamic imaging and can be used at the bedside.
- MRI is excellent for diagnosing stress-related injuries to bone, such as proximal femoral stress fractures and thigh splints.
- Radiography is a useful first-line study to evaluate athletic injuries of the hip in the acute/emergent setting, such as hip dislocation.

INTRODUCTION

Hip pain is a common complaint among athletes, with a hip injury rate of 53.06 per 100,000 student athletes competing in National Collegiate Athletic Association (NCAA) collegiate sports.[1] Hip injuries account for 17.2% of all musculoskeletal injuries in ballet dancers.[2] Up to 59% of soccer players will experience hip pain during their competitive season,[3] and up to 18% of all time loss injuries in male soccer players are related to hip injuries.[4] Hip injuries can have immediate consequences for athletes,

[a] Diagnostic Radiology Resident, University of Michigan Medical Center, 1500 E Medical Center Drive, B1 D502, Ann Arbor, MI 48103, USA; [b] University of Michigan Medical Center, 1500 E Medical Center Drive, TC 2910, Ann Arbor, MI 48103, USA
* Corresponding author.
E-mail address: kgaetke@umich.edu

Clin Sports Med 40 (2021) 713–729
https://doi.org/10.1016/j.csm.2021.05.008
0278-5919/21/© 2021 Elsevier Inc. All rights reserved.

as well as serious long-term morbidity in the form of osteoarthritis. In recent years, there has been a growing interest in characterizing and diagnosing injuries in younger athletes given the advent of newer surgical techniques, such as surgical correction of femoroacetabular impingement (FAI),[5] to prevent future problems.

Multiple modalities are used in the evaluation of hip pathology including radiography, computerized tomography (CT), magnetic resonance imaging (MRI), and ultrasound (US). Radiographs and US can be used for immediate evaluation of athletes in collegiate and professional sports because they are often present at the sporting venue, while CT and MRI are better for a more thorough evaluation off-site. Magnetic resonance arthrography (MRA) is an additional tool ideal for the assessment of intra-articular pathology. In younger athletes, workup with MR and US is preferred to avoid excessive ionizing radiation. US has the additional benefit of allowing dynamic, real-time evaluation of the hip, which is especially useful in certain conditions, as discussed in the following sections.

Hip pain is a multifaceted issue in athletes, with numerous etiologies. It is important for clinicians to be aware of the different imaging options when evaluating an athlete with hip pain to expedite diagnosis and limit both cost and radiation dose to the patient. This article provides a review of common intra- and extra-articular causes of hip pain with imaging examples.

DISCUSSION
Intra-articular Causes

Femoroacetabular impingement
FAI is a relatively common cause of intra-articular hip pain caused by abnormal anatomy of the acetabulum, proximal femur, or both. Deep groin pain is the most common presenting complaint, although patients may also present with pain involving the low back, buttock, lateral hip, and posterior thigh.[6,7] Mechanical symptoms such as subjective instability, audible popping, and reduced range of motion are also common.

Radiographs are considered first line in the evaluation of FAI. They allow for evaluation of the femoral and acetabular morphology, can be used to calculate standard measurements, and provide additional information such as the presence of degenerative changes, an important surgical outcome predictor.[6] CT facilitates advanced measurements and presurgical planning. Dose-reduction methods should be optimized to minimize ionizing radiation during CT. MRI, including MRA, is most useful for evaluating soft tissue and/or intra-articular pathology that can result from FAI, including labral and cartilage injury.

Two primary types of FAI have been described: cam-type and pincer-type. The cam-type, or pistol-grip deformity, is defined as a loss of the normal femoral head-neck offset with resulting abnormal contact of the femoral head and acetabulum during flexion and internal rotation. In pincer-type, the abnormal contact results from overcoverage of the femoral head by the acetabulum.[6,8] Some patients have both entities, or mixed-type FAI. **Fig. 1** illustrates the different types.

Radiographs of cam-type FAI typically show an osseous prominence at the femoral head-neck junction that is often more apparent on frog or Dunn lateral or false profile views (**Fig. 2**A). Alpha angle is measured on lateral views with the leg in neutral position, between a line drawn along the femoral neck axis and a second extending from the center of the femoral head to the point at which the spherical shape of the femoral head is lost. This can also be measured on CT or MRI. An angle greater than 50° to 55° is consistent with cam-type morphology[6] (**Fig. 2**B).

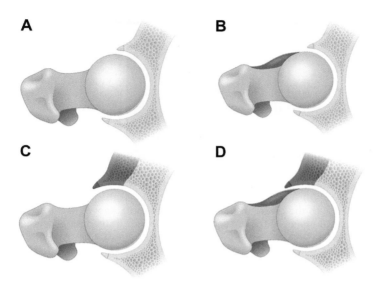

Fig. 1. Illustration of types of FAI. (*A*) Normal anatomy. (*B*) Cam-type deformity, with osseous protuberance along the lateral femoral head-neck junction shown in red. (*C*) Pincer-type deformity, with acetabular overcoverage highlighted in red. (*D*) Mixed-type, with both cam and pincer deformities. (From Gaetke-Udager K. Imaging of the Hip and Pelvis Gandikota G (Ed.), The Textbook of Radiology by Sutton. Eighth edition. Elsevier [In Press].)

Pincer-type FAI is best evaluated on a centered anteroposterior view of the pelvis. The crossover sign and posterior wall sign indicate acetabular retroversion. These, and lateral center-edge angle (Wiberg angle), are all helpful in assessing for pincer-type FAI.

- The crossover sign is present when the anterior acetabular rim crosses over the posterior rim on radiographs (**Fig. 3**A).

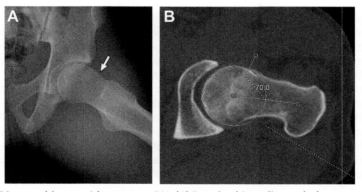

Fig. 2. A 20-year-old man with cam-type FAI. (*A*) Frog-leg hip radiograph shows osseous protuberance along the lateral femoral head-neck junction (*arrow*), consistent with a cam-type deformity. (*B*) Axial oblique CT image of the hip shows measurement of the alpha angle, which is found by drawing a line through the femoral neck axis and then drawing a line from the center of the femoral head through the point at which the sphericity of the femoral head is lost. An alpha angle greater than 50° is consistent with a cam-type deformity; in this case, the angle is 70°.

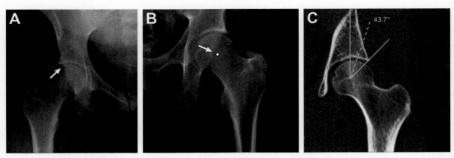

Fig. 3. A 25-year-old woman with pincer-type FAI. (*A*) Frontal radiograph of the hip shows the anterior acetabular wall (*arrow*) crossing over the posterior acetabular wall, known as the "crossover sign." (*B*) Frontal radiograph of the hip shows the posterior acetabulum (*arrow*) located medial to the center of the femoral head (dot), known as the "posterior wall sign." (*C*) Coronal CT image of the hip shows measurement of the lateral center-edge (Wiberg) angle. An angle greater than 40°, as in this case, suggests a pincer-type deformity.

- The posterior wall sign refers to a prominent posterior acetabular rim lying medial to the center of the femoral head (**Fig. 3**B).
- Measurement of the lateral center-edge (Wiberg) angle involves drawing a vertical line through the center of the femoral head. A second line is drawn from the center of the femoral head to the lateral edge of the acetabulum. An angle between 20° and 39° is considered within the normal rage. A measurement less than 20 is consistent with dysplasia, and an angle greater than 40 reflects overcoverage of the acetabulum seen in pincer-type FAI[6,8] (**Fig. 3**C).

Management of FAI can involve physical therapy, nonsteroidal anti-inflammatory (NSAID) medication, and corticosteroid therapeutic injections. Research has indicated that steroid injections may have the additional benefit of aiding in diagnosis of FAI.[9] The discussion of surgical management of FAI is beyond the scope of this article, but there has been considerable development in this field in recent years.

Labral tears

The labrum is a fibrocartilaginous ring that outlines the acetabulum, slightly deepening the acetabulum and adding to stability (**Fig. 4**). Labral tears are a common cause of hip pain, although they are most often seen in conjunction with other injuries or structural abnormalities, and only rarely seen in isolation.[10,11] The pathophysiology of labral tears is multifaceted and may be secondary to trauma, underlying structural abnormality, hip hypermobility, dysplasia, or degeneration.

While MR imaging is the gold standard for the diagnosis of labral tears, initial evaluation using radiography is useful. Radiographs may demonstrate structural or developmental abnormalities which predispose to labral tears. In addition, radiography may help identify os acetabuli or superolateral periacetabular ossicles suggestive of underlying labral pathology.[8] CT arthrography can identify tears with the help of contrast but is limited in the identification of subtle intrasubstance abnormalities.[12,13] MR imaging, specifically MRA, is the most sensitive and specific modality for the evaluation of labral tears. MRA achieves increased accuracy by distending the joint with contrast and allowing the labrum to be evaluated in exquisite detail. On MRA, a labral tear may be seen as high signal within the labral substance, a blunted or truncated labrum, contrast extension into the labral substance or infiltrating between labral attachments (**Fig. 5**), or a frank detachment. The orientation and length of the tear can be discerned.

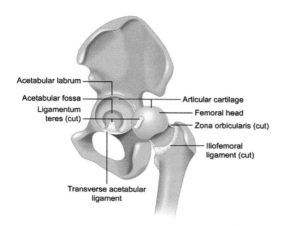

Fig. 4. Illustration of hip joint anatomy, including the labrum, with continuation of the labrum inferiorly as the transverse acetabular ligament. (From Gaetke-Udager K. Imaging of the Hip and Pelvis Gandikota G (Ed.), The Textbook of Radiology by Sutton. Eighth edition. Elsevier [In Press].)

In addition, the presence of a labral tear may be suggested by the presence of a paralabral cyst,[12] which can be seen adjacent to the labral tear, and sometimes extends into the adjacent bone.

Labral tears should be described in the radiology report in as much detail as possible. While Czerny and colleagues[14] created a detailed MRA radiologic classification system of labral tears, Blankenbaker and colleagues[15] showed poor correlation between the arthroscopic and MRA classification of labral tears. Blankenbaker's

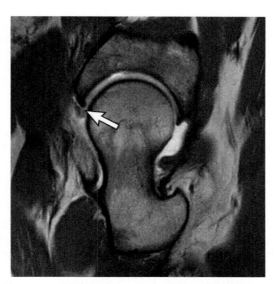

Fig. 5. A 21-year-old woman with labral tear. Sagittal T1-weighted image of the hip from an MR arthrogram shows a high-signal, cleft-like defect (*arrow*) in the anterior labrum, which has lost its normal triangular morphology.

group suggested a more simplified, four-part classification system for tear localization (**Table 1**).

Management of labral tears may be conservative or surgical. Conservative measures include rest and protected weightbearing,[16] although long-term consequences of nonsurgical treatment are not fully understood and may predispose to early onset degenerative disease.[17] Surgical treatment involves arthroscopy with debridement of the tear, which has been shown to result in both immediate symptom improvement and a decreased risk of future osteoarthritis.[18]

Cartilage defects

With the exception of the fovea capitus, a central depression which serves as the origin for the ligamentum teres, the entirety of the femoral head is covered with articular cartilage (**Fig. 4**).[19] Likewise, the acetabulum is covered with articular cartilage in a horseshoe configuration known as the "lunate".[19] This cartilage allows for smooth, gliding movements of the hip joint.

Defects involving the articular cartilage of the hip can be a result of direct trauma or degradation over time. In athletes, twisting injuries or direct impact to the hip joint can result in hyaline cartilage defects of either the acetabulum or femoral head.[20] Risk of chronic chondral injury is increased in the setting of anatomic abnormalities such as FAI,[21] in which the abnormal position of the femoral head in relation to the acetabulum leads to increased cartilaginous wear and tear. Specifically, defects along the anterosuperior acetabulum are often seen in cam-type FAI,[22] whereas posteroinferior acetabulum defects are associated with pincer-type FAI.[23]

MR is the most important modality in the detection of chondral defects, with evaluation greatly enhanced with MRA.[24] Normal articular cartilage is seen as an area of intermediate signal intensity outlining subchondral bone on fluid-sensitive sequences. Chondral injury is seen as full- or partial-thickness contour defects, thinning, fraying/fragmentation, or focal signal abnormalities (**Fig. 6**). On arthrography, defects may fill with contrast, increasing detection sensitivity.[25] Contrast may also be seen undermining the articular cartilage, which is highly specific for delamination/flap injury.[26] Visualization of loose interarticular chondral fragments is also improved with a contrast filled joint space. Chondral injury should be described thoroughly in the report; grading systems can be used, including the Noyes scale[24] (**Table 2**).

While radiography is not first-line in the evaluation of articular cartilage, it is useful in the assessment for secondary signs of cartilage loss including joint space narrowing, marginal osteophytes, and subchondral cysts/sclerosis.

Ligamentum teres injuries

The ligamentum teres is a band of tissue that originates at the acetabulum at the transverse acetabular ligament and inserts at the femoral head along the fovea capitis

Table 1	
Blankenbaker MR arthrography classification of labral tears[15]	
Type 1	Frayed: irregular margins of the labrum with a discrete tear
Type 2	Flap tear: contrast extending into or through the labral substance
Type 3	Peripheral longitudinal: contrast partially or completely between the labral base and acetabulum labral detachment
Type 4	Thickened and distorted and thus likely unstable

Data from Blankenbaker DG, De Smet AA, Keene JS, Fine JP. Classification and localization of acetabular labral tears. *Skeletal Radiol.* May 2007;36(5):391-7. doi:10.1007/s00256-006-0240-z

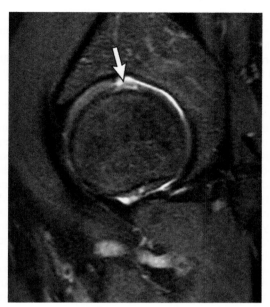

Fig. 6. A 44-year-old woman with cartilage abnormality. Sagittal proton density (PD) fat-saturated MR image of the hip shows a focal area of cartilage signal abnormality and irregularity (*arrow*), with a questionable flap-like configuration, along the superior femoral head.

(**Fig. 4**).[27] Although the exact function has been a subject of research, it may provide additional hip stabilization, especially during deep flexion.[27] Ligamentum teres injury is not frequently discussed but may contribute to hip pain in athletes, with the estimated prevalence on arthroscopy between 4% and 15%.[28,29] Etiologies of injury include traumatic or surgical dislocation, repetitive microtrauma, and underlying structural abnormality (eg, FAI).[27] Patients may present with complaints of groin pain, instability, or pain with physical examination maneuvers such as log-rolling or internal rotation while in flexion.[30]

MR is the most useful imaging technique in the workup of ligamentum teres injury, with MRA being more sensitive and specific than nonarthrographic technique.[31] A complete tear is seen as frank discontinuity of the ligamentum teres and high T2 signal within the distal and proximal stumps on fluid-sensitive sequences.[32] A partial-

Table 2	
Noyes scale for the evaluation of chondral defects[24]	
Grade 0	Normal
Grade 1	Heterogeneity, T2 hyperintensity
Grade 2	Partial-thickness defect <50% normal thickness
Grade 3	Partial-thickness defect >50% normal thickness
Grade 4	Full-thickness defect

Data from Hegazi TM, Belair JA, McCarthy EJ, Roedl JB, Morrison WB. Sports Injuries about the Hip: What the Radiologist Should Know. *Radiographics*. Oct 2016;36(6):1717-1745. doi:10.1148/rg.2016160012

thickness injury is identified as intermediate signal abnormality and/or thickening of the ligamentum teres (**Fig. 7**), possibly with a partial loss of continuity.[24] In both instances, a joint effusion may be seen.

Treatment options include debridement versus reconstruction, with surgical reconstruction reserved for instances of complete tear.[27]

Extra-articular Causes

Snapping hip syndrome/iliopsoas bursitis

Snapping hip syndrome refers to sudden painful and audible snapping of the hip during movement, most often from the frog leg position (flexion, abduction, and external rotation) to the neutral position.[33] Snapping hip syndrome is seen commonly in female athletes whose sports involve repetitive motion in exaggerated positions, particularly ballet dancers and gymnasts.[34] Both intra- and extra-articular causes have been described.[24] Extra-articular causes include snapping of a tendon while moving over bone, while intra-articular causes of painful snapping hip include intra-articular bodies and cartilage injury. Because extra-articular causes are more common and typically more symptomatic, it has been suggested that the term "snapping hip syndrome" be used exclusively in reference to the extra-articular type.[34,35] Of the extraarticular type, there are three main regions of tendon involvement: internal, external, and posterior. Internal, the most common, involves the musculotendinous iliopsoas unit, external involves the iliotibial band, and posterior involves the gluteus maximus tendon[36] and ischiofemoral region.[37]

US is the most useful modality to evaluate snapping hip syndrome given its capability to capture pathology in real time.[34] The most frequently described mechanism of snapping hip involves the iliopsoas tendon snapping on the superior pubic ramus after sudden movement of the iliacus muscle[33,34] (**Fig. 8**). When the hip moves into the frog leg position, the medial fibers of the iliacus displace and rotate into a position

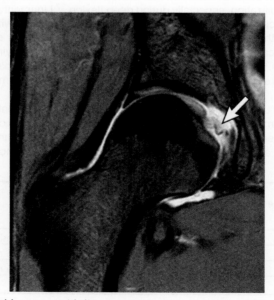

Fig. 7. A 36-year-old woman with ligamentum teres injury. Coronal T2-weighted, fat-saturated MR image of the hip shows diffuse thickening and high signal in the ligamentum teres (*arrow*), with areas of fiber loss but no discontinuity, consistent with a partial-thickness tear.

between the iliacus tendon and superior pubic ramus. When the hip then returns to a neutral position, the medial portion of the iliacus muscle releases suddenly from its position between the iliacus tendon and returns abruptly to the pubic ramus creating an audible and oftentimes painful snap.[33,34]

Management strategies include conservative measures such as rest, stretching exercises, corticosteroid injections, and NSAID medications. Surgery is indicated only if symptoms are refractory to typical conservative treatment.[34]

Femoral stress–related injuries

Femoral stress–related injuries are an important cause of hip pain, with femoral stress fractures comprising 3% of all stress fractures.[38] Patients often present with exercise-related, poorly-localized groin pain, commonly in the setting of a sudden increase in repetitive motion involving activities such as long-distance running and military training.[39,40] Pain is often of gradual onset and relieved by rest. In a healthy athlete, femoral stress fractures are "fatigue fractures" secondary to abnormal stress on normal bone leading to excessive cortical resorption and microfractures.[41] The initial microfracture will progress to an incomplete and finally a complete fracture, which, if untreated, may ultimately lead to displacement and avascular necrosis.[42,43] As such, early detection is paramount to avoid significant patient morbidity.

Radiography, although not particularly sensitive, is the preferred initial imaging evaluation tool. Anteroposterior views of the pelvis and lateral views of the proximal femur should be obtained to evaluate for periosteal reaction, linear sclerosis, and/or linear lucency.[40,44] These findings are often subtle, however, and some radiographs may appear normal even in the setting of a fracture. If there is high clinical suspicion for fracture and nothing is identified on radiographs, additional evaluation with MR should be recommended.

For the evaluation of femoral stress-related injury, MR imaging has near 100% specificity and sensitivity.[45] On fluid-sensitive sequences, stress reactions will appear as marrow and/or periosteal edema, while fractures appear as areas of linear, low signal on T1- and T2-weighted sequences (**Fig. 9**). The extent of marrow edema is directly related to stress fracture severity.[40] The Fredericson classification system for MRI is often used for grading tibial stress–related injuries and has been shown to be an important predictor of outcomes.[46,47] A similar classification system was recently proposed for femoral neck stress injuries[48] (**Table 3**). Of note, bone scans were commonly used in the workup of stress fractures in the past but have since fallen

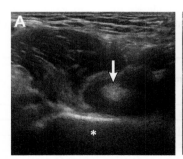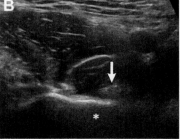

Fig. 8. A 24-year-old woman with snapping hip. (*A*) Transverse US image of the anterior hip region shows the iliopsoas tendon (*arrow*) over the iliopectineal eminence (*asterisk*); this image was taken before the "snap" occurred. (*B*) After the snap, the iliopsoas tendon (*arrow*) is seen inferomedial to its position in A.

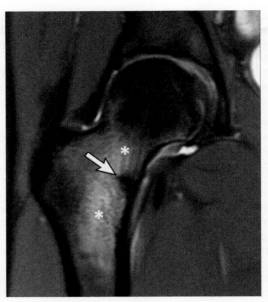

Fig. 9. A 25-year-old woman with proximal femoral stress fracture. Coronal short tau inversion recovery (STIR) MR image shows bone marrow edema in the femoral neck (*asterisks*) with linear, low signal (*arrowhead*) consistent with a stress fracture.

out of practice in favor of MRI, when possible, because of the better spatial resolution of MRI.[40,44]

Management of femoral stress fractures is highly dependent on the grade and fracture type. Lower grade injuries generally indicate a faster return to play,[24] while higher grade injuries result in increased rest time or more aggressive measures, including surgical fixation.[40]

Adductor insertion avulsion syndrome (thigh splints)

An important and sometimes overlooked cause of hip pain is adductor insertion avulsion syndrome, also referred to as "thigh splints." The adductor muscle group inserts along the mid-proximal aspect of the posteromedial femoral diaphysis.[24,49] Intense physical activity recruiting the adductors repetitively may lead to an avulsion-type injury in this area. The patient may present with posteromedial thigh pain that worsens

Table 3
Rohena-Quinquilla et al MRI classification system for femoral neck stress injuries[48]

Grade	MRI Findings
1 (Low grade)	Endosteal marrow edema less than or equal to 6 mm
2 (Low grade)	Endosteal marrow edema >6 mm, no fracture
3 (High grade)	Macroscopic fracture <50% femoral neck width
4 (High grade)	Macroscopic fracture greater than or equal to 50% of femoral neck width

Data from Rohena-Quinquilla IR, Rohena-Quinquilla FJ, Scully WF, Evanson JRL. Femoral Neck Stress Injuries: Analysis of 156 Cases in a U.S. Military Population and Proposal of a New MRI Classification System. *AJR Am J Roentgenol*. Mar 2018;210(3):601-607. doi:10.2214/AJR.17.18639

with intense physical activity and is relieved by rest.[24] Management involves rest and slow return to physical activity.

Radiography should be the first-line study and may be normal or show smooth periosteal reaction along the posteromedial femur. On MR imaging, fluid-sensitive sequences can show periosteal edema tracking along the medial mid-proximal femoral diaphysis and/or soft-tissue edema at the site of adductor muscle group insertion[24,49] (**Fig. 10**). There may be associated underlying bone marrow changes or cortical irregularity and linear signal abnormality, which indicates resulting stress fracture.[49] Bone scintigraphy is less frequently used in diagnosis but may show linear radiotracer uptake along the medial aspect of the mid-proximal femur, at the adductor muscle insertion.[50,51]

Athletic pubalgia/sports hernia: core muscle injuries

Athletic pubalgia or core muscle injuries, colloquially referred to as a "sports hernia," refers to a spectrum of injuries at the pubic symphysis and may be a cause of referred hip pain predominantly seen in soccer, ice hockey, and football athletes.[52,53] The rectus abdominus and adductor longus musculature attach at the pubic symphysis via their confluent anterior sheath, known as the rectus abdominus/adductor aponeurosis[52] (**Fig. 11**), and acute or chronic injury can lead to tears at this attachment site and injury to the underlying pubic tubercle.

MRI is preferred for imaging evaluation, and a specialized protocol with axial-oblique and sagittal sequences and small field of view, focused on the symphyseal area, is helpful. Positive findings on fluid-sensitive sequences may demonstrate a fluid-filled cleft within the aponeurosis, or between it and the pubic tubercle, often best seen on the sagittal sequences (**Fig. 12**). Osteitis pubis, which is a chronic, stress-related or inflammatory condition of the pubic symphysis, can also be seen on imaging. Radiographic changes of osteitis pubis are somewhat variable, including osteolysis or sclerosis with joint space widening or narrowing. Specialized flamingo views with the patient standing on one leg can demonstrate underlying instability if there is greater than 2 mm of vertical shift at the pubic symphysis.[54] Supportive findings on MRI include marrow edema in the pubic tubercles, edema in the periarticular soft tissues, articular surface irregularity, and periarticular fatty marrow metaplasia.[55]

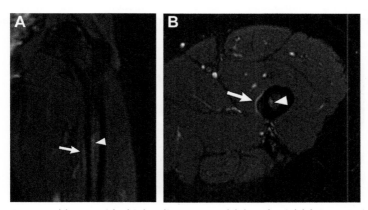

Fig. 10. A 36-year-old man with thigh splints. Coronal (*A*) and axial (*B*) STIR MR images of the proximal femur shows periosteal edema (*arrows*) at the adductor insertion site, with underlying bone marrow edema (*arrowheads*).

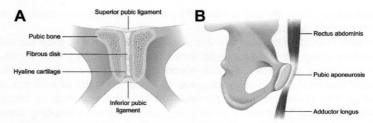

Fig. 11. Illustration of pubic symphysis. (*A*) Coronal view of symphyseal joint, including fibrous disk and hyaline cartilage. (*B*) Sagittal view of rectus abdominis and adductor longus muscle attachments. (From Gaetke-Udager K.Imaging of the Hip and Pelvis Gandikota G (Ed.), The Textbook of Radiology by Sutton. Eighth edition. Elsevier [In Press].)

Avulsion injuries

Avulsion injuries involve separation of osseous fragments at the insertion of tendons or ligaments. These may occur in adolescents with avulsion of an apophysis before ossification of the physis, or in adults along an enthesis when bone is overcome by force at the site of tendon attachment.[56] Common sites of avulsion injuries involving the hip and pelvis are included in **Table 4**. Of these, the anterior inferior iliac spine is the most common, comprising 33.2% of avulsion injuries.[57]

Imaging evaluation should begin with radiographs of the pelvis, which may be normal initially or may show the ossific fragment which has avulsed (**Fig. 13**). In addition to avulsed osseous fragments, MR can show associated soft-tissue injuries such as tendinosis or muscle strain, bone marrow edema, hematoma, or retraction of the tendon.[56] CT is optimal for identification of displaced apophysis or bone fragments and will also show callus formation and heterotopic ossification of chronic avulsion injuries. US may show widening of the physis or physeal hyperemia on Doppler imaging in adolescent patients.[58]

Management includes NSAIDs, physical therapy, and rest.[59] Avulsion fractures may be treated surgically if displaced more than 2 cm,[24] depending on their location.

Hip dislocation

Hip dislocation requires excessive force in the athletic setting but is a true emergency, necessitating urgent orthopedic evaluation and reduction.[60] Treatment by the orthopedic team is performed in two stages with the first stage being rapid closed reduction

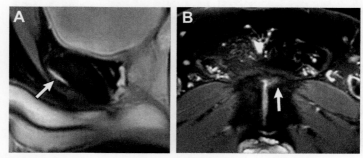

Fig. 12. A 44-year-old man with athletic pubalgia. Sagittal (*A*) and axial (*B*) proton density (PD) fat-saturated MR images of the pubic symphyseal region show a fluid-filled defect (*arrows*) at the rectus aponeurosis attachment site.

Table 4
Common sites of hip and pelvis avulsion injury

Avulsion Site	Musculotendinous Insertion
Ischial tuberosity	Hamstrings
Iliac crest	Abdominal muscles
Anterior superior iliac spine	Sartorius
Anterior inferior iliac spine	Rectus femoris

of the hip.[61] As such, prompt diagnosis with the aid of imaging is essential to reduce the risk of long-term morbidity including avascular necrosis and osteoarthritis.[62]

An anteroposterior radiograph of the pelvis with a cross-table lateral view is usually the most appropriate first-line imaging technique to determine if the dislocation is anterior or posterior, with posterior comprising 90% of all traumatic dislocations.[63] On frontal radiographs, posterior dislocation is typically present if the femoral head is displaced superolateral to the acetabulum with hip in flexion, adduction, and internal rotation[61] (**Fig. 14**), while in anterior dislocations, the femoral head will appear inferomedial to the acetabulum, with the hip fixed in external rotation.[61] The cross-table view can confirm the femoral head location.

The second stage of treatment is definitive management. After reduction, CT is used to assess for secondary injuries including acetabular or femoral head fractures, impaction injuries, intra-articular fragments, and soft-tissue injuries; to evaluate joint congruency; and to assess the size of acetabular fracture which may imply joint instability.[61]

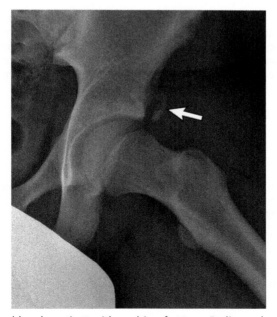

Fig. 13. A 16-year-old male patient with avulsion fracture. Radiograph of the hip shows a displaced osseous fragment (*arrow*) consistent with an avulsion fracture at the anterior inferior iliac spine.

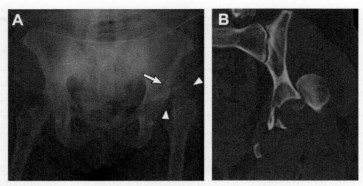

Fig. 14. A 40-year-old woman with hip dislocation. (*A*) Frontal radiograph of the pelvis shows superior-posterior dislocation of the femoral head (*arrow*) from the acetabulum. (*B*) Coronal CT image of the pelvis shows these findings with increased osseous detail and intra-articular osseous fracture fragments (*arrowheads*).

MRI is useful in the evaluation of nerves, labrum, bone contusions, and articular cartilage,[64] with sciatic nerve injury being a common complication of posterior dislocations and ischemia secondary to neurovascular bundle injury, a common complication of anterior dislocations.[65]

SUMMARY

Hip pain in athletes is a common and complex clinical entity. There are numerous etiologies, both intra- and extra-articular, including FAI, labral tears, cartilage defects, ligamentum teres injuries, snapping hip syndrome, femoral stress injuries, thigh splints, athletic pubalgia, avulsion injuries, and hip dislocation. Imaging allows for timely and thorough evaluation of pathologic hip conditions and may assist clinicians in attaining a prompt diagnosis. Knowledge of basic imaging principles during the evaluation of hip pain can be useful to the sports medicine clinician.

DISCLOSURES

The authors have nothing to disclose.

REFERENCES

1. Kerbel YE, Smith CM, Prodromo JP, et al. Epidemiology of hip and groin injuries in collegiate athletes in the United States. Orthop J Sports Med 2018;6(5). 2325967118771676.

2. Trentacosta N, Sugimoto D, Micheli LJ. Hip and groin injuries in dancers: a systematic review. Sports Health 2017;9(5):422–7.

3. Harøy J, Andersen TE, Bahr R. Groin problems in male soccer players are more common than previously reported: response. Am J Sports Med 2017;45(13): NP32–3.

4. Mosler AB, Weir A, Eirale C, et al. Epidemiology of time loss groin injuries in a men's professional football league: a 2-year prospective study of 17 clubs and 606 players. Br J Sports Med 2018;52(5):292–7.

5. Martin RK, Dzaja I, Kay J, et al. Radiographic outcomes following femoroacetabular impingement correction with open surgical management: a systematic review. Curr Rev Musculoskelet Med 2016;9(4):402–10.

6. Menge TJ, Truex NW. Femoroacetabular impingement: a common cause of hip pain. Phys Sportsmed 2018;46(2):139–44.

7. Philippon MJ, Maxwell RB, Johnston TL, et al. Clinical presentation of femoroacetabular impingement. Knee Surg Sports Traumatol Arthrosc 2007;15(8):1041–7.

8. Armfield DR, Towers JD, Robertson DD. Radiographic and MR imaging of the athletic hip. Clin Sports Med 2006;25(2):211–39, viii.

9. Khan W, Khan M, Alradwan H, et al. Utility of intra-articular hip injections for femoroacetabular impingement: a systematic review. Orthop J Sports Med 2015;3(9). 2325967115601030.

10. Bharam S. Labral tears, extra-articular injuries, and hip arthroscopy in the athlete. Clin Sports Med 2006;25(2):279–92, ix.

11. Kemp J, Grimaldi A, Heerey J, et al. Current trends in sport and exercise hip conditions: intra-articular and extra-articular hip pain, with detailed focus on femoroacetabular impingement (FAI) syndrome. Best Pract Res Clin Rheumatol 2019; 33(1):66–87.

12. Thomas JD, Li Z, Agur AM, et al. Imaging of the acetabular labrum. Semin Musculoskelet Radiol 2013;17(3):248–57.

13. Llopis E, Fernandez E, Cerezal L. MR and CT arthrography of the hip. Semin Musculoskelet Radiol 2012;16(1):42–56.

14. Czerny C, Hofmann S, Neuhold A, et al. Lesions of the acetabular labrum: accuracy of MR imaging and MR arthrography in detection and staging. Radiology 1996;200(1):225–30.

15. Blankenbaker DG, De Smet AA, Keene JS, et al. Classification and localization of acetabular labral tears. Skeletal Radiol 2007;36(5):391–7.

16. Narvani AA, Tsiridis E, Tai CC, et al. Acetabular labrum and its tears. Br J Sports Med 2003;37(3):207–11.

17. Seldes RM, Tan V, Hunt J, et al. Anatomy, histologic features, and vascularity of the adult acetabular labrum. Clin Orthop Relat Res 2001;(382):232–40.

18. Hase T, Ueo T. Acetabular labral tear: arthroscopic diagnosis and treatment. Arthroscopy 1999;15(2):138–41.

19. Chang CY, Huang AJ. MR imaging of normal hip anatomy. Magn Reson Imaging Clin N Am 2013;21(1):1–19.

20. Byrd JW. Lateral impact injury. A source of occult hip pathology. Clin Sports Med 2001;20(4):801–15.

21. Kaya M, Suzuki T, Emori M, et al. Hip morphology influences the pattern of articular cartilage damage. Knee Surg Sports Traumatol Arthrosc 2016;24(6): 2016–23.

22. Schmid MR, Nötzli HP, Zanetti M, et al. Cartilage lesions in the hip: diagnostic effectiveness of MR arthrography. Radiology 2003;226(2):382–6.

23. Pfirrmann CW, Mengiardi B, Dora C, et al. Cam and pincer femoroacetabular impingement: characteristic MR arthrographic findings in 50 patients. Radiology 2006;240(3):778–85.

24. Hegazi TM, Belair JA, McCarthy EJ, et al. Sports injuries about the hip: what the radiologist should know. Radiographics 2016;36(6):1717–45.

25. Agten CA, Sutter R, Buck FM, et al. Hip imaging in athletes: sports imaging series. Radiology 2016;280(2):351–69.

26. Pfirrmann CW, Duc SR, Zanetti M, et al. MR arthrography of acetabular cartilage delamination in femoroacetabular cam impingement. Radiology 2008;249(1): 236–41.

27. Kraeutler MJ, Garabekyan T, Pascual-Garrido C, et al. Ligamentum teres tendinopathy and tears. Muscles Ligaments Tendons J 2016;6(3):337–42.

28. Byrd JW, Jones KS. Traumatic rupture of the ligamentum teres as a source of hip pain. Arthroscopy 2004;20(4):385–91.

29. Rao J, Zhou YX, Villar RN. Injury to the ligamentum teres. Mechanism, findings, and results of treatment. Clin Sports Med 2001;20(4):791–9, vii.

30. de SA D, Phillips M, Philippon MJ, et al. Ligamentum teres injuries of the hip: a systematic review examining surgical indications, treatment options, and outcomes. Arthroscopy 2014;30(12):1634–41.

31. Datir A, Xing M, Kang J, et al. Diagnostic utility of MRI and MR arthrography for detection of ligamentum teres tears: a retrospective analysis of 187 patients with hip pain. AJR Am J Roentgenol 2014;203(2):418–23.

32. Cerezal L, Kassarjian A, Canga A, et al. Anatomy, biomechanics, imaging, and management of ligamentum teres injuries. Radiographics 2010;30(6):1637–51.

33. Deslandes M, Guillin R, Cardinal E, et al. The snapping iliopsoas tendon: new mechanisms using dynamic sonography. AJR Am J Roentgenol 2008;190(3): 576–81.

34. Bureau NJ. Sonographic evaluation of snapping hip syndrome. J Ultrasound Med Jun 2013;32(6):895–900.

35. Byrd JW. Evaluation and management of the snapping iliopsoas tendon. Instr Course Lect 2006;55:347–55.

36. Allen WC, Cope R. Coxa saltans: the snapping hip revisited. J Am Acad Orthop Surg 1995;3(5):303–8.

37. Ali AM, Whitwell D, Ostlere SJ. Case report: imaging and surgical treatment of a snapping hip due to ischiofemoral impingement. Skeletal Radiol 2011;40(5): 653–6.

38. Hulkko A, Orava S. Stress fractures in athletes. Int J Sports Med 1987;17(5): 221–6.

39. Winkelmann ZK, Anderson D, Games KE, et al. Risk factors for medial tibial stress syndrome in active individuals: an evidence-based review. J Athl Train 2016; 51(12):1049–52.

40. Robertson GA, Wood AM. Femoral neck stress fractures in sport: a current concepts review. Sports Med Int Open 2017;1(2):E58–68.

41. Matcuk GR, Mahanty SR, Skalski MR, et al. Stress fractures: pathophysiology, clinical presentation, imaging features, and treatment options. Emerg Radiol 2016;23(4):365–75.

42. Michael RH, Holder LE. The soleus syndrome. A cause of medial tibial stress (shin splints). Am J Sports Med 1985;13(2):87–94.

43. Johansson C, Ekenman I, Törnkvist H, et al. Stress fractures of the femoral neck in athletes. The consequence of a delay in diagnosis. Am J Sports Med 1990;18(5): 524–8.

44. Bencardino JT, Palmer WE. Imaging of hip disorders in athletes. Radiol Clin North Am 2002;40(2):267–87, vi-vii.

45. Shin AY, Morin WD, Gorman JD, et al. The superiority of magnetic resonance imaging in differentiating the cause of hip pain in endurance athletes. Am J Sports Med 1996;24(2):168–76.

46. Arendt E, Griffiths H. The use of MR imaging in the assessment and clinical management of stress reactions of bone in high-performance athletes. Clin Sports Med 1997;16(2):291–306.
47. Kijowski R, Choi J, Shinki K, et al. Validation of MRI classification system for tibial stress injuries. AJR Am J Roentgenol 2012;198(4):878–84.
48. Rohena-Quinquilla IR, Rohena-Quinquilla FJ, Scully WF, et al. Femoral neck stress injuries: analysis of 156 cases in a U.S. military population and proposal of a new MRI classification system. AJR Am J Roentgenol 2018;210(3):601–7.
49. Anderson MW, Kaplan PA, Dussault RG. Adductor insertion avulsion syndrome (thigh splints): spectrum of MR imaging features. AJR Am J Roentgenol 2001; 177(3):673–5.
50. Singh AK, Dickinson C, Dworkin HJ, et al. Adductor insertion avulsion syndrome. Clin Nucl Med 2001;26(8):709–11.
51. Mahajan MS. Bone scanning in the adductor insertion avulsion syndrome. World J Nucl Med 2013;12(2):73–5.
52. Cohen B, Kleinhenz D, Schiller J, et al. Understanding athletic pubalgia: a review. R Med J (2013) 2016;99(10):31–5.
53. Meyers WC, Foley DP, Garrett WE, et al. Management of severe lower abdominal or inguinal pain in high-performance athletes. PAIN (Performing Athletes with Abdominal or Inguinal Neuromuscular Pain Study Group). Am J Sports Med 2000;28(1):2–8.
54. Johnson R. Osteitis pubis. Curr Sports Med Rep 2003;2(2):98–102.
55. Cunningham PM, Brennan D, O'Connell M, et al. Patterns of bone and soft-tissue injury at the symphysis pubis in soccer players: observations at MRI. AJR Am J Roentgenol 2007;188(3):W291–6.
56. Albtoush OM, Bani-Issa J, Zitzelsberger T, et al. Avulsion injuries of the pelvis and hip. Rofo 2020;192(5):431–40.
57. Eberbach H, Hohloch L, Feucht MJ, et al. Operative versus conservative treatment of apophyseal avulsion fractures of the pelvis in the adolescents: a systematical review with meta-analysis of clinical outcome and return to sports. BMC Musculoskelet Disord 2017;18(1):162.
58. Lazović D, Wegner U, Peters G, et al. Ultrasound for diagnosis of apophyseal injuries. Knee Surg Sports Traumatol Arthrosc 1996;3(4):234–7.
59. Paluska SA. An overview of hip injuries in running. Sports Med 2005;35(11): 991–1014.
60. Epstein HC, Wiss DA, Cozen L. Posterior fracture dislocation of the hip with fractures of the femoral head. Clin Orthop Relat Res 1985;201:9–17.
61. Mandell JC, Marshall RA, Weaver MJ, et al. Traumatic hip dislocation: what the orthopedic surgeon wants to know. Radiographics 2017;37(7):2181–201.
62. Brooks RA, Ribbans WJ. Diagnosis and imaging studies of traumatic hip dislocations in the adult. Clin Orthop Relat Res 2000;377:15–23.
63. Sahin V, Karakaş ES, Aksu S, et al. Traumatic dislocation and fracture-dislocation of the hip: a long-term follow-up study. J Trauma 2003;54(3):520–9.
64. Laorr A, Greenspan A, Anderson MW, et al. Traumatic hip dislocation: early MRI findings. Skeletal Radiol 1995;24(4):239–45.
65. Stein MJ, Kang C, Ball V. Emergency department evaluation and treatment of acute hip and thigh pain. Emerg Med Clin North Am 2015;33(2):327–43.

3-T MRI of the Ankle Tendons and Ligaments

Parham Pezeshk, MD[a], Christine Rehwald, MD[b], Iman Khodarahmi, MD, PhD[c], Filippo Del Grande, MD[d], Parisa Khoshpouri, MD[e], Felix Chew, MD, MBA[b], Majid Chalian, MD[e],*

KEYWORDS

- Ankle • Sports injury • MRI • Ligament • Tendon

KEY POINTS

- High resolution 3T MRI of the ankle could visualize different degrees of ankle tendon and ligament injuries and provide valuable information for interventions.
- Familiarity of radiologists and surgeons with normal anatomic variants of the ankle is crucial to avoid unnecessary imaging and procedures.
- MRI could depict posterior tibialis tendon dysfunction at different clinical stages.

INTRODUCTION

Ankle sprain accounts for up to 30% of sports injuries and is considered the most common injury in the athletic population.[1] Ligament and tendon pathologies of the ankle are common, ranging from traumatic injuries to degeneration leading to chronic pain and acquired foot deformities. The ankle ligaments are divided into three main groups: (1) the lateral ligament complex (anterior talofibular, posterior talofibular, and calcaneofibular ligaments), (2) the medial collateral ligament complex, and (3) the tibiofibular syndesmotic ligaments.[2] The tendons that cross the ankle joint are also divided into three main groups based on the leg compartment from which they originate: (1) the deep posterior compartment (tibialis posterior, flexor digitorum

[a] Division of Musculoskeletal Imaging, Department of Radiology, University of Texas Southwestern Medical Center, 5323 Harry Hines Blvd, Dallas, TX 75390-9316, USA; [b] Division of Musculoskeletal Imaging and Intervention, Department of Radiology, University of Washington, 4245 Roosevelt Way NE, Box 354755, Seattle, WA 98105, USA; [c] Division of Musculoskeletal Imaging, Department of Radiology, New York University Grossman School of Medicine, Center for Biomedical Imaging, 660 First Ave, Room 223, New York, NY 10016, USA; [d] Clinica di Radiologia EOC, Instituto di Imaging della Svizzera Italiana, Via Tesserete 47, 6900 Lugano, Switzerland; [e] Division of Musculoskeletal Imaging and Intervention, Department of Radiology, University of Washington Medical Center, UW Radiology-Roosevelt Clinic, 4245 Roosevelt Way Northeast, Box 354755, Seattle, WA 98105, USA
* Corresponding author.
E-mail address: mchalian@uw.edu

Clin Sports Med 40 (2021) 731–754
https://doi.org/10.1016/j.csm.2021.05.009
0278-5919/21/© 2021 Elsevier Inc. All rights reserved.

longus [FDL], and flexor hallucis longus [FHL] tendons), (2) the lateral compartment (peroneus longus and brevis tendons), and (3) the anterior compartment (tibialis anterior, extensor digitorum longus, and extensor hallucis longus tendons). The Achilles tendon is formed from contributions of the gastrocnemius and soleus tendons and is located in the superficial posterior compartment.[3] The plantaris tendon is also present in this compartment.

MRI is the imaging modality of choice when evaluating tendon and ligament pathology of the ankle. Relative to 1.5-T MRI, 3-T MRI provides increased signal-to-noise ratio, higher spatial resolution, improved fat suppression, and increased contrast-to-noise ratio, which improves the depiction of anatomic detail and pathology.[4] T1-weighted (T1W) and proton density-weighted (PDW) imaging are ideal for evaluating the small ankle anatomic features. Fluid-sensitive sequences (T2-weighted and PDW fat-suppressed images) are best used for detecting disease processes. In this article we review normal anatomy and pathologies of the ankle tendons and ligaments using high-resolution 3-T MRI.

3-T MRI PROTOCOL AND POSITIONING

Similar to imaging of the other joints, imaging of the ankle is performed in axial, coronal, and sagittal planes. Patients are positioned supine with the feet toward the magnet (feet first supine). Ideally foot and ankle coil should be used that keeps the ankle in a 90° position. Axial images are acquired in the plane parallel to the axis of calcaneus from distal tibia through the plantar soft tissues to the skin surface. Coronal images are obtained in a plane aligned along the medial and lateral malleoli, perpendicular to the axial imaging plane, from the metatarsal bases through the calcaneus to the posterior skin. Sagittal imaging is obtained perpendicular to the coronal plane. Different centers might use different sequences, such as T1W or PDW to evaluate anatomy and T2-weighted, short tau inversion recovery, or fat-saturated (FS) PDW for pathology. The preference of the sequences depends on the comfort level and training of the interpreters and the time slot available for each scan. Dixon imaging is also used in some centers and has the advantage of shortening the scan time. Three-dimensional imaging is one of the advantages of 3-T MRI that can provide thin isotropic images that could be used to generate reconstructed images in different planes. If FS fails for any reason, such as artifacts from foreign bodies, short tau

Table 1 Recommended 3-T MRI protocol of the ankle joint					
Sequence	Slice Thickness (mm)	Gap (%)	Voxel Size (mm)	TR (ms)	TE (ms)
Coronal PD FS	3.5	10	0.4 × 0.5	3000	35–40
Axial PD FS	3.5	10	0.4 × 0.5	3000	35–40
Sagittal PD FS	3.5	10	0.4 × 0.5	3000	35–40
Axial PD	3.5	10	0.4 × 0.5	3000	40–45
Coronal T2 mDixon	3–4	10	0.4 × 0.5	3000	55
Coronal 3D PD TSE	3D	0	0.7 × 0.7	11,000	40
STIR (if fat sat fails)	3–4	10	0.4 × 0.5	3000	60

Abbreviations: 3D, three dimensional; PD, proton density; STIR, short tau inversion recovery; TE, echo time; TR, repetition time; TSE, turbo spin echo.

inversion recovery imaging is helpful. **Table 1** shows the 3-T MRI protocol for ankle imaging at one of the authors' institutions.

ANKLE TENDON ANATOMY AND NORMAL MRI APPEARANCE

The normal ankle tendons are hypointense on all pulse sequences; however, their curved course lends them susceptible to magic angle artifact. Apart from the anterior tibialis tendon, high signal is seen in all ankle tendons as they curve around the ankle and hindfoot in most asymptomatic patients when imaged in the supine and neutral position. Additionally, the oblique orientation of the tendons relative to coronal and axial planes can result in partial volume averaging and cause the tendons to appear blurry with increased signal. To mitigate these effects, the patient may be imaged in the prone position with the ankle in plantar flexion and obliquely oriented sequences may be obtained.[3] Long TE sequences (T2-weighted) helps reduce magic angle artifact and should be included in all ankle MRI protocols.

Flexor and peroneal tendons are seen along the medial and lateral aspects of the ankle, respectively (**Fig. 1**). At the level of the lateral malleolus, the peroneal tendons course along the superior peroneal tunnel and may be somewhat flattened in appearance. This appearance is often more pronounced for the peroneus brevis tendon, where it can take on a crescentic shape and mimic a tear. Evaluation of tendon thickness is helpful to distinguish this normal appearance from pathology. The normal tendon should be the same thickness in the middle as it is in the periphery.[3] Additionally, the peroneus brevis tendon might be partially medial to the medial border of the fibular groove mimicking a pseudosubluxation, which is accentuated by foot supination. The superior retinaculum appears as a thin hypointense band overlying the superior peroneal tendons at the level of the distal fibula. Flexor tendons course along the tarsal tunnel underneath the flexor retinaculum. Note that the distal aspect of the posterior tibialis tendon (PTT) widens and is interspersed with connective tissue, causing the signal to become heterogeneous. The PTT is typically about twice the size of the adjacent FDL. The FHL communicates with the tibiotalar joint in 20% of the population and fluid is seen along the tendon sheath in the setting of effusion. By contrast, fluid is rarely seen in the extensor tendon sheaths.[5] The flexor retinaculum is a thin hypointense band along the medial aspect of the flexor tendons seen best of coronal and axial planes. Tendon sheaths line the flexor, peroneal, and extensor tendons. Small volume fluid within the flexor and peroneal tendon sheaths is commonly seen and should not be confused with pathology.

The Achilles tendon does not have a tendon sheath, but rather, is covered by a double-layered connective tissue membrane called a paratenon. The paratenon has a robust vascular supply, which nourishes the Achilles tendon. This blood supply diminishes with age leading to an avascular zone approximately 4 cm above the insertion that is prone to traumatic injuries.[6] On MRI, the Achilles tendon may be mildly heterogeneous on T1W or PDW sequences (**Fig. 2**).[3] Because of the fascicular anatomy, normal scattered high linear signal at the insertion is seen. The tendon typically measures 5 to 7 mm in thickness and has a flat or slightly concave morphology, although may be focally rounded at the insertion of the soleus.[6]

NORMAL VARIANTS (ACCESSORY MUSCLES)

There are multiple anatomic variants about the ankle, namely accessory or extra muscles. These are typically asymptomatic and incidentally noted on advanced imaging.[7] However, mass effect on adjacent structures could create symptoms related to tenosynovitis or neuropathy. These include: the peroneus quartus muscle (**Fig. 3**),

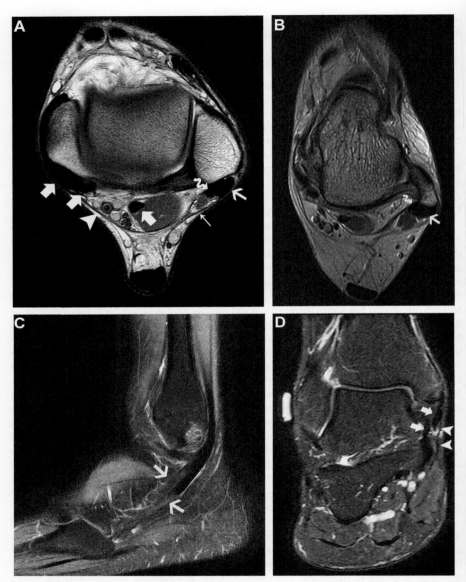

Fig. 1. Superior peroneal tunnel and tarsal tunnel. Axial proton density (PD) images (*A, B*) demonstrate the normal appearance of the peroneal tendons, the peroneus longus (*arrows*), and brevis (*curved arrows*) underneath the superior peroneal retinaculum (*thin arrow*). These tendons are closely associated as they cross the ankle and share a common tendon sheath. The peroneus brevis tendon runs slightly anteromedial to the peroneus longus tendon. The tendons take on a flattened morphology as they course behind the lateral malleolus (*B*). Note the intrinsic intermediate signal (*arrows*) on the sagittal PD FS image (*C*), because of magic angle artifact, a common finding as the tendons curve into the foot (*A*) and coronal T2 FS. (*D*) Note flexor retinaculum (*arrowheads*), which forms the medial border of the tarsal tunnel. This is a thin, hypointense structure lying just medial to the flexor tendons (*thick arrows*).

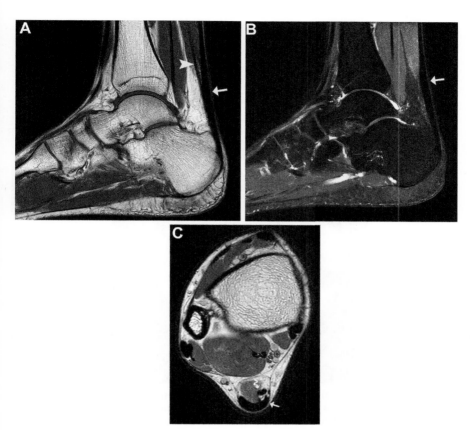

Fig. 2. Superficial posterior compartment. Sagittal T1 and PD FS images of the ankle (*A, B*) demonstrate the normal Achilles tendon (*arrows*), which is hypointense on all pulse sequences. Thin, hyperintense striations are allowed at the insertion. The soleus tendon (*arrowhead*) and gastrocnemius tendon combine to form the Achilles tendon approximately 5 to 6 cm above the calcaneus. Note the normal anterior concave morphology of the Achilles tendon on the axial PD image (*C*). *Curved arrow* represents plantaris tendon.

accessory soleus muscle (**Fig. 4**), flexor digitorum accessories longus (**Fig. 5**), peroneocalcaneus internus (**Fig. 6**), tibiocalcaneus internus, and peroneus tertius (**Fig. 7**). A low-lying peroneus brevis muscle is a rare anatomic variant with an elongated muscle belly usually extending below the level of retromalleolar groove (**Fig. 8**). Origin, course, and insertions of these anatomic variants are summarized in **Table 2**.

TENDON PATHOLOGIES

Pathology of the ankle tendons includes degeneration, tendinosis, partial or complete tear, tenosynovitis, deposition of lipid, uric acid tophi, or calcium, or rarely, tumors.

Tendinosis and Tears

In tendinosis, increased signal is seen in PDW and T1W and fluid-sensitive sequences. Initially, the tendon is thickened and chronically it can become thinned and attenuated.

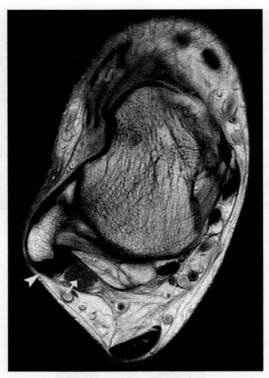

Fig. 3. Peroneus quartus (PQ) muscle. Axial PD image demonstrates a PQ muscle and tendon (*arrow*). The PQ muscle runs posteromedially to the other peroneal tendons (*arrowhead*). The tendon extends distally where it inserts on the lateral calcaneus.

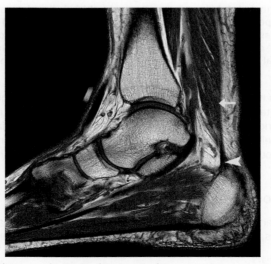

Fig. 4. Accessory soleus muscle. Sagittal T1 image demonstrating an accessory soleus muscle (*arrow*) in the posterior compartment lying anterior to the Achilles tendon location, with its tendinous insertion on the posteromedial calcaneus (*arrowhead*).

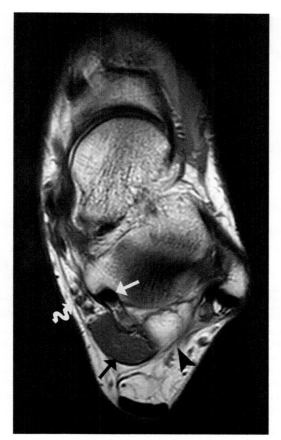

Fig. 5. Flexor digitorum accessorius longus (FDAL) muscle. Axial PD image of the ankle demonstrating an FDAL (*black arrow*) muscle and tendon. This muscle lies anterior to the Achilles tendon, but deep to the deep posterior retinaculum (*black arrowhead*), differentiating it from an accessory soleus muscle. It runs posterior to the FHL (*straight white arrow*) and closely follows the neurovascular bundle (*curved white arrow*) into the foot, where it spans onto either the FDL or quadratus plantae muscle (not shown).

Tendon tears are acute caused by trauma, chronic in the setting of underlying tendinosis, or a combination of the two. Tendon degeneration, tendinosis, and tear are different stages on a spectrum that can evolve depending on the severity, underlying cause, and duration of the insult (**Figs. 9** and **10**).

Tenosynovitis refers to inflammation of the tendon sheath, evidenced by accumulation of fluid and synovitis in the tendon sheath. As a rule of thumb, tenosynovitis is suggested if the surface area of the tendon sheath fluid in an axial image is equal or more than the surface area of the corresponding tendon, or if the fluid fully surrounds the tendon and contains debris. Tenosynovitis may be mechanical, inflammatory, or infectious in cause. Differentiation of septic and aseptic tenosynovitis is difficult based on imaging alone; however, it may be suggested in the setting of extensive surrounding soft tissue edema and enhancement. Stenosing tenosynovitis occurs when chronic inflammation results in scarring, fibrosis, and adhesion in a tendon sheath that restricts the smooth gliding of the tendon and presents as locking of the tendon clinically. On

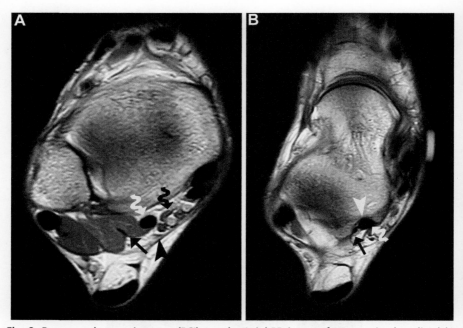

Fig. 6. Peroneocalcaneus internus (PCI) muscle. Axial PD images from proximal to distal (*A, B*) demonstrate a PCI muscle (*black arrows*). This muscle is situated deep to the deep posterior aponeurosis (*black arrowhead*) and lateral to the FHL (*white curved arrows*), running with the FHL in a slightly posterolateral fashion, through the calcaneal groove (*white arrowhead*), to eventually insert onto the medial base of the sustentaculum tali (insertion not shown). The PCI is not closely associated with the neurovascular bundle (*black curved arrow*), differentiating it from the FDAL.

MRI, the tendon sheath can look complex and loculated with asymmetric accumulation of fluid, internal debris, and scarring. Tenosynovitis is often associated with underlying tendinosis.

Posterior Tibial Tendon Dysfunction

PTT dysfunction is the most common cause of flatfoot deformity in adults. It is a degenerative process, which begins much earlier than onset of clinical symptoms, progresses to tendon tear, and eventually results in deformity and arthritis.[8] Presence of a watershed region in the retromalleolar portion of the tendon and its acute turn around the medial malleolus are among the factors that contribute to tendon insufficiency.[9] Also, presence of a type II accessory navicular may alter the PTT insertion point and contribute to tendinosis. Although radiographs are used to characterize foot alignment, MRI is superior to assess the abnormalities of the PTT, which range from tenosynovitis and tendinosis to partial or complete tears (**Table 3**).[10] Correlation between intraoperative and histologic findings and MRI staging of PTT tears is controversial, with some studies reporting no or fair correlation.[11,12]

The extra-articular lateral hindfoot impingement syndrome is a complication of PTT dysfunction when it is associated with pes planus and hindfoot valgus deformities. Common sites of impingement are between the calcaneus and fibula (subfibular impingement), the lateral talus and calcaneus (talocalcaneal impingement), or both.[13] On MRI, marrow edema pattern, cyst formation, and sclerosis may be seen

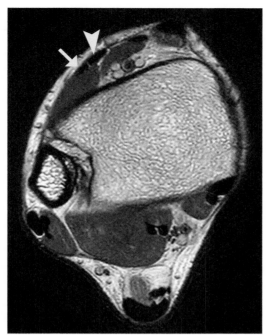

Fig. 7. Peroneus tertius (PT) muscle. Axial PD image demonstrates a PT muscle (*arrow*). This muscle and tendon run with the extensor digitorum longus (*arrowhead*) in the anterolateral ankle. It runs deep to the extensor retinaculum to insert onto the base of the 5th metatarsal (insertion not shown).

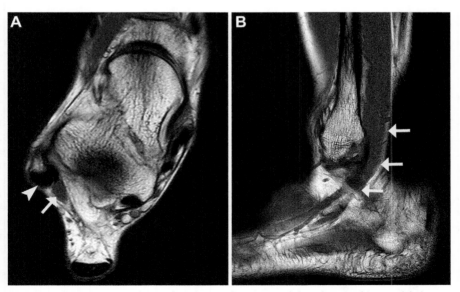

Fig. 8. Low-lying peroneus brevis muscle. Axial PD image (*A*) and sagittal image (*B*) demonstrate a low-lying peroneus brevis muscle (*arrows*), running posteromedially to the peroneus longus (*arrowhead*). In this case, the elongated peroneus muscle belly extends below the retromalleolar groove of the lateral malleolus.

Table 2
The course, function, and MRI appearance of the common accessory muscles and tendons of the ankle

Accessory Muscle	Origin	Insertion	Function	Normal MRI Appearance
Peroneus quartus	Peroneus quartus muscle arises from the posterior fibula, PL muscle, or PB muscle	Variable, but most commonly the retrotrochlear eminence of the calcaneus	Assists with hindfoot pronation	Tendon runs posteromedially to peroneal tendons
Low-lying PB	Same origin as the PB muscle	Same insertion as the PB tendon	Same function as PB	Musculotendinous junction forms low, approximately 1.6–2 cm above the distal tip of the fibula Best seen on sagittal and axial images, where muscle is seen at level of lateral malleolus
Accessory soleus	Arises from the fibula, soleal line of the tibia, or the soleus muscle	Variable, with both fleshy and tendinous insertions at superior calcaneus, medial calcaneus, or Achilles tendon	No significant function	Muscle located between FHL and Achilles tendon, superficial to the deep posterior aponeurosis Tendon runs anteromedially to the Achilles tendon
Flexor digitorum accessorius longus	FHL, deep posterior compartment fascia, medial or lateral aspects of fibula	Variable, with muscular, tendinous, or aponeurotic insertions at quadratus plantae or FDL	Assist in toe flexion	Muscle located deep to the deep posterior aponeurosis Tendon courses with posterior neurovascular bundle
Peroneocalcaneus internus	Peroneocalcaneus internus muscle arises from the lower third of the fibula	Medial base of the sustentaculum tali	No significant function	Muscle located deep to the deep posterior aponeurosis Tendon runs parallel to the FHL
Tibiocalcaneus internus	Tibiocalcaneus internus muscle arises from the medial crest of the tibia	Medial aspect of the calcaneus	No significant function	Muscle located deep to the deep posterior aponeurosis Tendon runs posterior to the FHL
Peroneus tertius	Peroneus tertius muscle arises from anterior distal third of the fibula	Dorsal base of the 5th metatarsal	Weak dorsiflexor of ankle Assists with ankle eversion	Muscle located in the anterolateral ankle Tendon runs with the EDL

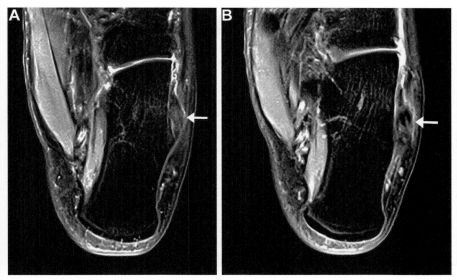

Fig. 9. Tendinosis and tendon tear. (*A*) Axial PD FS image of the ankle shows significant thickening of the peroneus longus tendon (*arrow*) below the retromalleolar grove consistent with tendinosis. (*B*) Axial PD FS of a separate patient shows longitudinal split tear of the peroneus longus (*arrow*).

at the opposing surfaces (see **Fig. 10**). In case of subfibular impingement, the calcaneofibular ligament and peroneal tendons may become entrapped.

Superior Peroneal Retinaculum Injuries and Peroneal Tendon Subluxations

The superior peroneal retinaculum (SPR) functions as the primary restraint to peroneal tendon subluxation and is also a secondary restraint to anterolateral ankle instability. The SPR creates a fibro-osseous tunnel for the peroneal tendons contained within their common tendon sheath. Injury of the SPR occurs with peroneal dislocation through forceful ankle dorsiflexion and concomitant reflex peroneal muscle

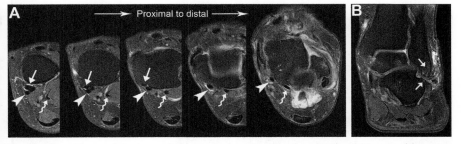

Fig. 10. Type III complete tear of the posterior tibial tendon (PTT). A 74-year-old woman with medial ankle pain. (*A*) Consecutive axial PD FS image of the ankle demonstrates splitting, attenuation, and finally disappearance of the PTT (*straight arrows*) on consecutive images, compatible with a complete tear. Flexor hallucis longus (*curved arrows*) and flexor digitorum longus (*arrowheads*) tendons are intact. (*B*) Coronal PD FS image of the ankle shows hindfoot valgus and findings of subfibular impingement, which include abutment of the distal fibula and lateral calcaneus associated with cystic formation and marrow edema pattern (*arrows*).

Table 3
Imaging spectrum of posterior tibialis tendon dysfunction on MRI

Tenosynovitis	Fluid or synovitis around the tendon distending a normal or thickened sheath. A threshold maximum fluid width ≥9 mm is proposed to represent those with clinical posterior tibialis tendon dysfunction.[37]
Tendinosis	Surface irregularity, thickening, and intrasubstance signal heterogeneity that is less intense than that of fluid. Motion of the type II accessory navicular (if present): increased signal intensity on fat-suppressed fluid-sensitive sequences at the synchondrosis between the accessory and native navicular bone.
Type I, partial tear	Fusiform enlargement, intrasubstance degeneration, and longitudinal splits. There is diagnostic overlap between this type of tendon tear and severe tendinosis.
Type II, partial tear	Stretching and elongation of the tendon (decreased tendon caliber equal to or less than that of the adjacent flexor digitorum longus tendon on axial images usually without signal intensity alterations).
Type III, complete tear	Tendon discontinuity with a gap filled with fluid or granulation tissue, depending on the chronicity of the injury.

contraction. This can occur in various sports-related injuries, such as skiing. SPR injury results in subluxation or dislocation of the peroneal tendons, which may result in tendon tear because of friction (**Fig. 11**). Early diagnosis is imperative for treatment. **Fig. 12** depicts Oden classification for assessment of SPR-associated injuries.

Cuboid Pulley Lesion

The cuboid acts as a pulley as the peroneus longus tendon passed underneath the bone through its course. This site undergoes mechanical stress and can cause

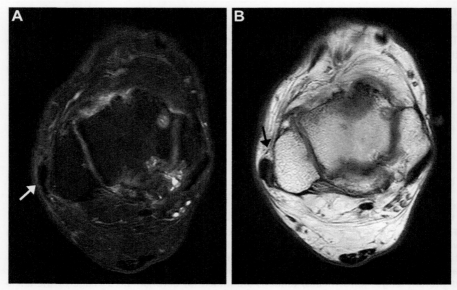

Fig. 11. Peroneal tendon dislocation. (*A*) Axial PD FS image at the level of the distal fibula shows lateral dislocation of the peroneus longus and brevis (*arrow*). (*B*) Note striping of the superior peroneal retinaculum (SPR) (*arrow*) on axial PD image.

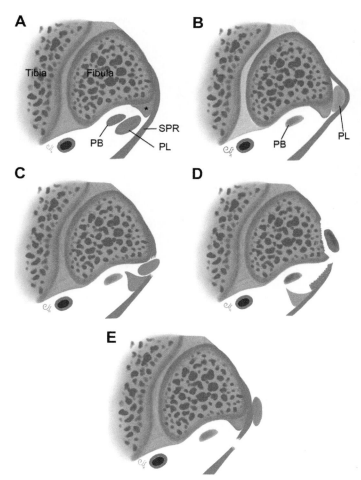

Fig. 12. Oden classification for injuries of the SPR. (*A*) Axial schematic image shows normal attachment of the SPR along the lateral aspect of distal fibula covering peroneus longus (PL) and brevis (PB) tendons. Note small fibrocartilaginous ridge (*asterisk*) at the osseous attachment of SPR. (*B*) Grade I SPR injury, most common type, shows striping and elevation of the SPR off the fibula with lateral subluxation of the tendons. (*C*) Grade II SPR injury with avulsion of the SPR from its fibular attachment. (*D*) Grade III SPR injury shows avulsion fracture at fibular attachment along with a small osseous fragment from the fibula. (*E*) Grade IV SPR injury with tear of the posterior fibers of SPR.

inflammation, which is known as cuboid pulley lesion. The peroneus longus tendon can show tenosynovitis, tendinosis, and tear with marrow edema present in the underlying cuboid bone (**Fig. 13**).

Achilles Tendon Pathologies and Haglund Syndrome

Paratenonitis is referred to the inflammation of the connective tissue membrane encasing the Achilles, which is seen as edema and enhancement around the tendon. Tears of the Achilles tendon are mostly seen at the insertion to the calcaneus and the relative avascular zone, which is approximately 4 cm proximal to the calcaneal

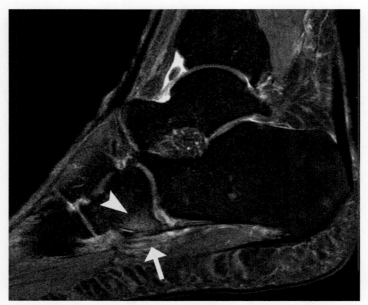

Fig. 13. Cuboid pulley lesion. Sagittal PD FS image at the level of cuboid demonstrates tendinosis and low-grade interstitial tearing of the peroneus longus (*arrow*) and mild edema in the underlying cuboid (*arrowhead*).

insertion site (**Fig. 14**). The gap of the tendon rupture should be measured for treatment planning. In the setting of rupture, care should be taken not to confuse an intact plantaris tendon with a partially intact Achilles tendon.

Haglund syndrome is a constellation of painful osseous and soft tissue abnormalities at the posterior heel. The Haglund lesion (retrocalcaneal exostosis) is a bony prominence at the posterosuperior aspect of the calcaneal tuberosity, which may cause mechanical inflammation of the retro-Achilles, retrocalcaneal bursae, and Achilles tendinosis, to form Haglund syndrome.[14,15] Radiography is often used to diagnose the bony Haglund lesion and sometimes the retrocalcaneal bursitis, which may be depicted as loss of the normal radiolucent retrocalcaneal recess. On MRI, the Haglund lesion is well visualized on sagittal T1W images, whereas fat-suppressed fluid-sensitive images may show marrow edema pattern at the calcaneal tuberosity. Excessive fluid in the retrocalcaneal and retro-Achilles bursa can also be seen on fat-suppressed fluid-sensitive images (**Fig. 15**).[16]

MRI of Postoperative Tendon

Surgical treatment of patients with ankle tendon pathologies is reserved for those who fail conservative measures, and is indicated to prevent progression to malalignment. Depending on the disease stage, the intervention includes soft tissue procedures that address the tendon pathology and/or osseous procedures to correct the malalignment.[17] Tendon debridement and repair is attempted in early clinical stages of the disease.[18] In cases of PTT dysfunction in the setting of an accessory navicular syndrome, a PTT advancement (Kidner) procedure is performed, which includes resection of the accessory navicular bone and anchoring the distal tendon fibers to the native navicular with suture anchors or screws. Pain following this procedure is often caused by PTT

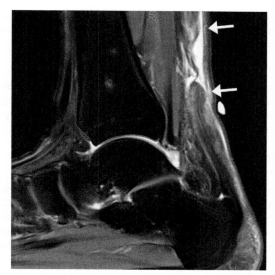

Fig. 14. Achilles tendon rupture. A 42-year-old man presented with acute ankle pain and popping during exercise. Sagittal PD FS image shows complete tear of the Achilles tendon at the myotendinous junction with 3 cm of gap filled with hemorrhage.

tendinosis.[19] In later clinical stages and often in conjunction with osteotomy and spring ligament reconstruction, an FDL tendon transfer may be performed to augment the PTT function.[17] The transferred FDL tendon is preferably attached to the remaining distal fibers of the PTT for better recreation of its function. If the residual PTT fibers are insufficient to interweave with the FDL tendon, a direct osseous attachment may be

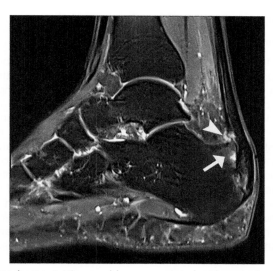

Fig. 15. Haglund syndrome. A 59-year-old man presented with posterior heel pain. Sagittal PD FS image shows marrow edema-like signal in the calcaneal tuberosity at a posterosuperior prominence consistent with a Haglund lesion (*arrow*), retrocalcaneal bursitis (*arrowhead*), and Achilles tendinosis characterized by tendon thickening and intrasubstance signal abnormality.

needed. Postoperative complications include avulsion of the transferred tendon resulting in acute recurrence of the flatfoot deformity, and tendinosis of the transferred FDL tendon or the residual PTT.

Tumors and Tumor-like Lesions of the Tendons

Different neoplastic or tumor-like pathologies can involve the ankle and foot tendons. The most common pathologies include ganglion cysts, xanthomas, giant cell tumors, and gout. Discussion on imaging appearance of tendon tumors is beyond the scope of this paper and can be found in the literature.[20]

ANKLE LIGAMENTOUS ANATOMY AND NORMAL MRI APPEARANCE
Lateral Ligamentous Complex

The lateral ligament complex includes the anterior talofibular ligament (ATFL), the posterior talofibular ligament (PTFL), and the calcaneofibular ligament (CFL). The ATFL is usually composed of two separate bands originating approximately 10-mm cranial from the lateral malleolar tip and extending to the anterior talus just adjacent the talofibular joint.[21] The ATFL is best imaged in the axial plane. The CFL originates from the distal fibular tip and runs posterior and inferior to insert onto the lateral calcaneus. The CFL is best imaged on the coronal and axial planes. The PTFL originates from the lateral malleolar fossa and runs obliquely to insert onto the posterolateral talus. The PTFL is best imaged on the axial and coronal planes.[22]

Medial Ligamentous Complex

The medial ligamentous complex is composed of six different bands (superficial posterior tibiotalar ligament [PTTL], tibiocalcaneal ligament, deep anterior tibiotalar ligament, tibiospring ligament, tibionavicular ligament, and deep PTTL). Only three of these bands are constant and usually visible on imaging: the two superficial bands (tibiospring and tibionavicular ligaments) and one deep band (deep PTTL).[2,23] The medial collateral ligaments are best imaged on coronal plane.

Syndesmotic Ligaments

The syndesmosis includes three main ligaments: (1) the anteroinferior tibiofibular ligament (AITFL), (2) posterior inferior tibiofibular ligament (PITFL), and the (3) distal interosseous ligament. The AITFL is made of three to four bands, originates from the anterior tubercle of the tibia 5 mm above the tibial surface, and extends laterally and caudally to the lateral malleolus. The PITFL run laterally and inferiorly from the posterior tubercle of tibia to the posterior tubercle of the lateral malleolus. AITFL and PITFL are best imaged on the axial plane. In light of the lateral and caudal course of the two ligaments, MRI sequences with axial oblique orientation or the use of axial oblique reconstructions allow visualization the whole course of both ligaments.[24,25] The distal interosseous ligament is considered the continuation of the interosseous membrane at the level of the syndesmosis and runs laterally and downward from the tibia to the fibula. The Basset ligament is an accessory AITFL, identified in up to 97% of ankles, which is located inferiorly to the AITFL and runs laterally and inferiorly.[26] Attention should be made not to misinterpret this as AITFL tear.

MIDTARSAL JOINT LIGAMENTS

From medial to lateral, the midtarsal joint includes three different ligaments. First, the talonavicular ligament extending from the neck of the talus to the dorsal surface of the navicular bone. Second, the V-shaped bifurcate ligament with two different bands (the calcaneonavicular and calcaneocuboideum ligament). Third, the dorsal calcaneocuboid ligament extending from the anterior process of the calcaneus to the lateral cuboid. The dorsal calcaneocuboid ligament shows several anatomic variants, such as bifurcate morphology, broadband morphology, or meniscoid morphology.[27]

LIGAMENT INJURIES

Acute tear of the ankle ligaments is classified according a three-grade scale. Grade 1 injuries represent stretching injuries with macroscopically intact ligament and soft tissue edema/hemorrhage around the ligament; grade 2 injuries represent partial discontinuity of the ligament, which is thinner or thicker than normal and soft tissue edema/hemorrhage around the ligament (**Fig. 16A**); grade 3 injuries are complete discontinuity of the ligament and soft tissue edema/hemorrhage around the ligament (**Fig. 16B**).[22] On MRI, acutely torn ligament is usually absent, partially or completely discontinuous, or wavy. In the acute stage, torn ligaments are surrounded by soft tissue edema/hemorrhage, which is seen as high signal intensity on fluid-sensitive sequences. In chronic injuries (after 6 weeks), ligaments are partially or completely resorbed or replaced by granulation tissue and/or scarring. On MRI ligaments are absent or are hypointense and thickened because of scar tissue.

The ATFL is the most commonly injured ligament of the ankle.[28] Approximately 20% of inversion injuries leads to tear of the ATFL and CFL (**Fig. 17**).[2] PTFL injuries usually happen because of major ankle traumas. Less than one-fifth to one-quarter of the patients show syndesmotic injuries after ankle sprain and ankle fractures, respectively. In high ankle sprain, the AITFL is generally injured (**Fig. 18**), whereas the PITFL and interosseous ligament (IOL) are torn with more severe injuries.[29] PITFL injury is the most reliable predictor of syndesmotic instability and longer disability.[14] When evaluating the injury on MRI, it is important to focus on soft tissue edema and direct signs of ligament rupture (discontinuation, absent or wavy appearance) rather than the classical indirect signs of syndesmotic rupture, such as tibiofibular widening and tibiofibular overlap. Severe joint effusion in the tibiotalar joint and the so-called lambda sign (fluid

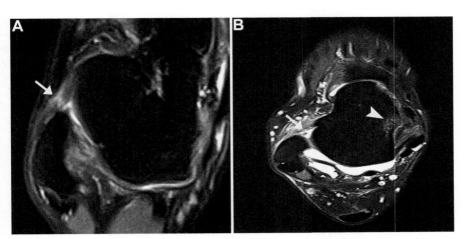

Fig. 16. ATFL injury. Axial PD FS images in two different patients. (*A*) Near complete tear (grade 2) (*arrow*) of ATFL following recurrent inversion injury. (*B*) Acute AFTL grade 3 (*arrow*) surrounded by soft tissue edema after inversion injury. Note the bone marrow edema on the talus (*arrowhead*).

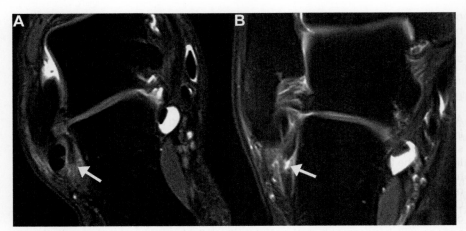

Fig. 17. CFL injury. A 29-year-old man with ankle instability after recurrent inversion injuries. Oblique axial T2 FS (*A*) and coronal PD FS (*B*) MRIs show complete (grade 3) CFL tear (*arrow*).

extension more than 10 mm cranial on the interosseous membrane) have been proposed in the literature as ancillary signs of syndesmotic rupture.[15,18]

Medial collateral ligament injuries are usually associated with ankle fractures. It is a strong ankle stabilizer and more than one-third of the patients with chronic medial ankle instability show deltoid ligament injuries. According to Chun and coworkers,[30] the sensitivity and the specificity for deltoid tear by MRI is 84% and 94%, respectively. Midtarsal sprains are common. Bone marrow edema on fluid-sensitive sequences at the attachment site of midtarsal ligaments, discontinuity or soft tissue edema surrounding the midtarsal ligaments, and bone fractures should be carefully scrutinized during MRI interpretation to rule out midtarsal sprain in patients undergoing MRI for persistent symptoms after ankle injuries.[31]

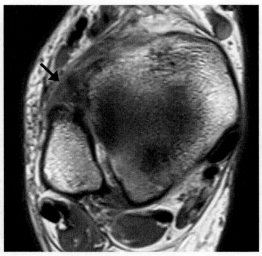

Fig. 18. AITFL injury. A 71-year-old woman with anterolateral pain after several inversion ankle injuries. Axial PD image shows thickening and scarring of the AITFL (*arrow*) representing grade II injury.

ANKLE IMPINGEMENT SYNDROMES

Impingement syndromes are characterized by pain and limitations in range of motion caused by pathologic abutment of bone, soft tissue, or both. Ankle impingement is primarily a clinical diagnosis; however, imaging may be used for confirmation, preoperative planning, and exclusion of alternate diagnoses. Because imaging findings do not always correlate with the patient's symptomatology, rather than making a diagnosis solely based on imaging, it is recommended to provide a detailed description of relevant imaging findings and their potential contribution to impingement.[21] Five spatial areas of impingement are delineated within the joint (discussed next).

Anterolateral Impingement

The anterolateral recess or gutter of the ankle joint is a pyramidal potential space, which is formed posteromedially by the tibia, laterally by the fibula, anteriorly by the ATFL and the joint capsule, inferiorly by the CFL, and superiorly by the AITFL.[13] Anterolateral impingement is thought to occur primarily after macrotrauma or microtrauma to the lateral ligament complex. Such trauma results in hemorrhage within the anterolateral gutter, which then evolves to reactive synovitis, organizing fibrosis, and eventually, mass-like scar formation. The contact between a post-traumatic thickened Basset ligament and talus may also contribute to symptoms of impingement.[32]

Spurring of the anterior tibial plafond or ossicles in the anterolateral gutter should raise a diagnosis of anterolateral impingement in the appropriate clinical setting. Synovitis of the anterolateral recess on MRI typically manifests as a nodular or mass-like area of intermediate signal on FS, fluid-sensitive sequences and intermediate to low signal on T1W or non-FS PDW sequences (**Fig. 19**). Other findings include post-traumatic changes of the ATFL and AITFL, and presence of a prominent Bassett ligament.

Anterior Impingement

The anterior recess is the anterior central portion of the tibiotalar joint, which is bordered by the anterior tibial plafond and talar dome posteriorly and joint capsule anteriorly. The recess contains fat, synovial lining, and a small amount of joint fluid. Anterior tibial and talar neck osteophytes through a cam-type mechanism with associated reactive capsular irritation and synovial inflammation can cause anterior impingement.[21] Originally, anterior osteophytes were attributed to traction-related spur formation associated with extreme plantar flexion of the ankle. However, these osteophytes are indeed intra-articular and far from the capsular attachment. More recent studies suggest direct microtrauma to the anterior joint as the cause.[33]

On radiographs, anterior osteophytes without significant joint space narrowing and decreased angle between the tibia and talus are the hallmark of anterior impingement. MRI depicts synovitis of the anterior recess as synovial thickening and hyperintensity on sagittal FS fluid-sensitive images (**Fig. 20**).[32]

Anteromedial Impingement

The anteromedial recess is demarcated medially by the medial malleolus, laterally by the talus, superficially by the anteromedial joint capsule, and inferiorly by the anterior tibiotalar fascicle of the deltoid ligament. Following an acute injury or repetitive microtrauma, thickening of the anterior tibiotalar fascicle of the deltoid ligament, synovitis, avulsion fragments, and bone spurring can contribute to anteromedial impingement.[34] Although conventional radiographs with frontal and exaggerated oblique projections better depict the medial talar, tibial plafond, and medial malleolar bone spurs, MRI is used to characterize ligamentous and synovial abnormalities (**Fig. 21**).[13]

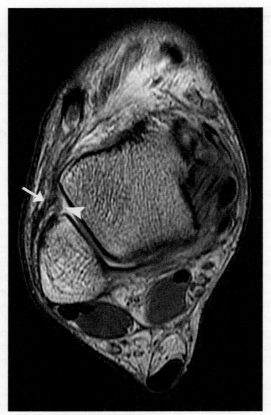

Fig. 19. Anterolateral ankle impingement. A 49-year-old woman who presented with anterolateral ankle pain during motion and remote history of ankle sprain. Axial PD image of the ankle demonstrates a thickened anterior talofibular ligament (*arrow*). There is scar tissue deep to the thickened ligament extending into the anterolateral gutter of the ankle (*arrowhead*).

Posteromedial Impingement

The posteromedial recess of the ankle is bound anteriorly by the medial malleolus and PTTL; laterally by the talar dome and posterior process of the talus; and posteriorly by the posteromedial joint capsule, FHL tendon, and the neurovascular bundle. This syndrome occurs infrequently after high-energy injuries to the PTTL, is often associated with osteochondral lesions, and manifests as pain over the posteromedial aspect of the ankle with passive and active movement.[32]

Because of the soft tissue nature of the pathology, conventional radiography is often of little utility. MRI may depict irregular synovial tissue in the posteromedial recess, which may encase the adjacent tendons and abnormalities of the PTTL including thickening, loss of the normal fibrillar pattern, and intermediate signal abnormality on fluid-sensitive sequences.[35]

Posterior Impingement

A secondary ossification center at the posterolateral aspect of the talus may form between the ages of 8 and 13 years. It may subsequently fuse within 1 year to form an

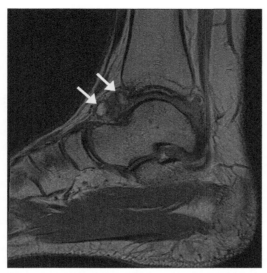

Fig. 20. Anterior ankle impingement. A 23-year-old man presented with anterior ankle pain and remote history of trauma. Sagittal T1W image of the ankle demonstrates multiple well-corticated osseous fragments in the anterior recess of the tibiotalar joint (*arrows*).

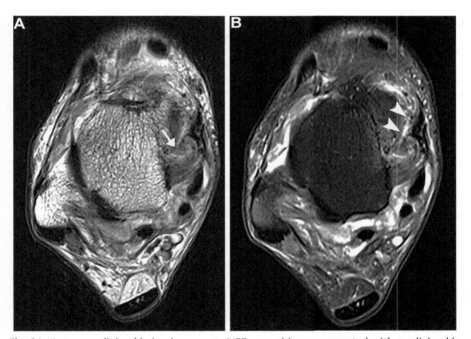

Fig. 21. Anteromedial ankle impingement. A 57-year-old man presented with medial ankle pain and remote history of ankle sprain. (*A*) Axial PD image of the ankle demonstrates tear of the anterior fascicles of the deltoid ligament (*arrow*), characterized by fiber discontinuity and wavy appearance. (*B*) Axial PD FS image shows scar tissue and extensive synovitis in the anteromedial recess (*arrowheads*).

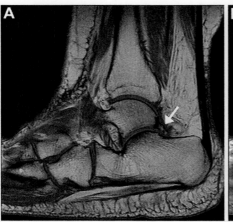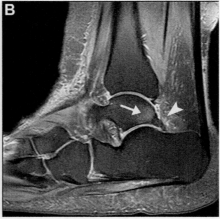

Fig. 22. Posterior ankle impingement. A 42-year-old woman presented with posterior ankle pain during plantar flexion. (*A*) Sagittal T1W image of the ankle demonstrates an os trigonum (*arrow*) at the posterolateral aspect of the talus. (*B*) Sagittal PD FS image of the ankle shows increased signal surrounding the synchondrosis (*arrow*) and mild synovitis (*arrowhead*) of the posterior joint recess.

elongated lateral tubercle known as the Stieda process or, in approximately 7% of cases, persist as an unfused ossicle, the os trigonum. Entrapment of a Stieda process or an os trigonum between the posterior tibial lip and the calcaneus during plantar flexion results in the clinical pain syndrome.

Although radiographs can adequately demonstrate the posterior talar process variants, these entities are common in asymptomatic individuals and are insufficient to make a diagnosis.[36] MRI is more valuable to diagnosis, by revealing marrow edema pattern in the os trigonum, posterior talus, and, less commonly, posterior tibial plafond and posterosuperior calcaneus (**Fig. 22**).[32] Other findings include synovitis and abnormalities of the posterior ligaments; increased signal at the synchondrosis; space-occupying lesions at the posterior ankle, such as ganglia; accessory muscles; or FHL tenosynovitis.[13]

SUMMARY

High-resolution 3-T MRI, as the modality of choice, can provide invaluable information about the anatomy and pathology of the ankle, specifically derangements of tendons and ligaments, which can help clinicians with management decision making.

CLINICS CARE POINTS

- Ankle sprain accounts for up to 30% of sport injuries and is the most common injury in the athletic population.
- MRI is the imaging modality of choice for evaluation of tendon and ligament pathologies of the ankle.
- 3T MRI is preferred for evaluation of fine soft tissue structures of the ankle due to highr signal-to-noise ration and better fat suppression, which improves visualization of anatomic detail and pathology.

DISCLOSURES

M. Chalian: Medical Advisor: Imagen Technologies Ltd. Other authors have nothing to disclose.

Conflicts of Interest: None.

The authors declare that they had full access to all the data in this study and the authors take complete responsibility for the integrity of the data and the accuracy of the data analysis.

REFERENCES

1. Waterman BR, Owens BD, Davey S, et al. The epidemiology of ankle sprains in the United States. J Bone Joint Surg Am 2010;92(13):2279–84.
2. Golanó P, Vega J, de Leeuw PA, et al. Anatomy of the ankle ligaments: a pictorial essay. Knee Surg Sports Traumatol Arthrosc 2010;18(5):557–69.
3. Tuite MJ. MR imaging of the tendons of the foot and ankle. Semin Musculoskelet Radiol 2002;6(2):119–31.
4. Chhabra A, Soldatos T, Chalian M, et al. Current concepts review: 3T magnetic resonance imaging of the ankle and foot. Foot Ankle Int 2012;33(2):164–71.
5. Schweitzer ME, van Leersum M, Ehrlich SS, et al. Fluid in normal and abnormal ankle joints: amount and distribution as seen on MR images. AJR Am J Roentgenol 1994;162(1):111–4.
6. Pierre-Jerome C, Moncayo V, Terk MR. MRI of the Achilles tendon: a comprehensive review of the anatomy, biomechanics, and imaging of overuse tendinopathies. Acta Radiol 2010;51(4):438–54.
7. Cheung Y, Rosenberg ZS. MR imaging of the accessory muscles around the ankle. Magn Reson Imaging Clin N Am 2001;9(3):465–73, x.
8. Schweitzer ME, Karasick D. MR imaging of disorders of the posterior tibialis tendon. AJR Am J Roentgenol 2000;175(3):627–35.
9. Knapp PW, Constant D. Posterior tibial tendon dysfunction. StatPearls. Treasure Island (FL): Stat Pearls Publishing Copyright © 2020, StatPearls Publishing LLC.; 2020.
10. Rosenberg ZS, Beltran J, Bencardino JT. From the RSNA Refresher Courses. Radiological Society of North America. MR imaging of the ankle and foot. Radiographics 2000;20(Spec No):S153–79.
11. Alaia EF, Rosenberg ZS, Bencardino JT, et al. Tarsal tunnel disease and talocalcaneal coalition: MRI features. Skeletal Radiol 2016;45(11):1507–14.
12. Braito M, Wöß M, Henninger B, et al. Comparison of preoperative MRI and intraoperative findings of posterior tibial tendon insufficiency. SpringerPlus 2016;5(1): 1414.
13. Berman Z, Tafur M, Ahmed SS, et al. Ankle impingement syndromes: an imaging review. Br J Radiol 2017;90(1070):20160735.
14. Park YH, Yoon MA, Choi WS, et al. The predictive value of MRI in the syndesmotic instability of ankle fracture. Skeletal Radiol 2018;47(4):533–40.
15. Crema MD, Krivokapic B, Guermazi A, et al. MRI of ankle sprain: the association between joint effusion and structural injury severity in a large cohort of athletes. Eur Radiol 2019;29(11):6336–44.
16. Lawrence DA, Rolen MF, Morshed KA, et al. MRI of heel pain. AJR Am J Roentgenol 2013;200(4):845–55.
17. Jesse MK, Hunt KJ, Strickland C. Postoperative imaging of the ankle. AJR Am J Roentgenol 2018;211(3):496–505.

18. Ryan LP, Hills MC, Chang J, et al. The lambda sign: a new radiographic indicator of latent syndesmosis instability. Foot Ankle Int 2014;35(9):903–8.

19. Dimmick S, Chhabra A, Grujic L, et al. Acquired flat foot deformity: postoperative imaging. Semin Musculoskelet Radiol 2012;16(3):217–32.

20. Wang C, Song RR, Kuang PD, et al. Giant cell tumor of the tendon sheath: magnetic resonance imaging findings in 38 patients. Oncol Lett 2017;13(6):4459–62.

21. Carreira DS, Ueland TE. Ankle impingement: a critical analysis review. JBJS Rev 2020;8(5):e0215.

22. Gonzalez FM, Morrison WB. Magnetic resonance imaging of sports injuries involving the ankle. Top Magn Reson Imaging 2015;24(4):205–13.

23. Perrich KD, Goodwin DW, Hecht PJ, et al. Ankle ligaments on MRI: appearance of normal and injured ligaments. AJR Am J Roentgenol 2009;193(3):687–95.

24. Sharif B, Welck M, Saifuddin A. MRI of the distal tibiofibular joint. Skeletal Radiol 2020;49(1):1–17.

25. Kalia V, Fritz B, Johnson R, et al. CAIPIRINHA accelerated SPACE enables 10-min isotropic 3D TSE MRI of the ankle for optimized visualization of curved and oblique ligaments and tendons. Eur Radiol 2017;27(9):3652–61.

26. Subhas N, Vinson EN, Cothran RL, et al. MRI appearance of surgically proven abnormal accessory anterior-inferior tibiofibular ligament (Bassett's ligament). Skeletal Radiol 2008;37(1):27–33.

27. Walter WR, Hirschmann A, Alaia EF, et al. Normal anatomy and traumatic injury of the midtarsal (Chopart) joint complex: an imaging primer. Radiographics 2019;39(1):136–52.

28. Boruta PM, Bishop JO, Braly WG, et al. Acute lateral ankle ligament injuries: a literature review. Foot & ankle. 1990;11(2):107–13.

29. McCollum GA, van den Bekerom MP, Kerkhoffs GM, et al. Syndesmosis and deltoid ligament injuries in the athlete. Knee Surg Sports Traumatol Arthrosc 2013;21(6):1328–37.

30. Chun KY, Choi YS, Lee SH, et al. Deltoid ligament and tibiofibular syndesmosis injury in chronic lateral ankle instability: magnetic resonance imaging evaluation at 3T and comparison with arthroscopy. Korean J Radiol 2015;16(5):1096–103.

31. Walter WR, Hirschmann A, Alaia EF, et al. JOURNAL CLUB: MRI evaluation of midtarsal (Chopart) sprain in the setting of acute ankle injury. AJR Am J Roentgenol 2018;210(2):386–95.

32. LiMarzi GM, Khan O, Shah Y, et al. Imaging manifestations of ankle impingement syndromes. Radiol Clin North Am 2018;56(6):893–916.

33. Tol JL, van Dijk CN. Etiology of the anterior ankle impingement syndrome: a descriptive anatomical study. Foot Ankle Int 2004;25(6):382–6.

34. Murawski CD, Kennedy JG. Anteromedial impingement in the ankle joint: outcomes following arthroscopy. Am J Sports Med 2010;38(10):2017–24.

35. Koulouris G, Connell D, Schneider T, et al. Posterior tibiotalar ligament injury resulting in posteromedial impingement. Foot Ankle Int 2003;24(8):575–83.

36. Yasui Y, Hannon CP, Hurley E, et al. Posterior ankle impingement syndrome: a systematic four-stage approach. World J Orthop 2016;7(10):657–63.

37. Gonzalez FM, Harmouche E, Robertson DD, et al. Tenosynovial fluid as an indication of early posterior tibial tendon dysfunction in patients with normal tendon appearance. Skeletal Radiol 2019;48(9):1377–83.

Imaging of Turf Toe

Michael T. Perry, MD*, Jennifer L. Pierce, MD

KEYWORDS

- Turf toe • Plantar plate • Metatarsophalangeal joint • Magnetic resonance imaging
- Ultrasonography • Forefoot • Hallux

KEY POINTS

- Turf toe, previously used to describe great toe injuries occurring on artificial turf, is now a term commonly used to describe hyperdorsiflexion injuries to the plantar plate complex.
- The most common injury of the plantar plate complex is sprain or tearing of the sesamoid-phalangeal ligaments.
- High-resolution MRI accurately assesses the presence and severity of sesamoid-phalangeal ligament tears and can provide additional evaluation of the MTP joint to guide management.
- Ultrasound assessment of turf toe injuries is highly accurate in identifying high-grade plantar plate complex injuries particularly when dynamic evaluation is used.

INTRODUCTION

Turf toe was originally described in collegiate football players in the 1970s and thought to be due to excessive hyperdorsiflexion of the hallux metatarsophalangeal (MTP) joint as a result of wearing soft-soled shoes on firm artificial playing surface.[1] Turf toe is now used to describe injuries to the plantar complex of the first MTP joint regardless of mechanism or playing surface where injury occurred.[2] The first MTP joint is a complex structure that must withstand forces up to 8 times the body weight with certain movements.[3] Both MRI and ultrasonography (US) can be used to accurately evaluate the integrity of the plantar plate complex and associated structures of the first MTP joint.[4] This article will discuss the normal anatomy of the first MTP joint with focus on the musculotendinous plantar plate complex. The normal appearance of the first MTP joint and plantar plate complex on MRI and ultrasound will be reviewed. Finally examples of turf toe pathology will be reviewed with illustrative examples including plain radiography, MRI, and US.

Department of Radiology and Medical Imaging, University of Virginia, PO Box 800170, Charlottesville, VA 22908, USA
* Corresponding author.
E-mail address: mtp2a@virginia.edu

Clin Sports Med 40 (2021) 755–764
https://doi.org/10.1016/j.csm.2021.05.010
sportsmed.theclinics.com

DISCUSSION
Anatomy of Metatarsophalangeal Joint

The anatomy of the first MTP joint is comprised of osseous structures (metatarsal, proximal phalanx, and sesamoid bones), muscle and tendon complexes (extensor, abductor hallucis, and adductor hallucis with oblique/transverse heads), medial and lateral collateral ligaments, and the musculotendinous plantar plate complex. The plantar plate complex and its role in stability of the first MTP joint will be the main focus of this article.

The first metatarsal head has unique anatomic features with two articular grooves along the plantar surface separated by a sagittally oriented crest ("crista") that articulate with the medial and lateral hallux sesamoid bones. The medial groove is larger and deeper as the medial hallux sesamoid is typically larger than the lateral.[5-8] Up to a third of all sesamoids are partite with bilateral involvement seen in 50% to 85% of cases.[9] The base of the first proximal phalanx is a broad concavity that allows for wide range of motion in the sagittal plane but relatively restricted motion in the coronal plane to varus and valgus forces.[2]

Stability of the hallux MTP joint in the sagittal plane is provided by the plantar plate complex that includes the joint capsule, ligaments, flexor hallucis brevis (FHB) tendon, and adductor/abductor hallucis tendons. Unlike the lesser MTP joints, the hallux MTP joint does not have a robust central plantar plate structure. Rather the plantar plate of the first MTP joint is a fibrocartilage thickening of the joint capsule that is thought to allow for smooth sliding of the hallux sesamoids. There is a stronger proximal attachment to the plantar base of the proximal phalanx and thinner attachment to the metatarsal head or intersesamoid ligament (ISL). The first MTP joint is primarily stabilized by the short flexor complex composed of the FHB tendons, sesamoid bones, sesamoid-phalangeal ligaments (SPLs), and abductor and adductor hallucis tendons.[3] The hallux sesamoid bones are invested within FHB tendon slips with strong connection to the proximal phalanx by the SPL. The FHB and adductor/abductor tendons predominantly insert on the respective proximal sesamoids with some fibers attaching to the joint capsule. The metatarsal-sesamoid ligaments (MTSLs), with the ISL, help stabilize the sesamoids by serving as suspensory connections between the metatarsal neck and the sesamoids. The flexor hallucis longus (FHL) tendon courses between the sesamoids and plantar to the ISL. The ISL is a thick band of tissue connecting the medial and lateral sesamoids allowing the plantar plate complex to function as a unit. Proximal to the ISL and between the medial and lateral SPLs, there is no true structure and only joint capsular tissue.[1-3,6,10]

Mechanism of Injury

The term turf toe was originally used to describe first MTP joint injuries in football players wearing flexible soled shoes on hard artificial surfaces resulting in excessive dorsiflexion of the first MTP joint.[11] Turf toe is now used in common practice to refer to injuries of the plantar plate complex without regard to the surface when injury occurred.[2] The mechanism of injury is hyperextension of the hallux MTP joint with fixed plantar flexion of the foot during axial loading. During hyperextension, force is predominantly applied to the SPLs making them the most vulnerable to injury.[3] Tearing of the SPLs may be unilateral or bilateral. When unilateral, tears are more often medial than lateral.[12] Injuries are typically graded by severity with the most common scheme created by Anderson.[1]

Grade I injuries consist of stretching of the plantar complex or mild sprain. Clinically patients experience focal tenderness and mild swelling without bruising. There may be mild restriction of range of motion and decreased performance. Grade II injuries reflect partial ligament tear that results in diffuse tenderness, moderate swelling, soft-tissue ecchymosis, and restricted range of motion of the MTP joint. Grade III injuries represent complete disruption of the plantar complex typically involving complete ligament tears. Sesamoid fracture or diastasis of partite sesamoid can also be present in grade III injuries. These patients present in severe pain and diffuse tenderness at the MTP joint. There is marked soft-tissue swelling and bruising with severe limitation of range of motion.[1,3,13]

IMAGING FINDINGS
Radiographs

First-line imaging is typically standard weight-bearing radiographs (**Fig. 1**). In ligamentous injuries, bony structures are typically intact although subtle avulsion could be seen at the capsular insertions of the plantar plate complex. Comparison to the contralateral uninjured foot may be useful to evaluate for proximal retraction of one or both sesamoid bones in the setting of complete ligamentous tear.[3] Sesamoid fracture may be difficult to distinguish from bipartite sesamoid on radiographs, particularly in the setting of chronic injury.[10] In the case of a bipartite sesamoid, forced dorsiflexion view should be performed to assess for diastasis. Live fluoroscopic evaluation can also be performed if grade III injury is suspected (**Fig. 2**). With complete disruption of the ligaments, the sesamoids will not track normally when the proximal phalanx is dorsiflexed.[3,10]

MRI

MRI is recommended in patients with radiographic abnormalities as well as cases of suspected grade II or grade III injury based on clinical examination to better define degree of soft-tissue injury as well as allowing assessment of the MTP joint cartilaginous and bony structures.[1] MRI protocol for evaluation of the first MTP joint should include at least one non–fat-suppressed T1-weighted (T1W) or proton-density-weighted (PDW) sequence for evaluation of osseous structures and overall anatomy. Axial, sagittal, and coronal fat-suppressed T2-weighted (T2W) images should be obtained for optimum assessment. These sequences could be short tau inversion recovery sequences, T2W fat-suppressed sequences, or fat-suppressed PDW sequences depending on institutional preference.[2,5,12]

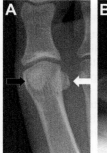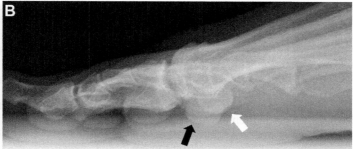

Fig. 1. Weight-bearing anterior-posterior (AP) radiograph (*A*) and lateral radiograph (*B*) of the hallux MTP joint demonstrates normal positioning of medial (*black arrow*) and lateral (*white arrow*) hallux sesamoid bones. Note the normal slightly more proximal position of the lateral sesamoid in relation to the medial.

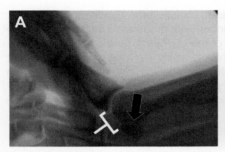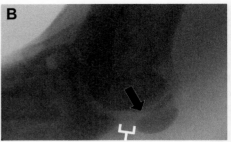

Fig. 2. Lateral intraoperative fluoroscopic image (*A*) reveals retraction of the sesamoid (*black arrow*) with dorsiflexion of the first MTP joint in keeping with full-thickness plantar plate complex tear. Intraoperative lateral fluoroscopic image made after turf toe repair (*B*) shows appropriate sesamoid positioning.

T1W sequences are important for assessing the marrow signal of the sesamoid bones for acute fracture or sclerosis. Normal sesamoids should follow normal marrow signal without increased edema signal on T2W fat-suppressed sequences (**Fig. 3**).[2]

The SPLs and joint capsule should be uniformly low signal intensity on PDW or T2W sequences (**Fig. 4**). The SPL and fibrocartilage plantar plate are best seen on sagittal images and should appear taut when imaged in neutral joint position.[2,5]

Musculotendinous structures including FHB, adductor, and abductor tendons are best seen on axial (long-axis) PDW or T2W FS sequences as low-signal linear structures inserting on the medial and lateral sesamoids. Muscle bulk and signal is best evaluated on coronal (short-axis) T1W sequence to assess for atrophy. The abductor hallucis tendon inserts on the proximal medial sesamoid to conjoin with the medial FHB tendon. The adductor hallucis tendon with oblique and transverse heads joins the lateral FHB tendon on the lateral sesamoid (**Fig. 5**).[6]

The ISL can be visualized best on coronal images extending between the sesamoid bones. The ISL typically spans the entire anterior-posterior length of the sesamoids. The FHL tendon is best seen in the coronal and sagittal planes as a uniformly low-signal tendon coursing immediately plantar to the ISL at the level of the sesamoids. MTSLs are also visualized on coronal images as thickened portions of the medial and lateral capsules extending from the first metatarsal neck to the plantar aspect of the sesamoids (see **Fig. 3**).[2,6]

Injuries of the plantar complex on MRI can be described as capsular or ligamentous sprain, partial thickness tears, or full-thickness disruption of the plantar mechanism.

Sprains of the plantar complex on MRI demonstrate mild soft-tissue edema surrounding the plantar aspect at the sesamoids, ligaments, and capsule. The SPLs remain intact with uniform low signal intensity as well as normal sesamoid bone marrow signal. Partial tearing of the SPLs is evidenced by attenuation or thinning of the ligament and surrounding soft-tissue edema in acute cases (**Fig. 6**). However, at least a few intact fibers should be visualized extending from the sesamoid to the base of the proximal phalanx on sagittal images. Complete disruption of the plantar complex most commonly involves full-thickness tear of one or both SPLs. Acute tears are best visualized on sagittal T2W sequence and evidenced by discontinuity of the normal low-signal ligament with intervening fluid signal and possible disruption of the joint capsule (**Fig. 7**). There may be proximal displacement of the sesamoid. Lack of contiguous fibers extending from the base of the proximal phalanx to the sesamoid confirms a full-thickness tear. Injury may be isolated to a single SPL or may involve both medial and lateral ligaments.[2,7,10,12]

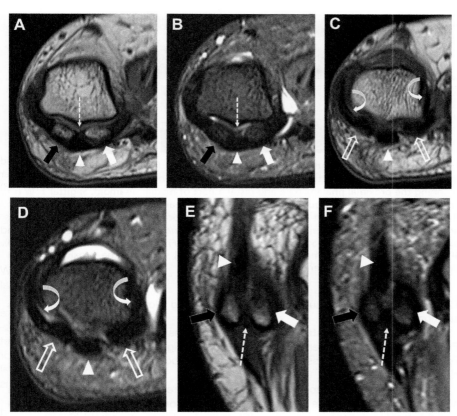

Fig. 3. Coronal (short-axis) T1W (*A*) and short tau inversion recovery (STIR) (*B*) MR images at the level of the hallux sesamoids show normal marrow signal intensity of medial (*black arrow*) and lateral (*white arrow*) hallux sesamoid bones. The ISL (*dashed arrow*) is seen between the sesamoids and immediately dorsal to the FHL (*arrowhead*). Coronal (short-axis) T1W (*C*) and STIR (*D*) MR images just distal to the hallux sesamoids show normal homogenous oval-shaped SPLs (*open arrows*). The FHL tendon courses between the SPLs along the plantar aspect of the MTP joint. The paired MTSLs (*curved arrows*) help stabilize the sesamoids and plantar plate complex. Axial (long-axis) T1W (*E*) and STIR (*F*) MR images show the normal location of the medial (*black arrow*) and lateral (*white arrow*) sesamoids with low signal interconnecting ISL (*dashed arrow*). The FHL tendon can be seen distally (*arrowhead*).

Grade III injury or complete disruption of the short flexor complex can also be the result of a fracture of the sesamoid or diastasis of the synchondrosis of a bipartite sesamoid (**Fig. 8**). On MRI, acute fractures are demonstrated by increased T2 signal at the fracture site with associated low T1 signal and distraction of the sesamoid fragments. Surrounding soft-tissue edema is also expected in acute injuries.[2,7,10] Chronic full-thickness tears may be more difficult to assess because of lack of soft-tissue edema. Heterotopic ossification in the region of the plantar plate complex has been associated with chronic injuries.[13]

Strains of the FHB, adductor, and abductor muscles may also be seen in acute injuries. Strains are diagnosed by seeing increased edema-like signal on fat-suppressed

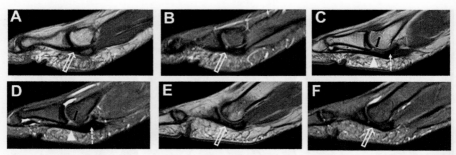

Fig. 4. Sagittal T1W (*A*) and short tau inversion recovery (STIR) (*B*) MR images through medial sesamoid show intact medial SPL (*open arrow*) with normal homogenous low signal spanning the proximal phalanx base and distal aspect of medial sesamoid. Sagittal T1W (*C*) and STIR (*D*) MR images through the first MTP joint reveal thin hypointense thickening of the plantar joint capsule that represents the central fibrocartilaginous plantar plate (*black arrow*). Normal intact FHL tendon (*arrowhead*) and ISL (*dashed arrow*) are seen along the plantar aspect of the joint. Sagittal T1W (*E*) and STIR (*F*) MR images show intact lateral SPL (*open arrow*) with normal homogenous low signal spanning the proximal phalanx base and distal aspect of lateral sesamoid.

T2W sequences in the muscle belly, often tracking along the musculotendinous junction.[7]

Cartilage loss or focal osteochondral injuries are best visualized on coronal T2W or PDW images as focal absence of normal cartilage signal replaced by fluid signal.[12] Full-thickness cartilage loss may have underlying bone marrow edema or cystic change.

Injuries to the ISL are uncommon and may be the result of severe trauma such as hallux dislocation. Tears are best visualized on T2W coronal images as demonstrated by fluid signal and discontinuity of the ISL at the level of the sesamoid.[12]

MTSL tears can occur at the proximal attachment at the first metatarsal neck, although they are less common than SPL tears. Tears can best be visualized on coronal T2W or PDW images.[2]

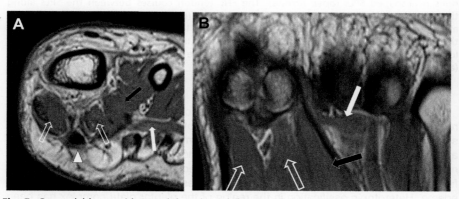

Fig. 5. Coronal (short-axis) T1W (*A*) and axial (long-axis) T1W (*B*) MR images demonstrate normal muscle bulk and signal of the adductor hallucis muscle (transverse head = *white arrow*; oblique head = *black arrow*), FHB muscle (*open arrows*), and normal FHL tendon (*arrowhead*).

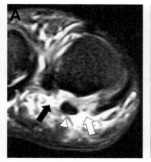
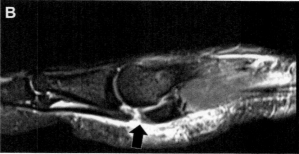

Fig. 6. Sagittal short tau inversion recovery (STIR) (*A*) MR image shows marked thinning and heterogenous signal intensity of the medial SPL with few intact fibers (*black arrow*). (*B*) Coronal (short-axis) MR image reveals high-grade partial thickness tear of the medial SPL (*black arrow*) with intact lateral SPL (*white arrow*). Arrowhead = FHL tendon.

Ultrasound

A high-frequency transducer such as a "hockey stick" probe is typically used to evaluate the plantar plate complex with ultrasound. The examination should begin in the transverse plane to first localize the sesamoid bones. The ISL is seen as a thick echogenic structure between the medial and lateral sesamoids. Just superficial to the ISL lies the ovoid-shaped echogenic FHL tendon (**Fig. 9**A). Then, the transducer is rotated to the longitudinal plane to visualize the SPLs and the FHL tendon. The SPLs are seen as hyperechoic structures between the sesamoid and proximal phalanx with clear broad attachments (**Fig. 9**B and D). The normal FHL tendon has a uniform echogenic fibrillary pattern and is positioned between the two sesamoids (**Fig. 9**C). After assessment of the SPLs, the transducer is slid proximally to assess the integrity of the FHB, adductor, and abductor tendons and muscles. The tendons broadly attach to the proximal aspect of the sesamoid with a somewhat echogenic appearance. The normal muscle bellies have a more hypoechoic appearance proximally. The medial sesamoid phalangeal ligament and medial capsule are assessed in the transverse plane. The

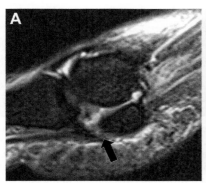
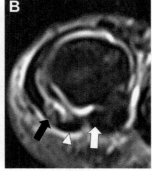

Fig. 7. (*A*) Coronal (short-axis) short tau inversion recovery (STIR) MR image reveals complete tear of both medial (*white arrow*) and lateral (*black arrow*) SPLs with normal low signal replaced by abnormal fluid signal intensity. FHL tendon (*arrowhead*) maintains normal signal and position. (*B*) Sagittal STIR MR image demonstrates gap in SPL with fluid signal cleft (*black arrow*) between the torn SPL and sesamoid bone.

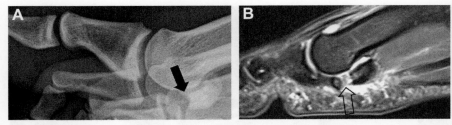

Fig. 8. (*A*) Lateral radiograph shows irregular distal cortex (*black arrow*) of the lateral hallux sesamoid with proximal retraction. (*B*) Sagittal short tau inversion recovery (STIR) MR image through the lateral sesamoid reveals a mildly distracted fracture (*open arrow*) through the distal aspect of the lateral sesamoid with bone marrow and surrounding soft-tissue edema.

medial SPL is seen as thickening of the joint capsule that extends from the dorsal aspect of the metatarsal to the medial aspect of the sesamoid.[14]

Plantar plate tears are diagnosed by ultrasound when the normal echogenic SPL is replaced by hypoechoic or heterogonous material. The torn irregular edges of the SPL may be visualized on longitudinal images (**Fig. 10**). Retraction of the sesamoid should be assessed in the setting of a full-thickness tear. Partial thickness tears typically occur along the articular surface of the SPL with remaining intact plantar fibers.[14]

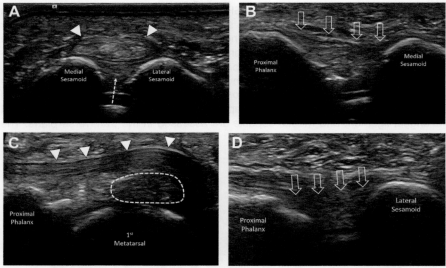

Fig. 9. Transverse US image (*A*) at the level of the sesamoids reveals normal echogenic oval-shaped FHL tendon (*arrowheads*). The ISL lies immediately deep to the FHL and is seen as a thick striated echogenic structure between the sesamoids (*dashed arrow*). Longitudinal US image (*B*) through the medial aspect of the first MTP joint reveals striated echogenic appearance of the normal SPL (*open arrows*) with broad attachment to the base of the proximal phalanx. Longitudinal US image (*C*) through the middle aspect of the first MTP joint shows uniform fibrillary pattern of the normal FHL tendon (*arrowheads*). The ISL ligament is seen deep to the FHL (*dashed circle*). Longitudinal US image (*D*) through the lateral aspect of the first MTP joint reveals echogenic appearance of the normal SPL (*open arrows*) spanning the base of the proximal phalanx and the lateral sesamoid.

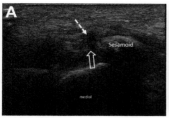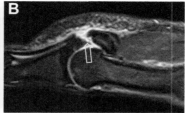

Fig. 10. Longitudinal US image (*A*) through the medial aspect of first MTP joint shows full-thickness tear of medial SPL with irregular torn edges (*open arrow*) and hypoechoic fluid filling the tear gap (*dashed arrow*). (*B*) Sagittal short tau inversion recovery (STIR) MR image of the same patient confirms full-thickness tear of SPL (*open arrow*) with fluid filled tear gap.

Studies have shown that dynamic evaluation of the plantar plate improves diagnostic accuracy of plantar plate tears complex. During passive dorsiflexion and plantar flexion of the MTP joint, a full-thickness defect in the SPL may become more apparent.[15,16]

US examination however is limited in certain aspects in evaluating turf toe injuries. Cartilage and osseous abnormalities are likely to be unappreciated on US when compared with high-resolution MRI.[5]

SUMMARY

Turf toe is an increasingly recognized injury of the first MTP joint that predominantly involves tearing of the sesamoid phalangeal ligaments of the plantar plate complex. Given the complex anatomy of the hallux MTP joint, MRI and US imaging can play an important role in the assessment of the integrity of the plantar plate complex and can assist in preoperative planning in the setting of high-grade injuries.

CLINICS CARE POINTS

- Turf toe is an acute injury of the plantar plate complex, typically the sesamoid-phalangeal ligaments, that results from hyperextension of the 1st MTP joint with fixed plantar flexion of the foot during axial loading.
- High resolution MR imaging is accurate in the diagnosis of high grade turf toe injuries as well as assessment of associated bone and cartilage injury.
- Dynamic evaluation to sonography improves diagnostic accuracy for high grade plantar plate complex tears.

DISCLOSURE

The authors have nothing to disclose.

REFERENCES

1. Anderson RB. Turf toe injuries of the hallux metatarsophalangeal joint. Tech Foot Ankle Surg 2002;1(2):102–11.

2. Hallinan JTPD, Statum SM, Huang BK, et al. High-resolution MRI of the first meta-tarsophalangeal joint: gross anatomy and injury characterization. Radiographics 2020;40(4):1107–24.
3. McCormick JJ, Anderson RB. Turf toe: anatomy, diagnosis, and treatment. Sports Health 2010;2(6):487–94.
4. Duan X, Li L, Wei DQ, et al. Role of magnetic resonance imaging versus ultrasound for detection of plantar plate tear. J Orthop Surg Res 2017;12(1):1–8.
5. Nery C, Baumfeld D, Umans H, et al. MR imaging of the plantar plate: normal anatomy, turf toe, and other injuries. Magn Reson Imaging Clin N Am 2017; 25(1):127–44.
6. Dietrich TJ, da Silva FLF, de Abreu MR, et al. First metatarsophalangeal joint- MRI findings in asymptomatic volunteers. Eur Radiol 2015;25(4):970–9.
7. Schein AJ, Skalski MR, Patel DB, et al. Turf toe and sesamoiditis: what the radiologist needs to know. Clin Imaging 2015;39(3):380–9.
8. Lucas DE, Philbin T, Hatic S. The plantar plate of the first metatarsophalangeal joint: an anatomical study. Foot Ankle Spec 2014;7(2):108–12.
9. Taylor JA, Sartoris DJ, Huang GS, et al. Painful conditions affecting the first metatarsal sesamoid bones. Radiographics 1993;13(4):817–30.
10. York PJ, Wydra FB, Hunt KJ. Injuries to the great toe. Curr Rev Musculoskelet Med 2017;10(1):104–12.
11. Bowers KD, Martin RB. Turf-toe: a shoe-surface related football injury. Med Sci Sports Exerc 1976;8(2):81–3.
12. Crain JM, Phancao JP. Imaging of turf toe. Radiol Clin North Am 2016;54(5): 969–78.
13. McCormick JJ, Anderson RB. The great toe: failed turf toe, chronic turf toe, and complicated sesamoid injuries. Foot Ankle Clin 2009;14(2):135–50.
14. Gregg JM, Silberstein M, Schneider T, et al. Sonography of plantar plates in cadavers: correlation with MRI and histology. Am J Roentgenol 2006;186(4):948–55.
15. Feuerstein CA, Weil L, Weil LS, et al. Static versus dynamic musculoskeletal ultrasound for detection of plantar plate pathology. Foot Ankle Spec 2014;7(4): 259–65.
16. Donegan RJ, Stauffer A, Heaslet M, et al. Comparing magnetic resonance imaging and high-resolution dynamic ultrasonography for diagnosis of plantar plate pathology: a case series. J Foot Ankle Surg 2017;56(2):371–4.

Stress Imaging of Bone

Maxine Ella Kresse, MD*, Nicholas C. Nacey, MD

KEYWORDS

- Stress fracture • Insufficiency fracture • Metabolic bone disease • Sports injury

KEY POINTS

- Stress injury is an umbrella term encompassing insufficiency (normal stress on an abnormal bone) and fatigue (abnormal stress on a normal bone) fractures.
- Radiographs followed by MRI are the imaging modalities of choice to evaluate potential stress injury/fracture.
- Being aware of the early imaging findings and the typical locations of stress injury aids in early detection and thus helps prevent the development of complications.
- The grade of stress injury is correlated with the time to return to sport.
- Because of the distribution of force, some stress injury locations are considered high risk, while others are low risk, a differentiation that is important in determining proper treatment.

INTRODUCTION/HISTORY/DEFINITIONS/BACKGROUND

Stress injury is an umbrella term that encompasses repetitive microtraumatic events that accumulate to surpass the threshold of bone failure with frank stress fracture as the end point.[1] Insufficiency and fatigue fractures fall under the umbrella term of stress injury/fracture. Insufficiency fractures result from normal stress on an abnormal bone (ie, an older patient with osteoporosis) and are more common in areas with a higher percentage of cancellous bone, such as vertebral bodies, the sacrum, and the subchondral regions of long bones. Fatigue fractures refer to an excessive/abnormal repetitive stress on a normal bone (ie, a military recruit starting training) and are more likely to be seen in weight-bearing bones with a higher percentage of cortical bone like the metatarsals.[1]

In order to understand the mechanism of stress injury, one must first consider the normal bone remodeling process given that stress injury is an accumulation of repetitive forces (because of excessive severity, duration, and/or frequency) that outweighs the normal bone remodeling process without enough time for repair.[2,3] Bone

The authors have nothing to disclose.
UVA Department of Radiology, 1215 Lee Street, Box 800170, Charlottesville, VA 22908, USA
* Corresponding author.
E-mail address: mk2fx@hscmail.mcc.virginia.edu

remodeling is a normal response to stress, including regular physical activity.[4] This complex process occurs over weeks to months and relies on an organized response of steps, including the creation of a microcrack, which is transformed into a cavity by osteoclast resorption, followed by new bone formation within this cavity by osteoblasts.[1,3] Greaney and colleagues found 64% of stress fractures in a military population begin within the first 7 days of training, supporting the idea that additional factors, such as decreased oxygen perfusion, likely play a role beyond sheer mechanical stress given the relatively rapid onset of symptoms.[4,5]

The specific composition of the bone in question alters this response to stress. For example, woven bone is mechanically weak because of an irregular orientation of collagen fibers and is primarily seen in fetuses and rapid bone turnover states like healing fractures, Paget disease, and hyperparathyroidism.[1,2] Conversely, lamellar bone is stronger and more organized; lamellar bone includes both cortical and cancellous (trabecular, medullary) bone. Compared with cancellous bone, cortical bone is stronger and more dense but less flexible with a slower turnover rate, making it more resistant to compressive loads and less resistant to tension forces.[1,2,4] During remodeling, cortical bone causes inflammation of the periosteum compared with trabecular bone, which reorients trabeculae in response to the direction of force[3]; these differences account for some of the imaging findings described in a dedicated section to follow.

DISCUSSION
Prevalence/Incidence

Several different factors weigh into this balance of stress and remodeling, making certain populations more at risk for stress injuries compared with others. Essential factors contributing to stress injury include a new or increased activity, repetition, and relatively strenuous nature of the activity.[2] A study by Goldberg and colleagues[6] emphasized this need for a change in activity by reporting 67% of 58 stress fractures in college varsity athletes occurred in freshmen, who are most likely to experience a significant change in exercise intensity and/or routine.

Furthermore, the tipping point of overwhelming the remodeling process can be altered by several intrinsic and extrinsic factors. Intrinsic factors include bone density, hormone levels, muscle strength, and anatomy/alignment, while extrinsic factors include training schedule, nutrition, sleep, equipment (ie, shoes), and training surfaces.[2,7] A unique risk factor for stress injuries is the so-called female athlete triad of energy deficiency, menstrual irregularity, and decreased bone mineral density; this triad has been shown to increase risk for stress fracture by 15% to 50%.[1,2]

The incidence and prevalence of stress injuries depends on these risk factors and particular activities. The incidence of stress fractures in the general athletic population may be less than 1% but could be as high as 20% in runners,[7] with the incidence of stress injury as high as 21% in track and field athletes and 31% in military recruits.[8] Stress fractures of the foot and ankle have been reported to account for up to 20% of sports medicine clinic visits.[9] In 370 athletes with stress fractures, the tibia was the most common bone at 49%, then the tarsal bones at 25%, followed by the metatarsals at 9%.[7] In military recruits, the tibia remains the most common bone at 24% to 73%, followed by the metatarsals at 17% to 35% and then the calcaneus at 21% to 28%.[9] In runners, the posteromedial tibia is most common followed by the distal fibula and navicular. In dancers, the metatarsals and anterior tibia are more commonly affected.[9]

Common locations of stress injury can be divided into high-risk and low-risk categories (**Fig. 1**). High-risk categories are in regions of tensile force and/or low vascularity locations.[2] Examples include the tension side of the femoral neck (convex surface), patella, anterior cortex of the tibia, medial malleolus, talus, tarsal navicular, proximal fifth metatarsal, and hallux sesamoids.[4,7] Treatment often needs to be more aggressive and may require restricted weight bearing and/or surgery because of the risk of fracture propagation, delayed union, and nonunion.[2,7,10]

Alternatively, low-risk categories are in regions of compressive forces.[2] Examples include the posteromedial tibial shaft, fibula, calcaneus, cuneiforms, cuboid, metatarsal necks or shafts, and the compressive side of the femoral neck (concave surface).[4,10] These injuries are more likely to heal with conservative treatment of activity and risk factor modification.[2,10] Typical treatment includes rest for 1 to 6 weeks with subsequent gradual increase in activity as tolerated in addition to modification of risk factors.[7]

Imaging Modalities

Radiographs are often the first imaging modality ordered for a suspected stress injury. However, 85% of radiographs are normal at the time of symptom onset[10] and can remain normal for weeks and even months after symptoms start.[7] Sensitivity of radiographs has been reported to be 15% to 35% in early stage and 30% to 70% in late-stage injuries.[3] Radiographic findings depend on the stage of injury and the type of bone involved. An early sign of stress injury in cortical bone is the gray cortex sign (**Fig. 2**), which is an often subtle area of decreased density within the cortex.[11] In bones with a higher percentage of trabecular bone, the earliest radiographic sign is subtle blurring and faint sclerosis of trabeculae.[3] Later signs include periosteal reaction and a frank fracture line. However, radiographs can at times be difficult to interpret, as there are many areas of physiologic cortical thickening or nutrient foramina that can mimic findings of a stress fracture (**Fig. 3**).

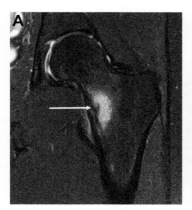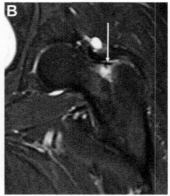

Fig. 1. (*A*) Coronal fluid-sensitive image depicts linear hypointense signal in the medial aspect of the basicervical femoral neck with surrounding edema (*arrow*), consistent with stress fracture and considered low risk because of presence on the compressive side of the femoral neck. (*B*) In contrast, this coronal fluid-sensitive image demonstrates similar findings along the lateral aspect of the femoral neck (*arrow*) from stress fracture, considered high risk for fracture propagation because of their presence on the tensile side of the femoral neck.

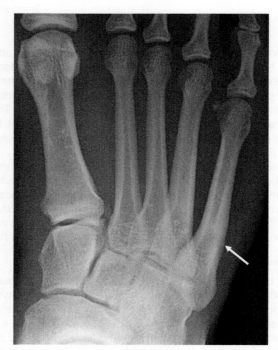

Fig. 2. Frontal radiograph in a 21-year-old collegiate athlete with foot pain demonstrates gray cortex along the proximal diaphysis of the fifth metatarsal (*arrow*) with associated adjacent medullary sclerosis and blurring of the endosteal margins, suspicious for developing stress fracture.

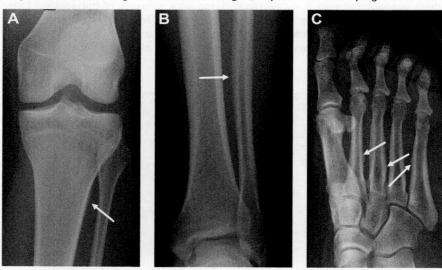

Fig. 3. Normal findings that may mimic stress changes on radiographs. (*A*) Frontal radiograph demonstrating a small portion of the tibial tuberosity (*arrow*), which is a common appearance depending on rotation of the radiograph but can mimic periosteal reaction. (*B*) Frontal radiograph of the tibia and fibula demonstrates a vague, fairly vertical linear lucency in the fibular cortex, which has sclerotic margins and an absence of periosteal reaction. This is consistent with a nutrient foramen for vessels penetrating the bone as opposed to fracture. (*C*) Oblique radiograph of the foot demonstrates multiple undulations in the metatarsal diaphyses that did not correlate with the patient's site of pain. This wavy appearance of the metatarsal cortices is a common finding in older patients and should not be confused with stress fracture.

Bone scans were traditionally used because of their increased sensitivity relative to radiographs and potential for earlier detection (**Fig. 4**). Bone scan has been shown to have near 100% sensitivity within 48 to 72 hours of symptom onset.[7,10] However, bone scans are less commonly used today due to lack of specificity and exposure to radiation compared with MRI, which is now the modality of choice if clinical suspicion remains high and radiographs are normal.

MRI is highly sensitive and specific for detection of stress injuries and also provides the additional benefit of evaluating for other causes of the patient's symptoms, such as bursitis, muscle injury, and tendon/ligament injury.[3,10] However, findings on MRI must be interpreted in correlation with the patient's symptoms to avoid overdiagnosis. Bergman and colleagues[12] found a tibial stress reaction in 43% of the 21 asymptomatic college distance runners studied; in addition to the lack of symptoms, none of these 9 patients developed a stress fracture on 12 to 48 months of follow-up imaging.

A specific classification system was developed by Fredericson and colleagues to grade tibial stress injuries and is often applied to other bones (**Fig. 5**). This initial classification includes grade 1 (periosteal edema with normal marrow signal), grade 2 (periosteal edema plus T2-weighted marrow edema), grade 3 (periosteal edema plus marrow edema on T1- and T2-weighted images), and grade 4 (grade 3 plus fracture line).[13] Kijowski and colleagues[14] later subdivided grade 4 into 4a (intracortical

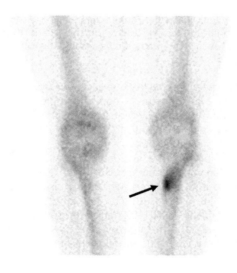

R ANTERIOR L

Fig. 4. Anterior image from a technetium 99 m methylene disphosphonate (MDP) bone scan in a 44-year-old female runner demonstrates focal increased uptake along the medial aspect of the proximal tibia. The imaging finding itself is nonspecific, but in the appropriate clinical context is consistent with a stress fracture.

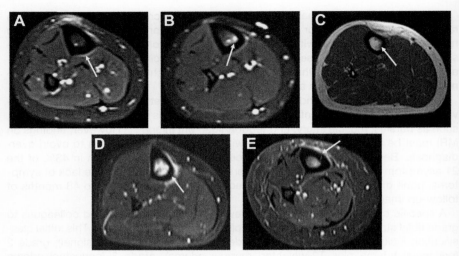

Fig. 5. (*A*) Axial STIR image demonstrates subtle periosteal edema along the posterior aspect of the tibia (*arrow*), consistent with grade 1 stress change. (*B*) This patient with grade 2 stress change has hyperintense signal in the medial tibial marrow on this STIR image (*arrow*), as well as underlying periosteal edema. Corresponding T1-weighted image (not shown) demonstrated normal hyperintense marrow signal from yellow marrow. (*C*) Axial T1-weighted image in a patient with grade 3 stress change shows hypointense signal (*arrow*) from more intensive marrow edema than is seen in patients with grade 2 stress change. (*D*) This patient with medullary and periosteal edema also has subtle intermediate signal within the normally hypointense cortex (*arrow*) on this axial STIR image, consistent with type 4a stress change. (*E*) Axial STIR image shows a frank linear fracture (*arrow*) in this patient with grade 4b stress change.

signal changes) and 4b (linear cortical fracture line). This classification has been further shown to be prognostic for time to return to sports for athletes with grade 1 showing an average of 16 days to return to sports, grade 2 to 4a with an average of 39 to 44 days, and grade 4b with an average of 71 days.[9,10,14]

When interpreting MRI of tibial stress injury, one must be cautious about the potential pitfalls of pretibial edema and islands of tibial red marrow. Periosteal edema is typically linear and closely approximates the outer periosteal layer of bone, as opposed to pretibial edema, which is more ill-defined and located in the adjacent subcutaneous fat. Red marrow can potentially be differentiated from areas of intramedullary STIR signal because of stress change by the absence of periosteal edema in red marrow and by occurring in a different location than the patient's reported pain, although in some cases, this may be a difficult differentiation to make.

Computed tomography (CT) is not routinely used in evaluation for potential stress injury but can be used as a problem-solving tool. It may be helpful in differentiating a stress fracture from malignancy by demonstrating a clear fracture line with careful attention to the possibility of a pathologic fracture. CT can also provide use in differentiating bone scan mimics like osteoid osteoma (**Fig. 6**) and osteomyelitis from stress fracture.[11]

Specific locations/scenarios
Pelvis. The pelvis is a common location for insufficiency fractures in elderly patients with osteoporosis.[15] Sacral insufficiency fractures are particularly common, and

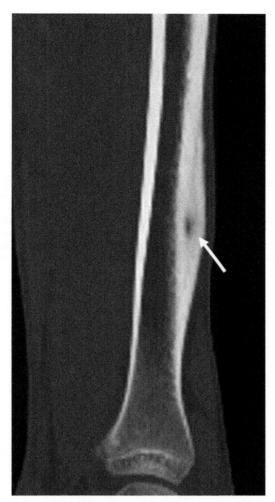

Fig. 6. Sagittal CT image in a 16-year-old boy with anterior tibial pain demonstrates a region of cortical thickening in the anterior distal tibia. There is an area of rounded lucency within the cortex (*arrow*) consistent with an osteoid osteoma, as opposed to the more linear appearance expected with a stress fracture.

may occur in a classic H-shaped distribution with vertical components in the bilateral sacral ala with a horizontal component in the midportion of the sacrum. These fractures are so common that sacral insufficiency fractures are a frequent unexpected finding when performing lumbar spine imaging (**Fig. 7**). T1-weighted images can be particularly helpful in differentiating insufficiency fractures from pathologic fractures caused by underlying neoplasm, with insufficiency fractures demonstrating a more ill-defined marrow abnormality with scattered areas of preserved hyperintense fat signal.[16] Pelvis insufficiency fractures are frequently multiple, and as such, the sacrum, parasymphseal region, pubic rami, and supra-acetabular region should be carefully scrutinized for other fractures whenever a pelvic insufficiency fracture is noted.

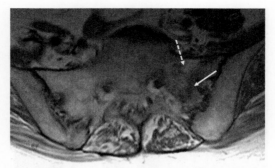

Fig. 7. Axial T1-weighted image from a lumbar spine MRI in a 77-year-old osteoporotic patient demonstrates linear T1 hypointensity (*arrow*) in the left sacral ala consistent with an insufficiency fracture. Slight decrease in T1 marrow signal (*dashed arrow*) is noted throughout the remainder of the left sacral ala relative to the other side, consistent with marrow edema. The absence of a well-defined T1 marrow low signal abnormality and scattered preservation of marrow fat makes underlying mass unlikely. Multiple vertebral body compression fractures were also seen on separate images of the lumbar spine.

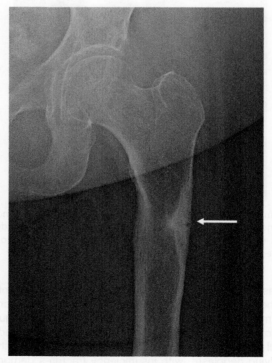

Fig. 8. A frontal radiograph from a 59-year-old woman on bisphosphonate therapy demonstrates significant cortical thickening in the lateral aspect of the subtrochanteric proximal femur, with an associated linear lucency compatible with developing insufficiency fracture. The location and appearance are the classic appearance for patients with bisphosphonate-related insufficiency changes, and place the patient at risk for progression to a complete fracture.

Bisphosphonate therapy. Bisphosphonates are a commonly prescribed medication class for patients with osteoporosis. However, bisphosphonates result in altered bone turnover, which in some patients can result in insufficiency changes. The typical location for these changes is in the lateral aspect of the proximal femoral diaphysis,[3] frequently in the subtrochanteric region (**Fig. 8**). These early insufficiency changes or even early fractures can be seen on radiographs in 2% of asymptomatic patients on bisphosphonates,[17] and are at risk of progressing to a complete transverse femoral fracture if the patient continues to bear weight and the medication is not stopped.

Subchondral location. Subchondral insufficiency fractures throughout the lower extremity have been increasingly recognized in recent years, in part as the improved resolution of current MRI scanners has allowed for improved visualization of subchondral fractures lines and differentiation from other diagnoses such as osteonecrosis.[18] These fractures typically occur in patients with a combination of overlying cartilage or meniscal damage and underlying osteoporosis. What had formerly been referred to as spontaneous osteonecrosis of the knee (SONK) in reality is caused by a subtle subchondral insufficiency fracture, typically in association with a posterior root meniscal tear (**Fig. 9**). The fracture may be so subtle that it is initially dismissed as being a slightly thickened area of subchondral bone plate, but is in reality a fracture immediately subjacent to the bone plate. Subchondral fractures in the

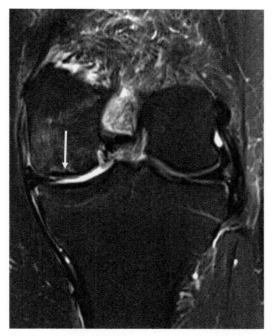

Fig. 9. Coronal T2-weighted fat-saturated image from a 69 year old woman with knee pain and osteoporosis demonstrates scattered marrow edema throughout the medial femoral condyle with subtle T2 hypointense signal along the subchondral bone plane consistent with subchondral insufficiency fracture (*arrow*). There is extrusion of the medial meniscal body secondary to a posterior root tear on other images, and scattered partial-thickness chondral loss is noted throughout the medial femoral condyle also.

femoral head are likely an underdiagnosed entity and may be confused with osteo-necrosis or transient bone marrow edema syndrome; however, visualization of the subchondral fracture line can help to confirm the diagnosis (**Fig. 10**). Subchondral insufficiency fractures in the talar dome, talar head, and metatarsal head have also been reported.

Foot/ankle. Stress fractures are particularly common in the foot and ankle. The meta-tarsal bones are the most common site for stress fractures after the tibia,[19] and are typically seen in the second and third metatarsals. Among the tarsal bones, the calca-neus is the most frequent to have a stress fracture, with the classic appearance being a sclerotic line perpendicular to the course of the normal bony trabeculae (**Fig. 11**). Navicular stress fractures are common in athletes; they are usually visualized in the sagittal plane and can be missed if the AP and oblique foot radiographs are not care-fully scrutinized (**Fig. 12**). A normal variant os supranaviculare has been reported as a risk factor for developing navicular fractures.[20]

Tibia. The tibia is the most common site of stress fracture in the body, and most of these fractures are on the compressive posteromedial side of the bone and have a good prognosis.[19] Anterior midtibial cortical stress fractures are challenging to treat and may present with multiple striations (**Fig. 13**). Plain radiographs should always be performed first in patients with anterior tibial pain, as there have been reported cases where MRI has been negative in the setting of radiographically clear anterior

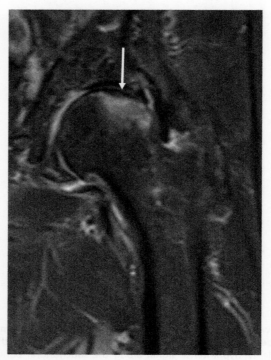

Fig. 10. Coronal T2 STIR image from a 61 year old female osteoporotic patient with hip pain demonstrates marrow edema in the superior femoral head with somewhat linear signal un-derlying the subchondral bone plate (*arrow*), consistent with insufficiency fracture.

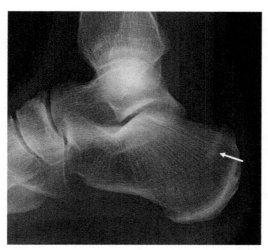

Fig. 11. Lateral radiograph from a 42-year-old woman demonstrates linear sclerosis along the calcaneal body in a perpendicular orientation to the dominant bony trabeculae (*arrow*), consistent with stress fracture.

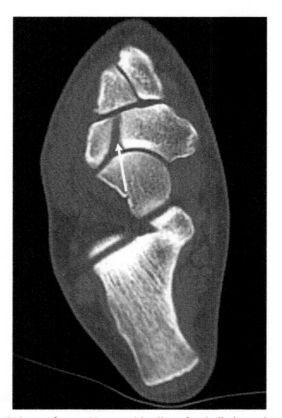

Fig. 12. Short axis CT image from a 22-year-old college football player demonstrates a sagittally oriented stress fracture through the midportion of the navicular bone.

tibial stress fractures.[21] Although most stress fractures are in a horizontal configuration in the tibia, some insufficiency fractures in the tibia have been reported to have a vertical configuration, often with a nearby nutrient foramen that may serve as a point of weakness for these fractures to develop.[22] Fibular fractures usually occur in runners in the distal third of the bone, but heal well because of the nonweight-bearing nature of the fibula.[19]

Upper extremity. Stress fractures are overall far more common in the lower extremity than the upper extremity because of weight bearing. However, upper extremity stress fractures can occur in athletes who engage in weight lifting, throwing, swinging, or weight bearing on the upper extremities through activities such as gymnastics.[23] Stress fractures of the humerus, olecranon (**Fig. 14**), and ulna have a tendency to occur in throwing athletes, particularly patients in their teens. Distal radial stress injuries have a tendency to occur in gymnasts because of bearing weight on their hands.

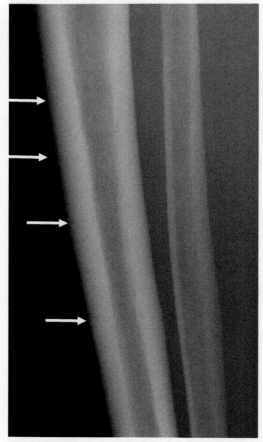

Fig. 13. Lateral radiograph from a 50-year-old man demonstrates multiple horizontal lucencies in the anterior tibia consistent with stress fractures (*arrows*). Anterior tibial stress fractures are considered high risk because of being on the convex, tensile side of the tibial bone, and may appear as multiple linear lucencies in some patients.

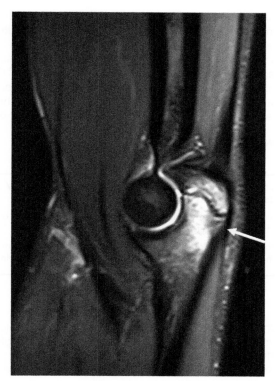

Fig. 14. Sagittal STIR MRI from a 17-year-old male athlete demonstrates significant marrow edema with a curvilinear hypointense fracture line consistent with a stress fracture.

Rib stress fractures may be seen in athletes with extensive torso rotation, such as rowing.[23]

SUMMARY

Stress injuries are a common occurrence in particular patient populations, including athletes, military recruits, and people with change in activity level, particularly if already predisposed to injury because of another risk factor like low bone mineral density. Early recognition and activity modification are important to prevent progression of the injury and to allow for quicker return to sport or normal activities. Radiographic imaging findings can be subtle and also delayed in onset relative to symptoms, making MRI a valuable tool in diagnosis of early stress injury.

Multiple factors, including the location of the injury (high-risk vs low-risk regions), underlying factors (eg, osteopenia), and severity of imaging findings can help predict recovery time. Like Fredericson and colleagues, Nattiv and colleagues found that higher MRI grade of injury correlated with longer time to return to sport. Nattiv and colleagues[8] also found lower total body density and trabecular bone stress injuries were associated with a longer time to return to sport.

An important differential consideration of a stress fracture is a pathologic fracture. On MRI, the most discriminating imaging finding of a pathologic fracture is a well-defined low signal intensity region surrounding a fracture on T1-weighted sequences representing the underlying tumor.[24] Follow up imaging in 2 to 3 weeks can also be helpful to discriminate, because a stress fracture should improve with rest while a tumor will not. CT can also help to delineate a frank fracture line.

Multiple studies suggest unrecognized stress injuries can progress to fracture, and preventative strategies may help prevent progression to fracture.[8,24] Given these findings, a low index of suspicion to pursue further evaluation with MRI should be considered in symptomatic patients with normal radiographs. This can help athletes and nonathletes progress quickly back to sports or other activities they enjoy.

CLINICS CARE POINTS

- Given the insensitivity of radiographs, especially early on, a low threshold to obtain an MRI should be considered in patients with symptoms of stress injury/fracture.

- Being aware of early, and often subtle, imaging features of stress injury can lead to earlier recognition and thus quicker return to sport/normal activity.

- Differentiating low-risk and high-risk fracture locations guides management and helps to stratify the urgency of treatment to prevent complications from developing.

REFERENCES

1. Pathria MN, Chung CB, Resnick DL. Acute and stress-related injuries of bone and cartilage: pertinent anatomy, basic biomechanics, and imaging perspective. Radiology 2016;280(1):21–38.
2. Mandell JC, Khurana B, Smith SE. Stress fractures of the foot and ankle, part 1: biomechanics of bone and principles of imaging and treatment. Skeletal Radiol 2017;46:1165–86.
3. Marshall RA, Mandell JC, Weaver MJ, et al. Imaging features and management of stress, atypical, and pathologic fractures. Radiographics 2018;38:2173–92.
4. Romani WA, Gieck JH, Perrin DH, et al. Mechanisms and management of stress fractures in physically active persons. J Athletic Train 2002;37(3):306–14.
5. Greaney RB, Gerber FH, Laughlin RL, et al. Distribution and natural history of stress fractures in U.S. Marine recruits. Radiology 1983;146:339–46.
6. Goldberg B, Pecora C. Stress fractures: a risk of increased training in freshman. Physician Sportsmed 1994;22(3):68–78.
7. Boden BP, Osbahr DC. High-risk stress fractures: evaluation and treatment. J Am Acad Orthop Surg 2000;8:344–53.
8. Nattiv A, Kennedy G, Barrack MT, et al. Correlation of MRI grading of bone stress injuries with clinical risk factors and return to play: a 5-year prospective study in collegiate track and field athletes. Am J Sports Med 2013;41(8):1930–41.
9. Mandell JC, Khurana B, Smith SE. Stress fractures of the foot and ankle, part 2: site-specific etiology, imaging, and treatment, and differential diagnosis. Skeletal Radiol 2017;4:1021–9.
10. Kaiser PB, Guss D, DiGiovanni CW. Stress fractures of the foot and ankle in athletes. Foot Ankle Orthop 2018;3:1–11.
11. Fredericson M, Jennings F, Beaulieu C, et al. Stress fractures in athletes. Top Magn Reson Imaging 2006;17(5):309–25.
12. Bergman AG, Fredericson M, Ho C, et al. Asymptomatic tibial stress reactions: MRI detection and clinical follow-up in distance runners. AJR Am J Roentgenol 2004;183(3):635–8.

13. Fredericson M, Bergman AG, Hoffman KL, et al. Tibial stress reaction in runners. Correlation of clinical symptoms and scintigraphy with a new magnetic resonance imaging grading system. Am J Sports Med 1995;23(4):472–81.
14. Kijowski R, Choi J, Shinki K, et al. Validation of MRI classification system for tibial stress injuries. Am J Roentgenol 2012;198(4):878–84.
15. Kreastan CR, Nemec U, Nemec S. Imaging of insufficiency fractures. Semin Musculoskelet Radiol 2011;15(3):198–207.
16. Fayad LM, Kamel IR, Kawamoto S, et al. Distinguishing stress fractures from pathologic fractures: a multimodality approach. Skeletal Radiol 2005;34:245–59.
17. La Rocca Vierira R, Rosenberg ZS, Allison MB, et al. Frequency of incomplete atypical femoral fractures in asymptomatic patients on long-term bisphosphonate therapy. AJR Am J Roentgenol 2012;198:1144–51.
18. Lee S, Saifuddin A. Magnetic resonance imaging of subchondral insufficiency fractures. Skeletal Radiol 2019;48:1011–21.
19. Berger FH, de Jonge MC, Maas M. Stress fractures in the lower extremity: the importance of increasing awareness amongst radiologists. Eur J Radiol 2007; 62:16–26.
20. Ingalls J, Wissman R. The os supranaviculare and navicular stress fractures. Skeletal Radiol 2011;40:937–41.
21. Smith R, Moghal M, Newton JL, et al. Negative magnetic resonance imaging in three cases of anterior tibial cortex stress fractures. Skeletal Radiol 2017;46: 1775–82.
22. Craig JG, Widman D, van Holsbeeck M. Longitudinal stress fracture: patterns of edema and the importance of the nutrient foramen. Skeletal Radiol 2003;32:22–7.
23. Jones GL. Upper extremity stress fractures. Clin Sports Med 2006;25:159–74.
24. Jones BH, Thacker SB, Gilchrist J, et al. Prevention of lower extremity stress fractures in athletes and soldiers: a systematic review. Epidemiol Rev 2002;24(2): 228–47.

Pediatric Sports Injuries

Jonathan D. Samet, MD

KEYWORDS

• Pediatric MSK • Musculoskeletal radiology • Physis

KEY POINTS

- Pediatric sports injuries are becoming more prevalent as children participate in sports.
- Pediatric injury patterns are unique because of the features of the growing skeleton including the growth plate, apophyses, cortex, and periosteum.
- This article will review the imaging appearances of the most commonly encountered pediatric sports injuries and highlight the important radiologic findings to recognize.

INTRODUCTION

Pediatric sports injuries are becoming more prevalent as children increase their participation in sports.[1] Pediatric injuries represent a unique constellation of injury due to inherent features of the growing skeleton. The physis (growth plate), cortex, and periosteum have unique properties in children. In addition, the ossifications centers, including the apophyses, serve as additional vulnerabilities in kids.

In growing bones, the physis, or growth plate, is a weak point in the bone which leads to special fractures unique to children. It is made of organized layers of chondrocytes that continuously produce a sliver of bone similar to a moving conveyer belt.

The cortex in kids is more malleable than adults and undergoes plastic deformities and buckle- or torus-type fractures with mild injury, before failing with a cortical disruption or complete fracture.[2]

Along the surface of the bone, the periosteum is an additional special feature in pediatrics. Owing to looser attachments in children, the periosteum can be stripped of the bone resulting in periosteal sleeve avulsion fractures, periosteal entrapment, and subperiosteal hemorrhages.[3]

By understanding these special features of pediatric bones, one will be prepared to predict the patterns of injury at multiple sites.

This article will focus on injuries that are unique to pediatrics and omit entities that are seen in both adults and children.

Pediatric Musculoskeletal Radiology, Department of Medical Imaging, Ann & Robert H. Lurie Children's Hospital of Chicago, Northwestern University Feinberg School of Medicine, 225 East Chicago Avenue, Chicago, IL 60614, USA
E-mail address: jonathansamet@gmail.com

Clin Sports Med 40 (2021) 781–799
https://doi.org/10.1016/j.csm.2021.05.012
0278-5919/21/© 2021 Elsevier Inc. All rights reserved.

PHYSIS

Physeal injuries can be grouped into acute and chronic. Acute injuries to the physis are characterized by the Salter-Harris (SH) classification, from 1 to 5.[4] These most often involve a part of the adjacent metaphysis or epiphysis and the physis. SH2 is the most common and involves the metaphysis and the growth plate[4] (**Fig. 1**). SH3 involves the epiphysis and growth plate (**Fig. 2**). SH4 affects the metaphysis, physis, and epiphysis. Salter-I involves the physis alone. SH5 is a crush injury to the physis and not as common. Injury to the growth plate is generally more severe as the SH number increases. Injury to the physis can lead to growth arrest. In the lower extremity, leg length discrepancy is the important complication that results. In the upper extremity, unequal bone lengths can lead to abnormal biomechanical stresses. A growth arrest will occur if there is focal sclerosis or bone bar that forms in a portion of the physis. This acts as a tether while the adjacent normal physis continues to grow leading to angular deformities. If the physeal bar is eccentric, the tethering may lead to varus or valgus deformities. A physeal bone bar can be seen on radiographs as a loss of the expected lucent line of the physis. Cross-sectional imaging with CT or MRI can more accurately depict the size of the physeal bar and allow the reader to calculate the percent of the affected physis (**Fig. 3**). In general, if the physeal bar is small, less than 50%, consideration can be made to resect the bar to restore growth potential. If the bar is extensive, epiphysiodesis of the contralateral side is considered to restore symmetric lengths.

Chronic physeal injuries result from chronic microtrauma to the growth plate and share a characteristic imaging appearance. With chronic physeal stress, a seemingly

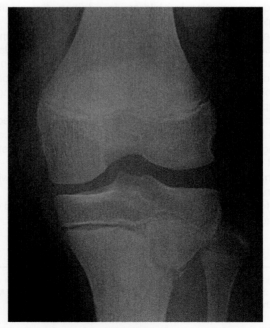

Fig. 1. AP radiograph of the knee demonstrating a fracture of the proximal tibial metaphysis extending to the medial physis where there is widening, compatible with a Salter-Harris (SH) type 2 fracture.

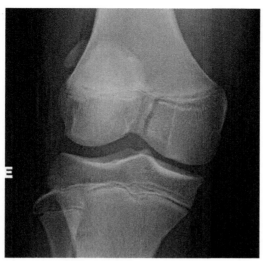

Fig. 2. AP radiograph of the knee demonstrating a fracture of the distal femoral epiphysis extending to the medial physis with widening, compatible with a Salter-Harris (SH) type 3 fracture.

counterintuitive process occurs; the physis thickens. This is thought to be due to a failure of chondrocyte apoptosis with stress that leads to a buildup of chondrocytes.[5] On imaging, the growth plate will look thicker and have irregular margins at its border with the adjacent bone. On radiographs, the lucent physis will be thicker and irregular, but the finding can be subtle and may need comparison radiographs to confirm. Similarly, on MRI, the T2 hyperintense growth plate will be thicker.

The classic examples of chronic physeal stress are "little league shoulder" and "gymnast wrist" (**Figs. 4** and **5**). But other sites can undergo similar stress responses as well, including the growth plates for the pelvic apophyses, medial epicondyle apophysis, and knee (**Fig. 6**).

Special Cases

Tibial tubercle fracture
The tibial tubercle ossification center has a physis that is continuous with the proximal tibial physis. In acute tibial tubercle fractures, there is a superiorly directed avulsion

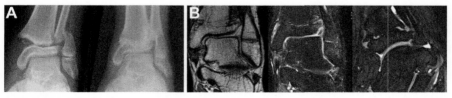

Fig. 3. (A) AP radiographs of the ankle after acute injury (*left*) and at 1-year follow-up (*right*). The acute injury shows an SH2 fracture of the distal tibia and fracture of the distal fibula. The 1-year follow-up shows narrowing and sclerosis of the distal tibial physis concerning for a growth arrest. (B) From left to right, coronal PD, coronal PDFS, and sagittal DESS MRI sequences. The coronal images show focal areas of tibial physeal bone bar formation medial and lateral. The sagittal DESS sequence clearly depicts disruption of the T2 hyperintense physis and formation of a bone bar. PD, proton density; PDFS, proton density fat suppression; DESS, dual echo steady state.

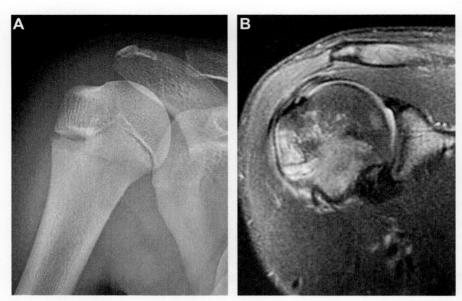

Fig. 4. (*A*) AP radiograph of the shoulder demonstrates widening and irregularity of the lateral proximal humeral physis. (*B*) T2FS coronal MRI image demonstrate widening of the T2 hyperintense lateral humeral physis with surrounding bone marrow edema. This represents a chronic physeal stress injury of the proximal humerus, compatible with "little league shoulder."

force of the patellar tendon on the tibial tubercle. In mild cases, there is widening of the tubercle physis alone. In severe cases, the physis opens similar to zipper and can extend into the proximal tibial physis and even the joint (**Fig. 7**).

The triradiate cartilage is the physis for the developing acetabulum and is y-shaped. Similar to other SH injuries, the triradiate cartilage can be fractured as well. On imaging, there may be subtle asymmetrical widening on one side (**Fig. 8**).

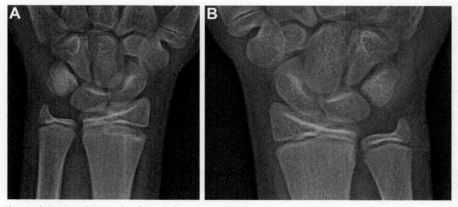

Fig. 5. (*A*) AP radiograph of the left wrist with widening and irregularity of the distal radial physis compatible with chronic physeal stress injury or "gymnast wrist." (*B*) AP radiography of the right wrist for comparison performed on the same day shows a normal distal radial growth plate.

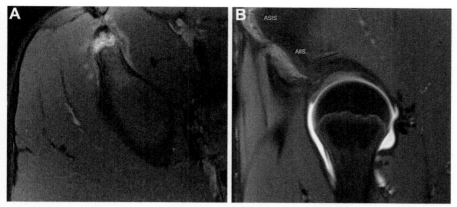

Fig. 6. (A) Axial PDFS MRI image of the right hip shows thickening of the physis for the anterior inferior iliac spine apophysis (AIIS). (B) Sagittal PDFS image of the same hip demonstrates thickening of the physis for the AIIS and anterior superior iliac spine apophyses. This is an example of chronic physeal stress injury.

CORTEX

In developing bones, the cortex is more malleable than the adult cortex.[2] The cortex is similar to an immature tree branch. A greenstick, or immature branch, is able to bend considerably before it cracks. With mild forces, the cortex wrinkles and gives rise to buckle- or torus-type fractures. The bone can also bend or bow, known as a bowing

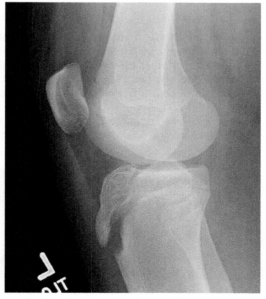

Fig. 7. Lateral radiograph of the knee with widening of the tibial tubercle physis, and intra-articular propagation of fracture into the anterior tibial epiphysis.

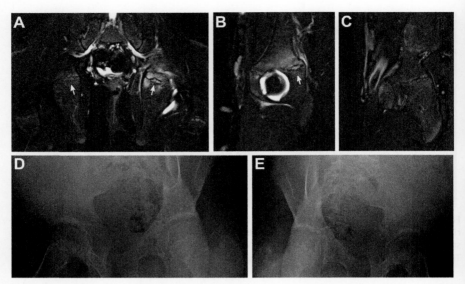

Fig. 8. (A, B) Coronal and Sagittal T2FS MRI images show asymmetrical thickening and T2 hyperintensity (arrows) of the left triradiate cartilage compatible with acute physeal fracture similar to an SH1. (C) Sagittal T2FS image of the unaffected normal right triradiate cartilage. (D, E) Right and left oblique views of the pelvis on follow-up demonstrate healing callus around the persistently widened left triradiate cartilage fracture.

fracture or plastic deformity. If part of the cortex breaks, but part is intact, this is known as a greenstick fracture, or incomplete fracture (**Fig. 9**).

APOPHYSIS

Apophyses are small rounded ossification centers that are attached to ends of long bones, pelvis, and other sites. They have a physis that attaches them to their parent bone. Often tendons attach to these small ossicles and exert an avulsion stress which can be acute or chronic, repetitive in nature. Unlike adults, where the tendon often fails before the bone, in pediatrics, the weaker physis and small apophyses are vulnerable to injury.[6]

In the elbow, the medial epicondyle apophysis is subjected to pull from the common flexor tendon origin. In acute injury, the tendon can avulse the medial epicondyle off

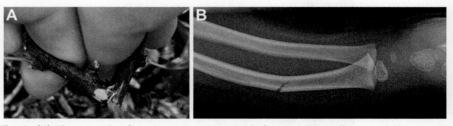

Fig. 9. (A) Photograph of an immature greenstick fracture. Note that one side remains intact. (B) Radiograph of an incomplete-type "greenstick" fracture of the distal radius. The cortex remains intact on one side in these unique pediatric fracture.

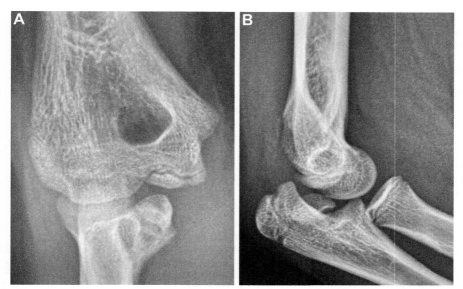

Fig. 10. (*A, B*) AP and lateral radiographs of the elbow. On the AP view, the expected medial epicondyle apophysis is missing but identified in the medial aspect of the ulnohumeral joint. On the lateral view, the medial epicondyle has been avulsed into the elbow joint.

the humerus. If severe, the apophysis can be displaced into the elbow joint (**Fig. 10**). With chronic microrepetitive trauma, such as in little league elbow, the valgus stresses can lead to sclerosis and fragmentation of the apophysis. The physis for the medial epicondyle can be thickened as a sign of physeal stress as well (**Fig. 11**).

In the pelvis, there are multiple apophyses from which tendons originate. Acute and chronic injuries can occur at each site producing characteristic injury patterns. The symmetry of the pelvis is very helpful in these cases. Common apophyses affected by injury are the anterior inferior iliac spine, anterior superior iliac spine, and ischial apophysis. Similar to other sites, these apophyses can be avulsed with displacement

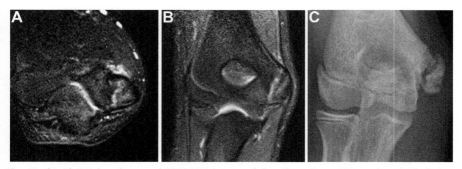

Fig. 11. (*A, B*) Axial and coronal T2FS MRI image of the elbow in an 18-year baseball pitcher. There is thickening of the physis for the medial epicondyle and bone marrow edema of the apophysis. (*C*) AP radiograph of the same elbow, with widening of the medial epicondyle physis. The apophysis is sclerotic and partially fragmented. These findings are compatible with chronic avulsion stress on the medial epicondyle apophysis and physis.

in acute injury, or affected by chronic microtrauma (**Fig. 12**). Sometimes there is a delay in presentation of a displaced apophyseal avulsion, and the hypertrophic healing bone can mimic a tumor (**Fig. 13**).

PERIOSTEUM

The periosteum is a two-layered structure that covers the surface of the cortex including an inner layer called the cambium and an outer fibrous layer.[7] It reacts to processes that affect the underlying bone, the most common of which being fractures. The younger a child is, the more robust a periosteal reaction occurs. Periosteal new bone formation appears typically 14 days after a fracture.[8] Therefore, if there is concern of a subtle occult fracture at the time of injury, it is common for a radiologist to recommend a 14-day follow-up to detect healing periosteal reaction (**Fig. 14**).

Periosteum can be stripped off the cortex in acute trauma because it has looser attachments to the cortex in children than in adults.[3] If it avulses with a sliver of bone, it is known as a periosteal sleeve avulsion fracture. The classic site is the inferior pole of the patella (**Fig. 15**). This can also occur at the distal clavicle.

In patients with neurogenic conditions, extensive subperiosteal hemorrhages can strip the periosteum off the bone for a long segment after an occult fracture (**Fig. 16**).

Rarely, the periosteal can become displaced and entrapped in the physis (**Fig. 17**).

KNEE
Osteochondritis Dissecans

Osteochondritis dissecans is a special pediatric type of osteochondral lesion that has predilection sites for the capitellum of the elbow, talar dome of the ankle, and medial femoral condyle of the knee. The pathophysiology is unclear but thought to be a combination of vascular insufficiency and overuse. While name implies inflammation, this has not been found on pathology. Fibrovascular tissue, similar to a healing fracture, has been reported.[9] Dissecans, from Latin *dissec*, meaning to separate, well describes the pathophysiology, as an osteochondral fragment has the potential to separate off the parent bone.

Attempts should be made to assess the stability of the lesion on MRI; however, correlation of imaging findings with arthroscopic findings is not as clear as that in adults.[9]

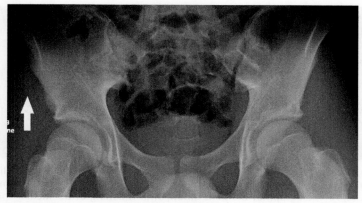

Fig. 12. Frog-leg lateral radiograph of the pelvis demonstrating an acute displaced avulsion fracture of the right anterior superior iliac spine.

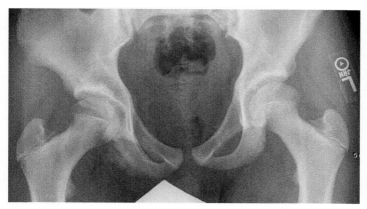

Fig. 13. AP radiograph of the pelvis with prominent ossification of the right ischial tuberosity which could be misinterpreted as osteosarcoma. This case was a healing avulsion fracture of the ischial apophysis.

Nevertheless, features of the lesion from superficial to deep can be described. This systematic outside-in approach is useful to characterize all the features. The overlying articular cartilage and subchondral bone plate should be assessed for fissures, defects, and disruption. The lesion will typically have a "sequestered" fragment which is a piece of subchondral bone that can be readily identified and measured. Deep margin features can include a fluid cleft and cyst formation. The greater the number and size of perilesional cysts, the poorer the healing potential of the OCD.[10] Well-formed fluid clefts bounded by hypointense sclerotic lines are associated with instability. Disruption in the subchondral bone plate is also an unstable finding. The lesions will sometimes be partially detached, a clear finding of instability. The most severe instance is when the osteochondral fragment separates completely of the parent bone and becomes a loose body, leaving a defect (**Fig. 18**).

Anterior cruciate ligament tears occur in pediatrics and adult medicine; however, anterior cruciate ligament tears (ACL) footplate avulsion fractures are unique to children. In this entity, the often intact ACL will avulse a fragment of bone off the tibial eminence.[11] Treatment may involve internal fixation of the footplate. The radiographs can be deceivingly mild in appearance because there may be a small sliver of bone floating above the tibial eminence (**Fig. 19**).

DISCOID MENISCUS

Discoid meniscus is a developmentally enlarged meniscus, almost always the lateral meniscus. Discoid menisci are prone to intrasubstance degeneration and tearing (**Fig. 20**).[12] In pediatrics, no well-established criteria exist on MRI for measurement. However, if the inner margin of the meniscus at the level of the meniscal body extends beyond the midpoint of the femoral condyle on a coronal slice, or if the meniscus is seen on 3 consecutive slices of the sagittal, a discoid meniscus should be suspected. It may also be enlarged in the craniocaudal dimension as well.

PATELLOFEMORAL DISLOCATION

Patellofemoral dislocation and instability are a common entity in pediatric sports medicine.[13] Imaging findings after acute injury and chronic maltracking will be discussed.

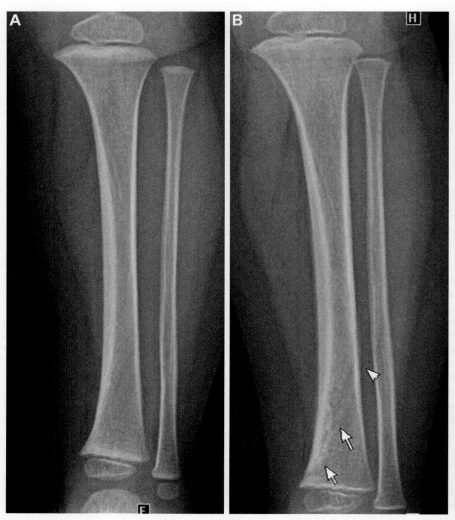

Fig. 14. (*A, B*) AP radiographs of the tibia/fibula at time of injury (*A*) and 2 wk later (*B*). On the initial film, there is no definite fracture. On the follow-up film, there is subtle periosteal reaction (*arrowhead*) along the lateral cortex, and an oblique partially sclerotic fracture line in the distal tibial metadiaphysis. This is a typical tibial spiral fracture (toddler's fracture).

In acute dislocation, the patella will translate laterally, and the medial patella will contuse the lateral femoral condyle before self-reduction. Radiographs are often normal, but MRI will show the bone contusions in these areas, alerting the radiologist of the patellofemoral dislocation relocation event. The medial patellar injury can be extra-articular or intra-articular, the latter of which can cause an osteochondral fracture. A thorough search must be made for an intra-articular body, reported in 12% to 42% of dislocations.[13] This results from an osteochondral fracture that detaches off the patella and into the joint. A loose body or intra-articular body is usually an indication for surgery.[14] In patients with chronic patellar instability, knee MRI is helpful to assess anatomy that may predispose to maltracking. Patella alta, trochlear dysplasia,

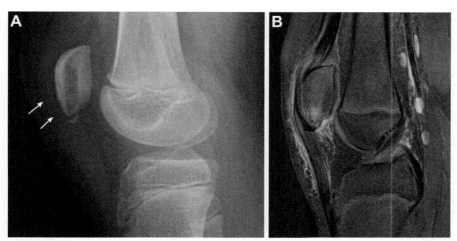

Fig. 15. (A) Lateral knee radiograph showing a thin crescentic bone fragment (arrows) avulsed off the anterior inferior patellar surface. (B) Sagittal PDFS MRI image demonstrating an avulsion fracture off the anterior patella including the hypointense periosteum, cortex, and piece of underlying unossified bone. There is associated strain of the extensor mechanism. Findings are classic for patellar sleeve avulsion fracture.

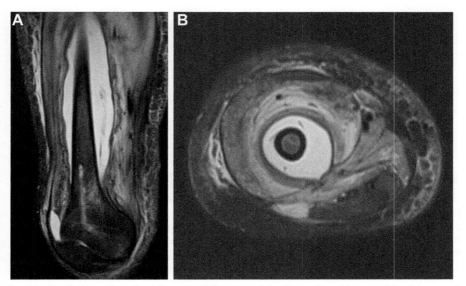

Fig. 16. (A, B) Coronal and axial T2FS MRI images of the femur in a 16 year with a history of spinal cord injury. There is a large subperiosteal fluid collection spanning most of the femur and circumferentially. The periosteum is the wavy T2 hypointense structure lifted off the cortex. After drainage and bone biopsy, no infection was found, and this was a chronic subperiosteal hemorrhage.

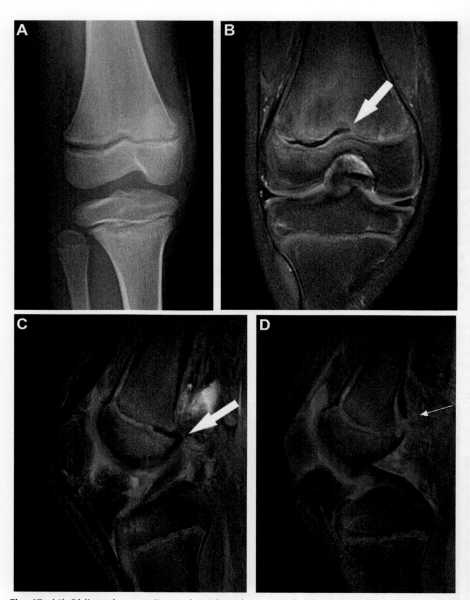

Fig. 17. (*A*) Oblique knee radiograph with widening and irregularity of the distal femoral physis compatible with an SH1 fracture. Coronal (*B*) and sagittal (*C, D*) PD FS images demonstrate a torn and displaced periosteum (*small white arrow*) that has become entrapped in the physis (*large white arrows*).

hypoplastic medial trochlear facet, lateral patellar tilt, elevated tibial tuberosity trochlear groove distance, and superolateral Hoffa's fat pad edema are findings associated with patellar maltracking and important to communicate to our orthopedic colleagues.[15]

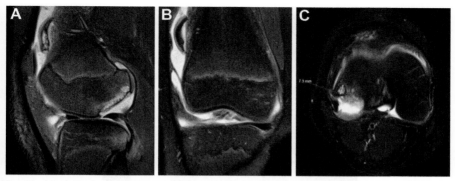

Fig. 18. (A–C) Sagittal (A), coronal (B), and axial (C) T2FS MR images demonstrating a detached osteochondral fragment from a pre-existing osteochondritis dissecans lesion in the medial femoral condyle. The large intra-articular body is clearly seen in the lateral superior joint recess. At the site of the osteochondral defect, note the large perilesional cyst which is a finding associated with instability.

ELBOW

Elbow fractures are common in the pediatric population. In descending order of prevalence, there is the supracondylar, lateral condyle, and medial epicondyle fractures.[16] The elbow development is complex with multiple ossification centers appearing sequentially in a relatively predictable pattern. These ossification centers can cause difficulty in interpretation, mimicking avulsion fractures. The trochlea can have a fragmented appearance as it develops. "CRITOE" is a helpful mnemonic for the order of appearance of the elbow ossification centers: Capitellum, Radial head, Internal condyle (medial epicondyle), Trochlea, Olecranon, and External condyle (lateral

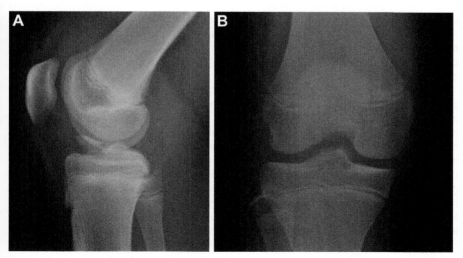

Fig. 19. (A, B) Lateral and AP radiographs of the knee show an anterior cruciate ligament footplate avulsion fracture, with a displaced tibial eminence fragment seen on the intercondylar notch.

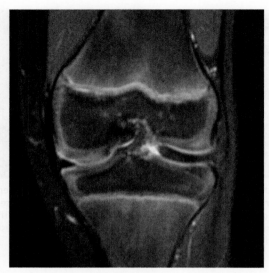

Fig. 20. Coronal T2FS MRI image of the knee in a 3-year-old demonstrating a very large lateral meniscus extending nearly to the intercondylar notch and with intrasubstance degenerative signal, compatible with discoid meniscus.

epicondyle). The mnemonic is most useful in the case of a medial epicondyle avulsion fracture because it alerts the observer that the expected apophysis is missing, therefore prompting a further search. Medial epicondyle avulsion fracture is discussed in detail under the apophysis section.

Supracondylar fractures of the distal humerus are most often due to a hyperextension mechanism, and the distal fragment becomes angulated and displaced posteriorly. In mild injury, there is posterior angulation but no cortical disruption. As severity increases, the anterior cortex will fracture, followed by the posterior cortex. The anterior humeral line is a useful tool to assess for subtle posterior angulation in mild fractures. The line is drawn along the anterior humeral cortex and should bisect the capitellar ossification center. If the line is entirely anterior to the capitellum, this is usually an indication for surgical fixation.[17]

Lateral condyle fractures can be an SH2 or SH4. The fracture is in the low metaphysis of the distal humerus and extends to the growth plate. If the fracture extends into the epiphysis, it is an SH4. The difficulty in interpretation is that the epiphysis, namely the trochlea, has not usually ossified at the age that lateral condyle fractures occur and therefore is invisible on radiographs. Therefore, the fracture gap in the metaphysis is used to guided management. If there is 2 mm or less of displacement, the fracture can be treated with casting alone, but under close follow-up. If there is greater than 2 mm displacement, there is more likely the possibility that the fracture had extended to the joint, and internal fixation is warranted (**Fig. 21**). Unrecognized SH4 lateral condyle fractures can lead to malunion or nonunion, and therefore, there is a low threshold to surgically intervene if there is a suggestion of displacement, defined as greater than 2 mm. Oblique views are essential to fully evaluate lateral condyle fractures.[18]

Monteggia fracture dislocation is a specific pattern of injury in which there is a radial head dislocation and proximal ulnar fracture (**Fig. 22**).

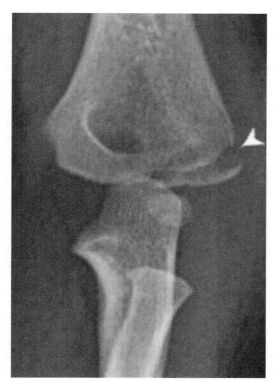

Fig. 21. AP elbow radiograph in a 2-year-old demonstrating a mildly displaced lateral condyle fracture. The displacement measured 3 mm, and this patient underwent internal fixation.

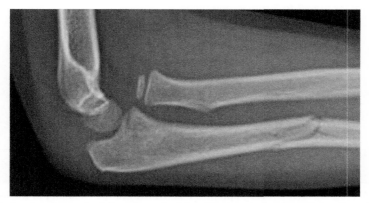

Fig. 22. Lateral radiograph of the elbow depicts a Monteggia fracture-dislocation characterized by anterior dislocation of the radial head and proximal ulna fracture.

HIP

Hip injuries specific to pediatrics include slipped capital femoral epiphysis (SCFE), stress fractures, and avulsion fractures (discussed previously). As labral tears, femoroacetabular and ischiofemoral impingement are also seen in adults, they will not be discussed here.

SCFE is a condition seen in adolescents, where the femoral neck displaces in relation to the head, therefore damaging the growth plate. The head remains articulated with the acetabulum, but the femur shifts. Obesity is the main risk factor, and it can be bilateral in up to one-third of patients. Anterior-Posterior and frog-leg lateral films will show SCFE which is characterized by widening of the physis and offset of the head and neck. Klein's line can be helpful to detect subtle slips, drawn along the lateral margin of the femoral neck and should intersect with the lateral femoral head. In early or subtle SCFE, MRI can be used for diagnosis and will show asymmetrical thickening of the T2 hyperintense physis (**Fig. 23**).

Femoral stress fractures occur along the medial and less frequently the lateral femoral neck. On radiograph, there may be a sclerotic line from the medial neck which terminates in the medullary space a short distance from the cortex. On MRI, the stress fracture will be hypointense on T1 and T2, and there will be surrounding bone marrow edema.

ANKLE

Ankle fractures specific to pediatrics are the juvenile Tillaux and triplane fractures. Juvenile Tillaux fracture is an SH3 fracture of the distal tibial epiphysis, caused by an avulsion of the anterior tibiofibular ligament. It is typically seen in adolescents aged approximately 12 to 14 years, as the child is nearing growth plate closure. The anterolateral tibial epiphysis is avulsed producing a characteristic imaging appearance (**Fig. 24**). Surgical fixation is indicated if the displacement is greater than 2 mm. This is distinguished from the triplane fracture which occurs in a slightly younger age group. It is an SH4-type fracture involving the distal tibial metaphysis, physis, and epiphysis. There is a vertically oriented sagittal plane fracture through the epiphysis, an axial plane fracture at the physis, and coronal plane fracture in the metaphysis. Therefore, on an AP view, Tillaux and triplane fractures can appear similarly. The lateral view, which identifies the coronal plane fracture of the metaphysis, is what distinguishes the triplane fracture (**Fig. 25**). Similarly, surgical intervention is indicated if displacement is greater than 2 to 3 mm in any plane.[19]

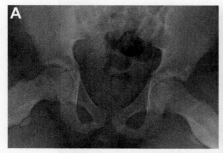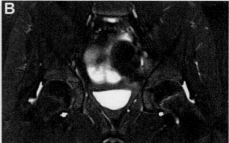

Fig. 23. (*A*) Frog-leg lateral radiograph of the pelvis with subtle widening of the left proximal femoral physis and suggesting of subtle slip. (*B*) MRI confirmed subtle SCFE with asymmetrical widening of the T2 hyperintense left proximal femoral physis.

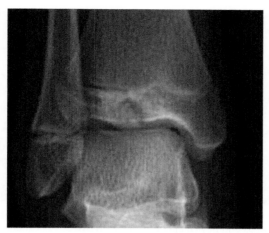

Fig. 24. AP radiograph of ankle with a vertically oriented fracture of the distal tibial epiphysis and widening of the lateral physis compatible with an SH3 juvenile Tillaux fracture.

Osteochondritis dissecans can affect the talar dome as mentioned previously, typically, medially. Evaluation of the lesion with MRI for signs of instability, similar to knee OCD, will help guide management.

Similar to adults, accessory ossicles can be incidental or potentially symptomatic including, os naviculare, os trigonum, and os peroneum.

Tarsal coalition can be a source of pain and limited range of motion. The two most common types are calcaneonavicular and talocalcaneal coalitions (**Fig. 26**). Coalitions

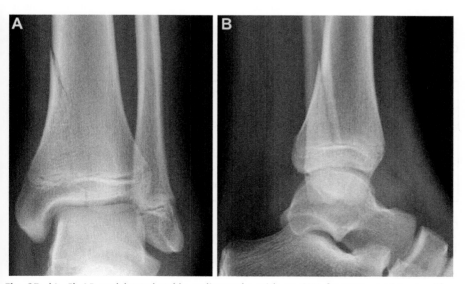

Fig. 25. (*A, B*) AP and lateral ankle radiographs with an SH4 fracture consistent with a triplane fracture. The AP and lateral views show the coronally oriented fracture of the metaphysis. The AP shows widening of the lateral physis and sagittal oriented fracture through the epiphysis.

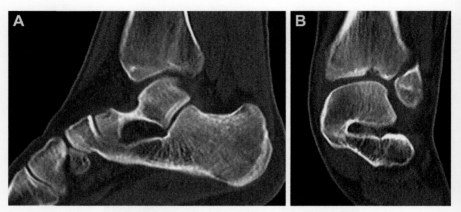

Fig. 26. (*A*) Sagittal CT image of the ankle with solid osseous bridging between the anterior process of the calcaneus and navicular consistent with osseous calcaneonavicular tarsal coalition. (*B*) Coronal CT image of the ankle with solid bridging of the medial subtalar joint between the talus and calcaneus, compatible with osseous talocalcaneal tarsal coalition.

are osseous or nonosseous. On radiographs, calcaneonavicular coalition is best identified on an oblique foot radiograph. Talocalcaneal coalition most commonly affects the middle facet of the subtalar joint and can be seen on a Harris view or on the lateral view of the ankle where there is sometimes a continuous "C" sign. CT and MRI are very helpful to confirm the diagnosis of coalition and guide operative management.

As in adults, anterior talofibular ligament is the most commonly injured ankle ligament. MRI can depict the ruptured ligament in acute injury with a fluid gap and retracted ligament seen. Ultrasound can also identify anterior talofibular ligament tears and may be useful in the setting of chronic tear and instability to identify ligament insufficiency with dynamic maneuvers.

CLINICS CARE POINTS

- Injury to the physis can be acute or chronic resulting in a spectrum of imaging abnormalities ranging from thickening to fusion.
- The pediatric cortex is more malleable than adults, which results in unique buckle and incomplete type fractures.
- Apophyses are small ossification centers that can avulse and be radiographically subtle, especially if displaced into the elbow joint.
- The periosteum has looser attachments in children and can be displaced from the cortex.

DISCLOSURE

The authors have nothing to disclose.

REFERENCES

1. Trentacosta N. Pediatric sports injuries. Pediatr Clin 2020;67(1):205–25.
2. Mabrey JD, Fitch RD. Plastic deformation in pediatric fractures: mechanism and treatment. J Pediatr Orthop 1989;9(3):310–4.

3. Bisseret D, Kaci R, Lafage-Proust M-H, et al. Periosteum: characteristic imaging findings with emphasis on radiologic-pathologic comparisons. Skeletal Radiol 2015;44(3):321–38.
4. Cepela DJ, Tartaglione JP, Dooley TP, et al. Classifications in brief: Salter-Harris classification of pediatric physeal fractures. Clinical Orthopaedics and Related Research 2016;474(11):2531–7.
5. Nguyen JC, Markhardt BK, Merrow AC, et al. Imaging of pediatric growth plate disturbances. Radiographics 2017;37(6):1791–812.
6. Bateni C, Bindra J, Haus B. MRI of sports injuries in children and adolescents: what's different from adults. Curr Radiol Rep 2014;2(5):45.
7. Laor T, Jaramillo D. It's time to recognize the perichondrium. Pediatr Radiol 2020; 50(2):153–60.
8. Rana RS, Wu JS, Eisenberg RL. Periosteal reaction. Am J Roentgenology 2009; 193(4):W259–72.
9. Kijowski R, Blankenbaker DG, Shinki K, et al. Juvenile versus adult osteochondritis dissecans of the knee: appropriate MR imaging criteria for instability. Radiology 2008;248(2):571–8.
10. Krause M, Hapfelmeier A, Möller M, et al. Healing predictors of stable juvenile osteochondritis dissecans knee lesions after 6 and 12 months of nonoperative treatment. Am J Sports Med 2013;41(10):2384–91.
11. LaFrance RM, Giordano B, Goldblatt J, et al. Pediatric tibial eminence fractures: evaluation and management. J Am Acad Orthop Surg 2010;18(7):395–405.
12. Rohren EM, Kosarek FJ, Helms CA. Discoid lateral meniscus and the frequency of meniscal tears. Skeletal Radiol 2001;30(6):316–20.
13. Zaidi A, Babyn P, Astori I, et al. MRI of traumatic patellar dislocation in children. Pediatr Radiol 2006;36(11):1163–70.
14. Farr J, Covell DJ, Lattermann C. Cartilage lesions in patellofemoral dislocations: incidents/locations/when to treat. Sports Med Arthrosc Rev 2012;20(3):181.
15. Earhart C, Patel DB, White EA, et al. Transient lateral patellar dislocation: review of imaging findings, patellofemoral anatomy, and treatment options. Emerg Radiol 2013;20(1):11–23.
16. Ladenhauf HN, Schaffert M, Bauer J. The displaced supracondylar humerus fracture: indications for surgery and surgical options a 2014 update. Curr Opin Pediatr 2014;26(1):64–9.
17. Iorio C, Crostelli M, Mazza O, et al. Conservative versus surgical treatment of Gartland type 2 supracondylar humeral fractures: what can help us choosing? J Orthop 2019;16(1):31–5.
18. Song KS, Waters PM. Lateral condylar humerus fractures: which ones should we fix? J Pediatr Orthop 2012;32:S5–9.
19. Crawford AH. Triplane and Tillaux fractures: is a 2 mm residual gap acceptable? J Pediatr Orthop 2012;32:S69–73.

Ultrasound in Sports Injuries

Cristy N. French, MD[a],*, Eric A. Walker, MD[b,c], Shawn F. Phillips, MD[d], Jayson R. Loeffert, DO[e]

KEYWORDS

• Ultrasound • Sports injuries • Tendon • Ligament • Muscle

KEY POINTS

• Utilization of musculoskeletal ultrasound in sports medicine has dramatically increased in the last two decades.
• Ultrasound can supplement the clinical examination to establish a diagnosis, estimate prognosis, and guide treatment of sports injuries.
• There are unique advantages of ultrasound over other imaging modalities for sports imaging.
• Musculoskeletal ultrasound can provide a detailed evaluation of muscles, tendons, ligaments, and nerves.
• Ultrasound guidance can also improve accuracy in targeted percutaneous injection therapies.

 Video content accompanies this article at http://www.sportsmed.theclinics. com.

INTRODUCTION

Nearly 20% of the United States population engaged in sports or exercise on a daily basis from 2010 to 2019.[1] As expected, exercise and sports-related injuries are common, both in the elite athlete and in the general population. These injuries frequently lead to sport participation absence or contact with the health care system.[1] A thorough history and physical examination of the injured athlete frequently establishes the source of pain or dysfunction. Imaging can afford additional diagnostic information

[a] Department of Radiology, Penn State Health Milton S. Hershey Medical Center, 500 University Drive, MB HG300T, Hershey, PA 17033, USA; [b] Department of Radiology, Penn State Health Milton S. Hershey Medical Center, 500 University Drive, MB HG300V, Hershey, PA 17033, USA; [c] Uniformed Services University of the Health Sciences, Bethesda, MD, USA; [d] Department of Family and Community Medicine, Penn State Health Medical Group Mount Joy, 201 Lefever Road, Mount Joy, PA 17552, USA; [e] Department of Family and Community Medicine, Penn State Health Medical Group Middletown, 3100 Schoolhouse Road, Middletown, PA 17057, USA
* Corresponding author.
E-mail address: Cfrench2@pennstatehealth.psu.edu

Clin Sports Med 40 (2021) 801–819
https://doi.org/10.1016/j.csm.2021.05.013
0278-5919/21/© 2021 Elsevier Inc. All rights reserved.

sportsmed.theclinics.com

when the clinical picture is unclear or further information is necessary for risk stratification and treatment planning.

Each imaging modality has certain advantages over others, and they are best used as complementary tools to provide the best care for the patient[2] (**Table 1**). MRI is particularly useful in cases of vague or diffuse pain, evaluation of deep soft-tissue structures and bones, and intra-articular structures. Propelled by advances in technology over the last 20 years, ultrasound (US) utilization in musculoskeletal imaging and, in particular, sports medicine has dramatically increased.[3] Compact portable US machines are becoming increasingly available, affording prompt diagnosis of sports injuries on the field.[3] With the development of high-frequency transducers, the spatial resolution of US is superior to MRI for superficial structures.[4] As a result, US can provide a detailed evaluation of targeted musculoskeletal structures.

The real-time nature of US provides the opportunity to interact with the athlete and correlate symptoms with sonographic findings, potentially rendering an immediate diagnosis. In addition, US affords the unique capability to dynamically evaluate structures. US guidance can also improve accuracy in targeted percutaneous injection therapies.[2] Some of the most significant disadvantages of US are the relatively long learning curve and inherent operator dependence. Dedicated training and standardized technique can minimize these limitations.

Most sports US evaluations entail a targeted regional examination relevant to the patient's clinical symptoms. A complete discussion of all injuries encountered in sports medicine is beyond the scope of this article. Instead, the aim is to provide a brief review of the general US appearance of soft-tissue injuries of muscles, tendons, ligaments, and nerves highlighting its use in the diagnosis of several sport-specific injuries.

Sonographic Equipment and Technique

Most musculoskeletal sports injuries are well-suited for US evaluation as most structures are superficial. High-frequency (9–18 MHz) linear array transducers with a small footprint provide excellent detail and spatial resolution. Lower frequency transducers (6 MHz) may be required to evaluate deeper structures, such as the hip joint, particularly in larger patients.[5] It is important to be familiar with common US parameters and machine operation. Proper patient positioning, transducer placement, and machine

Table 1 Advantages of musculoskeletal ultrasound and MRI	
Advantages of Ultrasound	**Advantages of MRI**
Low cost	Large field of view
No ionizing radiation	Superior contrast resolution
No hardware artifact	Bone marrow edema
MRI incompatible devices	Sensitive for subtle soft tissue edema
Increasing availability	Intra-articular structure evaluation
Portability	Surgical planning
Quick contralateral comparison	
Direct correlation with symptoms	
Immediate results	
Dynamic capability	
Procedure guidance	

settings are essential for optimal image acquisition. Owing to the limited field of view, accurate interpretation requires detailed knowledge of the relevant musculoskeletal anatomy and awareness of potential artifacts and pitfalls. A standardized protocol for assessment of structures in both the transverse and longitudinal planes ensures a complete examination. Sonographic palpation can be used to correlate the site of pain with the US images, which further increases the sensitivity of US. Doppler imaging is also helpful to assess tissue vascularity in the setting of acute inflammation or chronic neovascularization.[6]

Normal Sonographic Appearance of Musculoskeletal Structures

On US, normal muscles are hypoechoic relative to subcutaneous fat with internal hyperechoic septations representing perimysium connective tissue surrounding the bundles of muscle fibers. In the transverse plane, the alternating hypoechoic muscle fibers and hyperechoic perimysium result in the so-called pennate or "starry sky" appearance.[6] In long axis, muscles appear striated (**Fig. 1**).

A tendon consists of a tightly packed parallel array of collagen fibers with supporting connective tissue.[4] On US, tendons are hyperechoic with an organized fibrillar pattern in longitudinal axis or a "paint brush" appearance in short axis due to visualization of individual tendon fibers.[6] This normal sonographic appearance occurs when the US beam is 90° to the tendon. As the tendon is imaged at increasing or decreasing angles relative to the perpendicular, it appears progressively hypoechoic. This artifact, known as anisotropy, represents a potential pitfall in US imaging and may be misinterpreted for pathology. Other musculoskeletal structures manifest anisotropy but to a lesser degree[6] (**Box 1**). A heel-toe or toggle maneuver of the transducer when in the longitudinal or transverse plane, respectively or beam steering, performed by advanced US machines/transducers may be helpful to eliminate anisotropy.[6]

Similar to tendons, normal ligaments are also hyperechoic, but the fibrillar echotexture is more compact.[6] When surrounded by echogenic fat, ligaments may appear relatively hypoechoic.[6] Nerves demonstrate a fascicular pattern on US. The normal appearance of a nerve in short axis is that of hypoechoic fascicles separated by echogenic perineurium resulting in a "honey-comb" appearance. The long-axis appearance has been likened to a bundle of straws. Nerves are less prone to anisotropy, which can aid in differentiating nerve from tendon or ligament.[6]

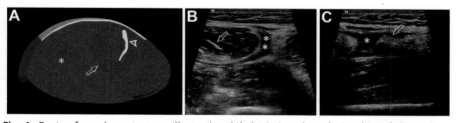

Fig. 1. Rectus femoris acute tear. Illustration (*A*) depicting the relationship of the indirect and direct heads of the rectus femoris muscle. Shown are the inner/central indirect (*arrow*) head with tendon (*arrowhead*) and superficial direct (*asterisk*) head. Ultrasound transverse (*B*) and longitudinal (*C*) images with 9-MHz transducer of a patient with left thigh pain after a strenuous martial arts session. Peripheral myofascial partial thickness tear (grade II) along the medial margin of the superficial direct head rectus femoris with interposed hematoma (*asterisks*). Note the mild hypoechoic edema around the inner/central indirect head tendon (*arrow*) compatible with grade I strain. Long-axis image (*C*) shows retracted tendon stump (*arrow*) and interposed hematoma (*asterisk*).

Box 1
Order of sonographic anisotropy of musculoskeletal structures

Tendons > Ligaments > Muscles > Nerves

Sports Injuries

Muscles

Evaluation of muscles and tendons for strain or tear is one of the most common applications of musculoskeletal US in sports medicine. Acute muscle injuries can be divided into two general categories based on the mechanism of injury. The first category involves direct impact or crush injury, resulting in muscular contusion or laceration. Initially, the intramuscular hematoma often appears as a heterogeneous hyperechoic, ill-defined region or collection that becomes more hypoechoic over time.[7]

The second category is an indirect injury caused by excessive stretching of the muscle, often during concomitant muscle contraction. These stretch or strain injuries frequently occur at the musculotendinous junction and have a predilection for myotendinous units that span two joints, such as the rectus femoris, hamstrings, or gastrocnemius muscles. Tears can be intramuscular or occur at the myofascial junction and, in some cases, avulse directly from bone.[7] Clinically, these injuries are graded on degree of severity from "strain" (grade I) to essentially complete tear (grade III), and this grading system provides important information on prognosis and expected recovery times[8] (**Table 2**). US injury grading matches the clinical grading scale.[8] An area of healed tear with fibrotic scar tissue may be isoechoic or frequently hyperechoic to the surrounding musculature, often with associated muscular volume loss (see **Fig. 1**). The US appearance of muscular fatty degeneration includes abnormal architecture with loss of the muscle pennate pattern and increased echogenicity. In severe cases, decreased muscle bulk can be seen in the setting of atrophy. Occasionally, heterotopic ossification may occur at the site of prior injury, presenting as a hyperechoic focus with posterior acoustic shadowing.

Table 2
Grading of muscle injuries

Grade	% Muscle Involvement (Cross-Sectional Diameter)	Ultrasound Findings	Average SPA
I	<5%	Normal Focal/regional areas hyperechogenicity Perifascial fluid without fiber interruption	~2 wk
II	5%–50%	Partial fiber disruption Hypoechoic/anechoic fluid in gap + Hypervascularity around injury	~2–6 wk
III	>50%	Extensive to complete fiber disruption with retraction Extensive hematoma (hypoechoic/anechoic fluid in gap) + Hypervascularity around injury	~6–12 wk +

Abbreviation: SPA, sport participation absence.

Rectus Femoris Tear

The rectus femoris is the most commonly injured quadriceps muscle.[7,9] Injuries are common in sprinters, soccer, football, and martial arts athletes. Although the typical tendon pathology (tendinosis, calcific tendinosis, tear, avulsion) involving the proximal or distal tendon is common, the distinctive anatomy of the rectus femoris musculotendinous unit leads to a unique pattern of injury.[10] A unipennate muscle arises from the direct head and surrounds an inner bipennate muscle arising from the indirect head (see **Fig. 1**). This unique anatomy predisposes to central aponeurosis and myotendinous junction tears isolated to the substance of the muscle.

These injuries manifest with various US appearances based on the location of injury and degree of severity. Mild strain may reveal fluid surrounding the central indirect head tendon, the interface between the inner and outer rectus femoris muscles, or the myofascial junction of the peripheral direct head component[9,10] (see **Fig. 1**; **Fig. 2**). More severe injuries will result in partial or complete disruption of muscle fibers. Comparison with the contralateral side may be helpful to discern subtle abnormalities. Follow-up studies often show an ill-defined hyperechoic scar centered on the central aponeurosis with associated muscle atrophy resulting in a palpable depression in the muscle[9,10] (see **Fig. 2**). Contraction of the normal muscle surrounding the atrophic scar tissue may even clinically mimic a mass.[10,11]

Tennis Leg

Recent studies have revealed that medial head gastrocnemius tears are more common than plantaris rupture as a cause of tennis leg.[12,13] The classic history is acute medial calf pain in a middle-aged athlete during active ankle plantar flexion and knee extension, such as running up a hill. Some patients experience a "pop" or sensation of being directly impacted by a projectile.[13,14] Medial gastrocnemius tears occur at the distal myotendinous junction and are best visualized in longitudinal orientation on US. Findings include fiber interruption of the tapered, triangular interface at the gastrosoleus aponeurosis with surrounding hypoechoic hemorrhagic fluid (**Fig. 3**). Larger

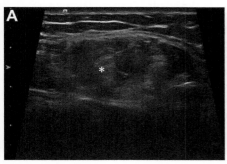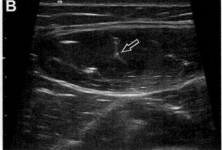

Fig. 2. Rectus femoris chronic central myotendinous tear. A 14-year-old female with a history of a focal depression in the anterior mid-right thigh. She recalls "pulling a quadriceps muscle" approximately 9 months prior. Ultrasound transverse (*A*) image with 14-MHz transducer of the right thigh reveals an indistinct hyperechoic tendon of the inner/central indirect head (*asterisk*) of the rectus femoris muscle with generalized blurring of the interface between hypoechoic muscle fibers and echogenic connective tissue septa. Transverse image (*B*) obtained through the normal left side for comparison demonstrates normal thin echogenic central tendon (*arrow*) within the rectus femoris muscle indirect head component.

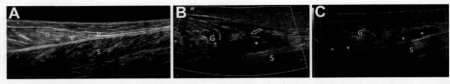

Fig. 3. Acute medial head of gastrocnemius tear. Ultrasound images of the mid-calf in a 45-year-old patient who experienced a popping sensation while running hill sprints. Long-axis ultrasound image (*A*) of a normal gastrocnemius (G) and soleus (S) aponeurosis (*arrowheads*). Long-axis Doppler ultrasound (*B*) with 15-MHz transducer shows fiber disruption at the gastrosoleus myotendinous aponeurosis (*arrow*) with surrounding anechoic or hypoechoic hemorrhage (*asterisk*). Extended field of view long-axis image (*C*) demonstrates the extent of hemorrhage (*asterisks*) between the medial head gastrocnemius (G) and soleus (S) muscles.

tears are characterized by retraction and heterogeneous fluid extending proximally, between the muscle bellies of the medial head of the gastrocnemius and the soleus.[14] This tubular hematoma between the muscles may mimic a plantaris myotendinous junction rupture; however, this injury is rare in isolation.[13] On follow-up imaging, heterogeneous hyperechoic scar tissue can be identified at the gastrocnemius myotendinous junction as the tear heals.[14]

Muscle Hernia

Muscle hernias result from the protrusion of muscle through an acquired or congenital fascial defect into the overlying subcutaneous fat. They often present a diagnostic dilemma, as young athletes may present with exercise-induced pain, cosmetic mass, or a concern for tumor. In many cases, the fascial defect is due to perforating vessels; however, other implicated causes include trauma and chronic exertional compartment syndrome.[15] Most muscle hernias occur in the lower leg and affect the tibialis anterior muscle.[15,16]

The classic history is a mass that appears or enlarges when the affected muscle is contracted and is effaced or shrinks when the muscle is relaxed. Dynamic US with provocative maneuvers (dorsiflexion, standing, squatting) for tibialis anterior herniations is often necessary to visualize the muscle hernia and is more sensitive than MRI.[15–17] The liberal use of gel as a standoff enables light pressure during scanning, ensuring the hernia is not reduced or obscured.[6] Frequently, the mushroom-shaped muscle protrusion is hypoechoic compared with the adjacent normal muscle and is accompanied by a herniated blood vessel traversing the fascial defect (**Fig. 4**). For athletes with activity-related pain that hinders sports participation, surgical fasciotomy may be necessary. Many patients are able to return to sports; however, residual symptoms are common in runners.[17]

Tendons

Tendon injuries can be divided into acute and overuse injuries. Acute injuries are often encountered in sports with high-speed, explosive forces and contact (skiing, football). Tendon injuries can occur at the musculotendinous junction, within the tendon substance, at the bony attachment, or as an apophyseal avulsion in adolescent athletes. Acute tendon tears may be partial or complete, and the tendon ends may be separated by hypoechoic blood or herniated adjacent soft-tissue structures. Dynamic imaging and the presence of refraction shadowing at the retracted tendon stump can be particularly useful in determining if a tendon tear is partial or complete.[18]

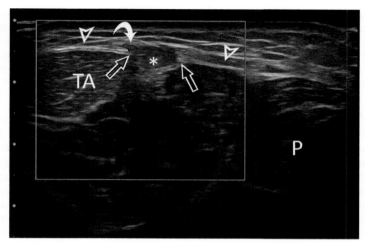

Fig. 4. Muscle herniation. A 12-year-old male with intermittent bulge in the anterior calf during exercise. Ultrasound short-axis Doppler image of the tibialis anterior muscle (TA) and peroneus longus (P) with 18-MHz transducer reveals a defect (between open *arrows*) in the hyperechoic muscle fascia (*arrowheads*) with focal muscle herniation (*asterisk*). Note the perforating vessel (*curved arrow*) at the fascial defect site.

Tendon overuse injuries are perhaps a more frequent source of pain for athletes participating in sports requiring repetitive motions such as distance running, racquet sports, and kicking. Recurring, low-magnitude microtrauma in the absence of sufficient repair time may result in tendon damage. Initially, there may be a painful, inflammatory phase characterized on US by increased vascularity, hypoechoic edematous tissue, and possible small tears. Over time, this maladaptive healing response may lead to tendon degeneration or tendinosis. At this stage, histopathologic examination of the tendon reveals myxoid degeneration, neovascularization, and disruption of collagen fibers without inflammatory cells.[19] The US findings of tendinosis are nearly universal throughout the body and appear as hypoechogenicity, thickening, and loss of the fibrillar architecture (**Fig. 5**). Often, there are enthesopathic changes at the bony attachment or intratendinous microcalcifications. Intratendinous hyperemia on Doppler imaging has been shown to represent neovascularity, rather than inflammation, often with accompanying neural in-growth which explains the occurrence of pain.[19]

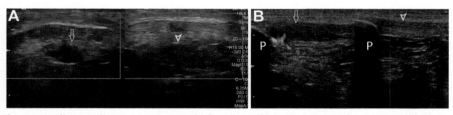

Fig. 5. Patellar tendinosis. A 17-year-old female volleyball player with anterior right knee pain. Short-axis (*A*) and long-axis (*B*) ultrasound evaluation with 15-MHz transducer demonstrates thickening and decreased echogenicity in the deep aspect of the right proximal patellar tendon (*open arrow*) with associated neovascularity and the normal left patellar tendon (*arrowhead*) for comparison.

The diagnostic utility of US for the diagnosis of common tendon pathology throughout the body (achilles,[20,21] distal biceps,[18,22] rotator cuff,[23,24] peroneal tendons[25,26]) has been well-described in the literature. Although these tears can be seen in the athlete, they are also frequently found in the general population. The following are other tendon pathologies found in athletes and sports injuries that can be assessed by US.

Jumper's Knee

Young athletes participating in sports requiring repetitive jumping, such as basketball and volleyball, are at risk for patellar tendinosis. Often colloquially referred to as "jumper's knee," patellar tendinosis is a chronic overuse injury associated with overloading of the knee extensor mechanism. It presents as pain and tenderness at the inferior pole of the patella. Not surprisingly, the deep aspect of the proximal patellar tendon is the most common site of involvement.[27,28] US features include a thickened, hypoechoic tendon with loss of the normal organized fibrillar pattern. Coexisting interstitial tears appear as anechoic clefts in the tendon. Irregularity of the inferior patellar cortex and calcifications within the tendon are not uncommon. Intratendinous blood flow may be seen within the areas of tendon abnormality on Doppler imaging[28] (see **Fig. 5**). Sonographic findings of patellar tendinopathy are common in elite athletes even in the absence of symptoms but may be a harbinger for development of jumper's knee during the season.[27] When conservative treatment fails, these areas of tendinosis can be specifically targeted during US-guided percutaneous therapy.[29,30]

Athletic Pubalgia or Core Muscle Injury

Groin injuries are common in athletes involved in cutting sports such as soccer, lacrosse, rugby, and hockey. Athletic pubalgia is increasingly recognized as a cause of chronic groin pain in these patients. The colloquial term "sports hernia" is a misnomer as the pathophysiology represents a constellation of overuse core muscle injuries about the pubic symphysis rather than a true hernia.[31] The most frequently implicated pathology involves injury to the rectus abdominis-adductor longus aponeurosis, which attaches to the periosteum of the anterior pubic bones and the capsule and disc of the pubic symphysis[32] (**Figs. 6** and **7**).

US features of athletic pubalgia include tendinosis or tearing of the distal rectus abdominis or proximal adductor longus often accompanied by irregularity of the pubic cortex.[33,34] In severe injuries, there may be complete avulsion of the common adductor tendon origin with retraction and interposed hematoma or granulation tissue that may mimic a mass[33] (see **Figs. 6** and **7**). To assess the adductor longus, the transducer should be placed in an oblique sagittal orientation. Abduction and external rotation of the hip helps to lengthen the adductor longus tendon and stresses the aponeurotic plate at its pubic attachment.[33] In turn, this may make some detachments more conspicuous.[34] Of note, the proximal adductor tendon is prone to anisotropy. Therefore, heel-toe maneuver is necessary to maintain parallel transducer orientation, and comparison with the contralateral side may be helpful to discriminate normal tendon from pathology.[34] Identifying the source of groin pain can be challenging in these athletes, and US evaluation of additional regional structures should be considered using a routine protocol[33] (**Box 2**). In the absence of US findings, MRI of the pelvis, using a dedicated athletic pubalgia protocol, can be considered to evaluate for subtle injuries or marrow edema in the setting of stress reaction.[32]

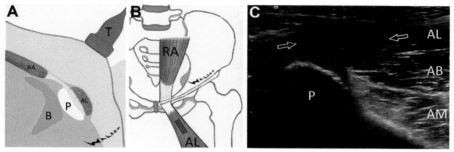

Fig. 6. Athletic Pubalgia. Graphical illustrations demonstrating transducer position for scanning the rectus abdominis-adductor aponeurosis. Illustration (*A*) shows a long-axis scanning position of the rectus abdominus (RA) tendinous attachment just lateral to midline. Note the oblique orientation of the adductor longus (AL) tendinous attachment to the pubic body (P). Transducer (T) and bladder (B) are also shown. Illustration (*B*) reveals the rectus abdominus (RA) and adductor longus (AL) attachment to the left pubic body. The gray dotted box shows a long-axis scanning position of the adductor longus (AL). (*C*) Long-axis ultrasound image with an 18-MHz transducer in a 20-year-old male hockey player with left groin pain demonstrates a full-thickness tear of the adductor longus (AL) origin with interposed hypoechoic hemorrhage (between *arrows*). Pubic bone (P), adductor brevis (AB), and adductor magnus (AM).

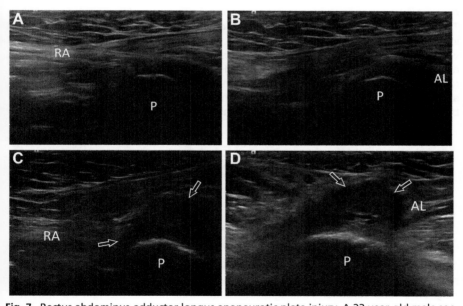

Fig. 7. Rectus abdominus-adductor longus aponeurotic plate injury. A 22-year-old male soccer player with left groin pain. Long-axis ultrasound images (*A, B*) with a 9-MHz transducer reveal a normal right rectus abdominus (RA) and adductor longus (AL) with aponeurotic plate attachment to the pubis (P). Figures (*C, D*) demonstrate hypoechoic thickening of the common aponeurosis between the left rectus abdominus (RA) and adductor longus (AL) indicating interruption of the aponeurosis fibers and partial avulsion with hematoma (between *arrows*) in the gap.

Box 2
Common causes of groin pain in athletes

Athletic Pubalgia

Anterior labral tear

Inguinal hernia

Inguinal ligament avulsion

Pubic stress fracture

Osteitis pubis

Iliopsoas impingement

Nerve injury (ilioinguinal, iliohypogastric, genitofemoral, obturator, lateral femoral cutaneous nerve)

Snapping Hip Syndrome

Athletes, particularly young female athletes, may experience symptomatic snapping of the hip. Snapping hip syndrome can refer to several distinct entities broadly divided into intra-articular and extra-articular types. The intra-articular type is not well evaluated on US; however, US is ideal to evaluate the extra-articular causes, which are further subtyped as external or internal based on location.[35]

Anterior Snapping Hip

Anterior (internal) snapping hip is due to abnormal movement of the iliopsoas complex. To evaluate with US, the transducer is placed just proximal and medial to the anterior inferior iliac spine in the axial oblique plane. At this level, the psoas major tendon is visualized medial to the iliacus muscle fibers (**Fig. 8**). As the patient flexes, abducts, and externally rotates the hip, the psoas tendon normally glides laterally over the pubic ramus and smoothly returns to position as the patient straightens the leg; however, in anterior snapping hip, the medial fibers of the iliacus become temporarily entrapped between the psoas tendon and bone. As the hip returns to the neutral position, the

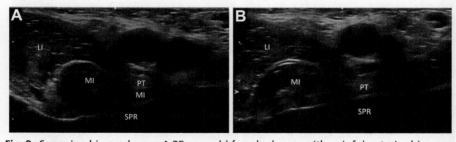

Fig. 8. Snapping hip syndrome. A 25-year-old female dancer with painful anterior hip snapping. Ultrasound transverse (*A*) image with 18-MHz transducer of the right hip in flexion/abduction (frog leg) position demonstrates entrapment of the medial fibers of the iliacus muscle (MI) between the psoas major tendon (PT) and the superior pubic ramus (SPR). Transverse image (*B*) is obtained as the hip is slowly extended. As the hip is moved from flexion/abduction to extension, the medial fibers of the iliacus (MI) slide laterally, and there is sudden rapid motion of the psoas major tendon (PT) toward the superior pubic ramus (SPR) producing a snapping sensation. Also shown are the lateral fibers of the iliacus muscle (LI).

psoas tendon quickly flips over the medial iliacus muscle onto the subjacent pubic bone (see **Fig. 8**) (Video 1). Additional causes of snapping iliopsoas include bifid psoas tendon heads flipping over one another or an anterior paralabral cyst.[35] It is important to remember occasional painless snapping phenomena can occur in asymptomatic people and application of excessive transducer pressure during the ultrasound examination can prevent snapping.[35,36] An assistant can be beneficial to facilitate the dynamic hip motion and allow the scanner to focus on maintaining appropriate positioning and visualization of the psoas tendon. Even if the snapping tendon is not visualized sonographically, pain relief after iliopsoas bursa steroid injection may be long term and is a predictor of good outcome after surgical release of the iliopsoas tendon.[37]

Lateral Snapping Hip

Lateral, or external, snapping hip results from abnormal movement of the iliotibial band or anterior gluteus maximus muscle over the greater trochanter during hip flexion and extension[36] (Video 2). Occasionally, the patient can reproduce the symptoms while lying in the decubitus position, but frequently dynamic scanning must be performed with the patient in the standing position.[38] US may show thickening and decreased echogenicity of the iliotibial band. There may be associated greater trochanteric bursitis.[36]

Ultrasound Guided Percutaneous Tendon Treatment Strategies

Initial treatment for tendinosis is primarily conservative. Surgery is indicated in a small percentage of recalcitrant cases after conservative management is exhausted. Unfortunately, clinicians often encounter a treatment gap for a substantial percentage of young, active patients with a strong desire to return to activity, yet for whom conservative measures have failed and surgery is not indicated. US can provide target localization during image-guided percutaneous therapy. Steroid injections have been shown to temporarily improve pain in the short term, but there is limited evidence that they are efficacious in the long term and may even be harmful in some cases.[39] Percutaneous tenotomy for the treatment of tendinopathy has been used throughout the body with success.[40] The premise of percutaneous tenotomy or "dry needling" is to convert a chronic degenerative process to an acute inflammatory condition that will progress to the repair phase of healing.[40] US guidance for the procedure is useful to accurately target areas of tendon abnormality and importantly the tendon enthesis.[40] This treatment technique has few contraindications (recent steroid injection, infection, tears > 50%), and negligible complications (tendon tear, infection) have been described. There is also limited evidence for the efficacy of percutaneous ultrasonic tenotomy (Tenex).[41,42]

In recent years, the field of orthobiologics has exploded. US can provide target localization during administration of a wide array of injectable agents (prolotherapy, autologous whole blood, and platelet-rich plasma). The premise of platelet-rich plasma injection is to deliver a high concentration of growth factors to the poorly vascularized tendon in an effort to promote tendon healing. Currently, there is mixed evidence regarding the superiority and cost-effectiveness of platelet rich plasma (PRP) over tendon fenestration.[30,43–46] Future research requires standardization in study protocols, PRP preparation techniques, and outcomes measures.

Ligaments

Ligaments are typically injured after an acute trauma, unlike tendons where overuse injuries are more prevalent. Ligament injuries can occur at the midsubstance, at the ligament-bone interface, or as an osseous avulsion injury. Ligament injuries are classified similar to tendon tears as grade I-III.[47] Sprain or grade I injuries are interstitial tears without macroscopic disruption. The ligament may appear thickened and hypoechoic, often with fluid and inflammatory change in the adjacent tissues. Higher grade tears involve increasing percentages of fiber interruption, sometimes accompanied by an osseous avulsion. The ligament may remain sonographically abnormal in remote injuries with resolution of the inflammatory change in the surrounding tissues. Perhaps the most beneficial aspect of US imaging of ligaments is the dynamic evaluation.[48] By stressing a ligament under US, the clinician may be able to identify laxity or small tears that would otherwise be missed by static US evaluation and even MRI. It can be beneficial to compare with the contralateral side when comparing laxity.

Ulnar Collateral Ligament of the Elbow

Sports that require repetitive throwing, such as javelin, tennis, softball, and baseball (particularly high velocity pitchers), impart high valgus loads to the athlete's elbow.[49] The ulnar collateral ligament (UCL) is the primary soft-tissue stabilizer against valgus stress in the medial elbow. The clinical diagnosis of acute, complete tears is often straightforward, but partial tears and chronic ligament overuse injury often present a considerable diagnostic challenge.[50] Imaging can afford additional information when the clinical picture is unclear or further information is necessary for risk stratification and treatment planning. Although, MR arthrogram has the best sensitivity and specificity for evaluating the UCL, US has been shown to be accurate (sensitivity, 81%; specificity, 91%) and reproducible.[51]

To image the UCL, it is important to place the elbow in 30° of flexion. The US findings of pathology are similar to aforementioned findings in other ligaments[51] (**Fig. 9**). Multiple studies have demonstrated the added value US provides during dynamic valgus stress imaging to demonstrate medial joint gapping in the setting of a subtle partial-

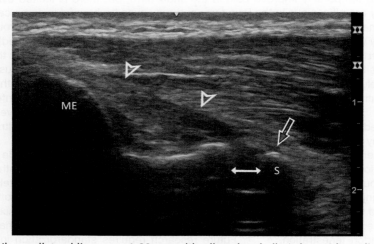

Fig. 9. Ulnar collateral ligament. A 20-year-old college baseball pitcher with medial elbow pain in the late cocking stage of throwing and accompanying decrease in pitch velocity. Long-axis ultrasound image of the UCL anterior band (*arrowheads*) demonstrates a near-complete tear with a few thin superficial fibers (*arrow*) attached to sublime tubercle (S). Note the medial joint gapping between the humerus and medial ulna (*double head white arrow*). ME, medial epicondyle.

thickness UCL tear[52,53] (see **Fig. 9**). It is important to remember UCL thickening, cal-cifications, and asymmetric laxity with valgus stress are common findings in the domi-nant elbow of asymptomatic high-level throwers and represent chronic adaptive changes of the ligament.[53] A greater than 2-mm change in joint space gapping on dy-namic US should raise suspicion for UCL tear.[54]

Surgical reconstruction of the UCL is indicated for the throwing athlete with a com-plete tear or partial-thickness tear that has failed a comprehensive rehabilitation pro-gram. US-guided PRP injection may improve nonoperative outcomes in athletes with partial UCL ears.[55]

Ankle Sprain

Ankle sprains are one of the most common injuries in sports.[48] While most ankle sprains are treated conservatively, recurrent ankle sprains due to chronic ligamentous instability occasionally require more prolonged rehabilitation or even operative man-agement. US has similar reliability to MRI when screening for complete discontinuity of the anterior talofibular ligament (ATFL) and anterior inferior tibiofibular ligament (AITFL)[47,56] (**Fig. 10**). For evaluation of the lateral ligaments, the patient is positioned in the contralateral decubitus position with a towel roll just proximal to the ankle to take advantage of gravity stress on the ligaments and to eliminate redundancy. When a normal ATFL is identified, an isolated tear of the calcaneofibular ligament is

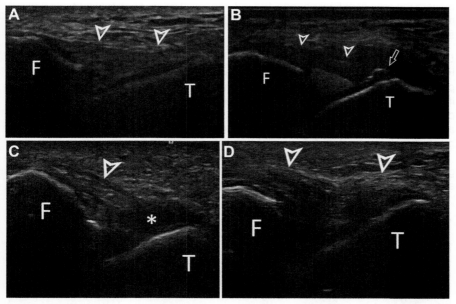

Fig. 10. Anterior talofibular ligament. Ultrasound (*A*) image of the normal anterior talofib-ular ligament (ATFL) with a 14-MHz transducer reveals a thin ligament (*arrowheads*) be-tween the fibular tip (F) and the talus (T). Long-axis ultrasound (*B*) of a 22-year-old basketball player with persistent pain 8 weeks after ankle sprain shows avulsion (*arrow*) of the ATFL ligament (*arrowheads*) off of the talus (T). Image (*C*) demonstrates a subacute complete tear of the ATFL (*arrowhead*) in a different patient with a hypoechoic focus of hemorrhage (*asterisk*) within the ligament discontinuity at the talar attachment. (*D*) Chronic ATFL injury with a thickened and hypoechoic ligament (*arrowheads*) with ligamentous laxity.

unlikely.[47] Dynamic inversion stress maneuvers and the anterior drawer test improve detection of tears on US.[48,56]

Ankle syndesmotic injuries (high ankle sprain) are important to identify as they are often misdiagnosed as a lateral ankle sprain and require a more prolonged course of rehabilitation.[56] Furthermore, they are frequently missed in the absence of distal fibular fracture. The AITFL is the first ligament disrupted in high ankle sprains, and US is approximately 85% accurate for the diagnosis[56] (**Fig. 11**). Of note, the AITFL consists of multiple fascicles that should not be confused with injury on US.[47] A dynamic US evaluation of the AITFL with the ankle in eversion can show widening of the tibiofibular clear space and ligament fiber discontinuity[48,56] (Video 3). In the setting of an AITFL tear, the interosseous membrane should also be investigated for a concomitant tear.

Nerves

The diagnosis of nerve injury is primarily clinical with electromyography used for confirmation as well as to counsel the patient regarding the expected course of recovery. US can be used to look for a site of compression, but more importantly, a potential etiology. It is well suited to evaluate peripheral nerve abnormalities due to its high spatial resolution and ability to follow the course of the nerve throughout the extremity.[5] The nerve may become enlarged, edematous, and hypoechoic proximal to the site of compression.[57] Long-axis extended field-of-view technique can be helpful to discern the area of caliber change, but differences in cross-sectional area are typically measured in short axis (**Fig. 12**). Dynamic US can be used to look for abnormal nerve subluxation or dislocation.

Ulnar neuritis

In high-level throwing sport athletes, ulnar neuritis is a frequent cause of medial elbow pain accompanied by ring and small finger numbness. It can result from chronic repetitive neuropraxic injury or compression of the ulnar nerve in the cubital tunnel by osteophytes related to valgus extension overload. On short-axis US, a cross-sectional nerve area greater than 9 mm^2 at the site of maximal enlargement, or an increase in caliber by a ratio of greater than 2.8 is considered abnormal[58,59] (see **Fig. 12**).

There are several pitfalls in ulnar nerve imaging at the elbow. First, mild hypoechogenicity alone may be normal as the curvilinear course of the nerve predisposes it to anisotropy at the cubital tunnel. The nerve should be measured in elbow extension,

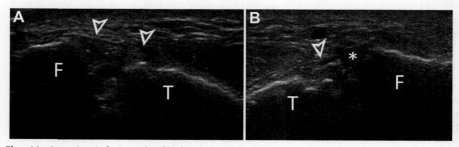

Fig. 11. Anterior inferior tibiofibular ligament. A 25-year-old football player with high ankle sprain on the left. Ultrasound (*A*) image of the normal anterior inferior tibiofibular ligament (AITFL) on the right with a 14-MHz transducer reveals an intact ligament (*arrowheads*) between the fibula (F) and the tibia (T). Ultrasound image (*B*) on the symptomatic left side demonstrates a tear (*asterisk*) of the AITFL (*arrowhead*).

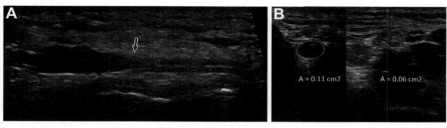

Fig. 12. Ulnar nerve enlargement. A 19-year-old male baseball pitcher with medial elbow pain and 4th and 5th digit numbness. Longitudinal ultrasound image (*A*) with 14-MHz transducer reveals ulnar nerve enlargement with a swollen, hypoechoic nerve proximal to the cubital tunnel with sharp transition (*arrow*) to normal caliber within the cubital tunnel indicating ulnar nerve entrapment. Ultrasound transverse (*B*) image demonstrates cross-sectional areas (*yellow circles*) of the ulnar nerve in the upper arm and at the cubital tunnel. Greater than 9 mm² or a caliber change of greater than 2.8 is reported to be sensitive for neuritis.

and only the inner hypoechoic part of the nerve should be measured to avoid overestimation of pathology. Finally, physiologic side-to-side variability exists, and it may reach values near 20% of the cross-sectional area of the nerve.[57]

Ulnar Nerve Dislocation and Snapping Triceps

Ulnar nerve examination in throwing athletes should also include dynamic imaging of the cubital tunnel during end-range elbow flexion to evaluate for transient anterior dislocation of the nerve over the medial epicondyle.[60] The ulnar nerve is most easily evaluated by placing the patient in the ipsilateral decubitus position with the arm abducted, hanging over the edge of the table.[60] This position is helpful to maintain skin contact, particularly during dynamic maneuvers. A generous amount of gel and small footprint transducers can help to improve the transducer contact and avoid excessive pressure, which may prevent nerve dislocation from the tunnel.[57] It should be emphasized that the anterior end of the transducer must maintain visualization of the medial epicondyle to avoid a false-positive diagnosis of apparent dislocation. It is also important to note that the ulnar nerve can dislocate in up to 20% of asymptomatic individuals.[60] Nerve dislocation may also be accompanied by subluxation of the medial head of the triceps tendon, known as snapping triceps syndrome[60] (Video 4). Undiagnosed snapping of the medial triceps is a recognized cause for continuous snapping and pain after ulnar nerve transposition.[60]

FUTURE DIRECTIONS

In recent years, quantitative US methods, such as shear-wave elastography (SWE) and contrast-enhanced US, have moved from research to practical applications as an adjunct tool to standard techniques in the evaluation of various musculoskeletal structures throughout the body. In particular, SWE has seen an exponential increase in the number of musculoskeletal applications and publications in the past two decades. By quantifying mechanical and elastic tissue properties, SWE may provide important information about preclinical injuries in musculoskeletal tissues and tissue healing after injury.[61] Although SWE is Food and Drug Administration-approved on most US platforms for diagnostic imaging, future research requires standardization in study protocols, techniques, and outcomes measures. Nonetheless, this technology is promising for the future of ultrasonography in sports medicine and may help practitioners to individualize the retraining plan for the injured athlete.

SUMMARY

US is an important adjunct tool to physical examination and other imaging modalities in evaluation and management of the injured athlete. It offers unique advantages in specific clinical scenarios. Dedicated training and a standardized scanning technique are important to overcome the inherent operator dependence and avoid pitfalls that can lead to misdiagnosis. US guidance can also improve accuracy in targeted percutaneous injection therapies.

CLINICS CARE POINTS

- Tendon, ligament, and muscle injuries often appear on ultrasound as decreased echogenicity with loss of the normal architecture and varying degrees of fiber discontunity.
- Ultrasound has comparable accuracy to MRI for the diagnosis of many sports injuries in the hands of an experienced operator.
- Ultrasound offers the advantage of dynamic imaging.
- Ultrasound guidance improves accuracy for many percutaneous procedures.

DISCLOSURE

The authors have nothing to disclose.

SUPPLEMENTARY DATA

Supplementary data related to this article can be found online at https://doi.org/10.1016/j.csm.2021.05.013.

REFERENCES

1. Hauret KG, Bedno S, Loringer K, et al. Epidemiology of Exercise- and Sports-Related Injuries in a Population of Young, Physically Active Adults: A Survey of Military Servicemembers. Am J Sports Med 2015;43(11):2645–53.
2. Nazarian LN. The top 10 reasons musculoskeletal sonography is an important complementary or alternative technique to MRI. AJR Am J Roentgenol 2008; 190(6):1621–6.
3. Kanesa-Thasan RM, Nazarian LN, Parker L, et al. Comparative Trends in Utilization of MRI and Ultrasound to Evaluate Nonspine Joint Disease 2003 to 2015. J Am Coll Radiol 2018;15(3 Pt A):402–7.
4. Erickson SJ. High-resolution imaging of the musculoskeletal system. Radiology 1997;205(3):593–618.
5. Klauser AS, Tagliafico A, Allen GM, et al. Clinical indications for musculoskeletal ultrasound: a Delphi-based consensus paper of the European Society of Musculoskeletal Radiology. Eur Radiol May 2012;22(5):1140–8.
6. Jacobson JA. Ultrasound in sports medicine. Radiol Clin North Am 2002;40(2): 363–86.
7. Draghi F, Zacchino M, Canepari M, et al. Muscle injuries: ultrasound evaluation in the acute phase. J Ultrasound 2013;16(4):209–14.
8. Peetrons P. Ultrasound of muscles. Eur Radiol 2002;12(1):35–43.

9. Bianchi S, Martinoli C, Waser NP, et al. Central aponeurosis tears of the rectus femoris: sonographic findings. Skeletal Radiol 2002;31(10):581–6.

10. Balius R, Maestro A, Pedret C, et al. Central aponeurosis tears of the rectus femoris: practical sonographic prognosis. Br J Sports Med 2009;43(11): 818–24.

11. Walker E, Brian P, Longo V, et al. Dilemmas in distinguishing between tumor and the posttraumatic lesion with surgical or pathologic correlation. Clin Sports Med 2013;32(3):559–76.

12. Delgado GJ, Chung CB, Lektrakul N, et al. Tennis leg: clinical US study of 141 patients and anatomic investigation of four cadavers with MR imaging and US. Radiol 2002;224(1):112–9.

13. Bianchi S, Sailly M, Molini L. Isolated tear of the plantaris tendon: ultrasound and MRI appearance. Skeletal Radiol 2011;40(7):891–5.

14. Kwak HS, Han YM, Lee SY, et al. Diagnosis and follow-up US evaluation of ruptures of the medial head of the gastrocnemius ("tennis leg"). Korean J Radiol 2006;7(3):193–8.

15. Beggs I. Sonography of muscle hernias. AJR Am J Roentgenol 2003;180(2): 395–9.

16. Kramer DE, Pace JL, Jarrett DY, et al. Diagnosis and management of symptomatic muscle herniation of the extremities: a retrospective review. Am J Sports Med 2013;41(9):2174–80.

17. Jarrett DY, Kramer DE, Callahan MJ, et al. US diagnosis of pediatric muscle hernias of the lower extremities. Pediatr Radiol 2013;43(Suppl 1):S2–7.

18. Lobo Lda G, Fessell DP, Miller BS, et al. The role of sonography in differentiating full versus partial distal biceps tendon tears: correlation with surgical findings. AJR Am J Roentgenol 2013;200(1):158–62.

19. Klauser AS, Miyamoto H, Tamegger M, et al. Achilles tendon assessed with sonoelastography: histologic agreement. Radiol 2013;267(3):837–42.

20. Hartgerink P, Fessell DP, Jacobson JA, et al. Full- versus partial-thickness Achilles tendon tears: sonographic accuracy and characterization in 26 cases with surgical correlation. Radiology 2001;220(2):406–12.

21. Aström M, Gentz CF, Nilsson P, et al. Imaging in chronic achilles tendinopathy: a comparison of ultrasonography, magnetic resonance imaging and surgical findings in 27 histologically verified cases. Skeletal Radiol 1996;25(7):615–20.

22. de la Fuente J, Blasi M, Martínez S, et al. Ultrasound classification of traumatic distal biceps brachii tendon injuries. Skeletal Radiol 2018;47(4):519–32.

23. Okoroha KR, Fidai MS, Tramer JS, et al. Diagnostic accuracy of ultrasound for rotator cuff tears. Ultrasonography 2019;38(3):215–20.

24. de Jesus JO, Parker L, Frangos AJ, et al. Accuracy of MRI, MR arthrography, and ultrasound in the diagnosis of rotator cuff tears: a meta-analysis. AJR Am J Roentgenol 2009;192(6):1701–7.

25. Grant TH, Kelikian AS, Jereb SE, et al. Ultrasound diagnosis of peroneal tendon tears. A surgical correlation. J Bone Joint Surg Am 2005;87(8):1788–94.

26. Lee SJ, Jacobson JA, Kim SM, et al. Ultrasound and MRI of the peroneal tendons and associated pathology. Skeletal Radiol 2013;42(9):1191–200.

27. Peace KA, Lee JC, Healy J. Imaging the infrapatellar tendon in the elite athlete. Clin Radiol 2006;61(7):570–8.

28. Khan KM, Bonar F, Desmond PM, et al. Patellar tendinosis (jumper's knee): findings at histopathologic examination, US, and MR imaging. Victorian Institute of Sport Tendon Study Group. Radiology 1996;200(3):821–7.

29. Kanaan Y, Jacobson JA, Jamadar D, et al. Sonographically guided patellar tendon fenestration: prognostic value of preprocedure sonographic findings. J Ultrasound Med 2013;32(5):771–7.

30. Dragoo JL, Wasterlain AS, Braun HJ, et al. Platelet-rich plasma as a treatment for patellar tendinopathy: a double-blind, randomized controlled trial. Am J Sports Med 2014;42(3):610–8.

31. Palisch A, Zoga AC, Meyers WC. Imaging of athletic pubalgia and core muscle injuries: clinical and therapeutic correlations. Clin Sports Med 2013;32(3):427–47.

32. Hegazi TM, Belair JA, McCarthy EJ, et al. Sports Injuries about the Hip: What the Radiologist Should Know. Radiographics 2016;36(6):1717–45.

33. Jacobson JA, Khoury V, Brandon CJ. Ultrasound of the Groin: Techniques, Pathology, and Pitfalls. AJR Am J Roentgenol 2015;205(3):513–23.

34. Morley N, Grant T, Blount K, et al. Sonographic evaluation of athletic pubalgia. Skeletal Radiol 2016;45(5):689–99.

35. Bureau NJ. Sonographic evaluation of snapping hip syndrome. J Ultrasound Med 2013;32(6):895–900.

36. Lungu E, Michaud J, Bureau NJ. US Assessment of Sports-related Hip Injuries. Radiographics 2018;38(3):867–89.

37. Blankenbaker DG, De Smet AA, Keene JS. Sonography of the iliopsoas tendon and injection of the iliopsoas bursa for diagnosis and management of the painful snapping hip. Skeletal Radiol 2006;35(8):565–71.

38. Chang CY, Kreher J, Torriani M. Dynamic sonography of snapping hip due to gluteus maximus subluxation over greater trochanter. Skeletal Radiol 2016;45(3):409–12.

39. Coombes BK, Bisset L, Vicenzino B. Efficacy and safety of corticosteroid injections and other injections for management of tendinopathy: a systematic review of randomised controlled trials. Lancet 2010;376(9754):1751–67.

40. Chiavaras MM, Jacobson JA. Ultrasound-guided tendon fenestration. Semin Musculoskelet Radiol 2013;17(1):85–90.

41. Seng C, Mohan PC, Koh SB, et al. Ultrasonic Percutaneous Tenotomy for Recalcitrant Lateral Elbow Tendinopathy: Sustainability and Sonographic Progression at 3 Years. Am J Sports Med 2016;44(2):504–10.

42. Koh JS, Mohan PC, Howe TS, et al. Fasciotomy and surgical tenotomy for recalcitrant lateral elbow tendinopathy: early clinical experience with a novel device for minimally invasive percutaneous microresection. Am J Sports Med 2013;41(3):636–44.

43. de Vos RJ, Weir A, van Schie HT, et al. Platelet-rich plasma injection for chronic Achilles tendinopathy: a randomized controlled trial. J Am Med Assoc 2010;303(2):144–9.

44. de Vos RJ, Windt J, Weir A. Strong evidence against platelet-rich plasma injections for chronic lateral epicondylar tendinopathy: a systematic review. Br J Sports Med 2014;48(12):952–6.

45. Peerbooms JC, Sluimer J, Bruijn DJ, et al. Positive effect of an autologous platelet concentrate in lateral epicondylitis in a double-blind randomized controlled trial: platelet-rich plasma versus corticosteroid injection with a 1-year follow-up. Am J Sports Med 2010;38(2):255–62.

46. Franchini M, Cruciani M, Mengoli C, et al. Efficacy of platelet-rich plasma as conservative treatment in orthopaedics: a systematic review and meta-analysis. Blood Transfus 2018;16(6):502–13.

47. Alves T, Dong Q, Jacobson J, et al. Normal and Injured Ankle Ligaments on Ultrasonography With Magnetic Resonance Imaging Correlation. J Ultrasound Med 2019;38(2):513–28.

48. Sconfienza LM, Orlandi D, Lacelli F, et al. Dynamic high-resolution US of ankle and midfoot ligaments: normal anatomic structure and imaging technique. Radiographics 2015;35(1):164–78.

49. Dugas J, Chronister J, Cain EL Jr, et al. Ulnar collateral ligament in the overhead athlete: a current review. Sports Med Arthrosc 2014;22(3):169–82.

50. O'Driscoll SW, Lawton RL, Smith AM. The "moving valgus stress test" for medial collateral ligament tears of the elbow. Am J Sports Med 2005;33(2):231–9.

51. Campbell RE, McGhee AN, Freedman KB, et al. Diagnostic Imaging of Ulnar Collateral Ligament Injury: A Systematic Review. Am J Sports Med 2020; 48(11):2819–27.

52. De Smet AA, Winter TC, Best TM, et al. Dynamic sonography with valgus stress to assess elbow ulnar collateral ligament injury in baseball pitchers. Skeletal Radiol 2002;31(11):671–6.

53. Nazarian LN, McShane JM, Ciccotti MG, et al. Dynamic US of the anterior band of the ulnar collateral ligament of the elbow in asymptomatic major league baseball pitchers. Radiol 2003;227(1):149–54.

54. Ciccotti MG, Atanda A Jr, Nazarian LN, et al. Stress sonography of the ulnar collateral ligament of the elbow in professional baseball pitchers: a 10-year study. Am J Sports Med 2014;42(3):544–51.

55. Podesta L, Crow SA, Volkmer D, et al. Treatment of partial ulnar collateral ligament tears in the elbow with platelet-rich plasma. Am J Sports Med 2013;41(7): 1689–94.

56. Baltes TPA, Arnáiz J, Geertsema L, et al. Diagnostic value of ultrasonography in acute lateral and syndesmotic ligamentous ankle injuries. Eur Radiol 2020. https://doi.org/10.1007/s00330-020-07305-7.

57. Tagliafico AS, Bignotti B, Martinoli C. Elbow US: Anatomy, Variants, and Scanning Technique. Radiol 2015;275(3):636–50.

58. Yoon JS, Walker FO, Cartwright MS. Ultrasonographic swelling ratio in the diagnosis of ulnar neuropathy at the elbow. Muscle Nerve 2008;38(4):1231–5.

59. Thoirs K, Williams MA, Phillips M. Ultrasonographic measurements of the ulnar nerve at the elbow: role of confounders. J Ultrasound Med 2008;27(5):737–43.

60. Jacobson JA, Jebson PJ, Jeffers AW, et al. Ulnar nerve dislocation and snapping triceps syndrome: diagnosis with dynamic sonography–report of three cases. Radiol 2001;220(3):601–5.

61. Snoj Ž, Wu CH, Taljanovic MS, et al. Ultrasound Elastography in Musculoskeletal Radiology: Past, Present, and Future. Semin Musculoskelet Radiol 2020;24(2): 156–66.

United States Postal Service — Statement of Ownership, Management, and Circulation (All Periodicals Publications Except Requester Publications)

1. Publication Title	2. Publication Number	3. Filing Date
CLINICS IN SPORTS MEDICINE	000 – 702	9/18/2021

4. Issue Frequency	5. Number of Issues Published Annually	6. Annual Subscription Price
JAN, APR, JUL, OCT	4	$364.00

7. Complete Mailing Address of Known Office of Publication (Not printer) (Street, city, county, state, and ZIP+4®)

ELSEVIER INC.
230 Park Avenue, Suite 800
New York, NY 10169

Contact Person
Malathi Samayan

Telephone (Include area code)
91-44-4299-4507

8. Complete Mailing Address of Headquarters or General Business Office of Publisher (Not printer)

ELSEVIER INC.
230 Park Avenue, Suite 800
New York, NY 10169

9. Full Names and Complete Mailing Addresses of Publisher, Editor, and Managing Editor (Do not leave blank)

Publisher (Name and complete mailing address)

TAYLOR BALL, ELSEVIER INC.
1600 JOHN F KENNEDY BLVD. SUITE 1800
PHILADELPHIA, PA 19103-2899

Editor (Name and complete mailing address)

LAUREN BOYLE, ELSEVIER INC.
1600 JOHN F KENNEDY BLVD. SUITE 1800
PHILADELPHIA, PA 19103-2899

Managing Editor (Name and complete mailing address)

PATRICK MANLEY, ELSEVIER INC.
1600 JOHN F KENNEDY BLVD. SUITE 1800
PHILADELPHIA, PA 19103-2899

10. Owner (Do not leave blank. If the publication is owned by a corporation, give the name and address of the corporation immediately followed by the names and addresses of all stockholders owning or holding 1 percent or more of the total amount of stock. If not owned by a corporation, give the names and addresses of the individual owners. If owned by a partnership or other unincorporated firm, give its name and address as well as those of each individual owner. If the publication is published by a nonprofit organization, give its name and address.)

Full Name	Complete Mailing Address
WHOLLY OWNED SUBSIDIARY OF REED/ELSEVIER, US HOLDINGS	1600 JOHN F KENNEDY BLVD. SUITE 1800 PHILADELPHIA, PA 19103-2899

11. Known Bondholders, Mortgagees, and Other Security Holders Owning or Holding 1 Percent or More of Total Amount of Bonds, Mortgages, or Other Securities. If none, check box ▶ ☐ None

Full Name	Complete Mailing Address
N/A	

12. Tax Status (For completion by nonprofit organizations authorized to mail at nonprofit rates) (Check one)
The purpose, function, and nonprofit status of this organization and the exempt status for federal income tax purposes:
☒ Has Not Changed During Preceding 12 Months
☐ Has Changed During Preceding 12 Months (Publisher must submit explanation of change with this statement)

PS Form 3526, July 2014 [Page 1 of 4 (see instructions page 4)] PSN: 7530-01-000-9931 PRIVACY NOTICE: See our privacy policy on www.usps.com.

---

13. Publication Title	14. Issue Date for Circulation Data Below
CLINICS IN SPORTS MEDICINE	JULY 2021

15. Extent and Nature of Circulation			Average No. Copies Each Issue During Preceding 12 Months	No. Copies of Single Issue Published Nearest to Filing Date
a. Total Number of Copies (Net press run)			179	171
b. Paid Circulation (By Mail and Outside the Mail)	(1)	Mailed Outside-County Paid Subscriptions Stated on PS Form 3541 (Include paid distribution above nominal rate, advertiser's proof copies, and exchange copies)	111	99
	(2)	Mailed In-County Paid Subscriptions Stated on PS Form 3541 (Include paid distribution above nominal rate, advertiser's proof copies, and exchange copies)	0	0
	(3)	Paid Distribution Outside the Mails Including Sales Through Dealers and Carriers, Street Vendors, Counter Sales, and Other Paid Distribution Outside USPS®	34	38
	(4)	Paid Distribution by Other Classes of Mail Through the USPS (e.g., First-Class Mail®)	0	0
c. Total Paid Distribution (Sum of 15b (1), (2), (3), and (4))		▶	145	137
d. Free or Nominal Rate Distribution (By Mail and Outside the Mail)	(1)	Free or Nominal Rate Outside-County Copies included on PS Form 3541	20	18
	(2)	Free or Nominal Rate In-County Copies Included on PS Form 3541	0	0
	(3)	Free or Nominal Rate Copies Mailed at Other Classes Through the USPS (e.g., First-Class Mail)	0	0
	(4)	Free or Nominal Rate Distribution Outside the Mail (Carriers or other means)	0	0
e. Total Free or Nominal Rate Distribution (Sum of 15d (1), (2), (3) and (4))		▶	20	18
f. Total Distribution (Sum of 15c and 15e)		▶	165	155
g. Copies not Distributed (See Instructions to Publishers #4 (page 83))		▶	14	16
h. Total (Sum of 15f and g)		▶	179	171
i. Percent Paid (15c divided by 15f times 100)		▶	87.87%	88.39%

* If you are claiming electronic copies, go to line 16 on page 3. If you are not claiming electronic copies, skip to line 17 on page 3.

PS Form 3526, July 2014 (Page 2 of 4)

16. Electronic Copy Circulation		Average No. Copies Each Issue During Preceding 12 Months	No. Copies of Single Issue Published Nearest to Filing Date
a. Paid Electronic Copies	▶		
b. Total Paid Print Copies (Line 15c) + Paid Electronic Copies (Line 16a)	▶		
c. Total Print Distribution (Line 15f) + Paid Electronic Copies (Line 16a)	▶		
d. Percent Paid (Both Print & Electronic Copies) (16b divided by 16c × 100)	▶		

☒ I certify that 50% of all my distributed copies (electronic and print) are paid above a nominal price.

17. Publication of Statement of Ownership
☒ If the publication is a general publication, publication of this statement is required. Will be printed
in the OCTOBER 2021 issue of this publication. ☐ Publication not required.

18. Signature and Title of Editor, Publisher, Business Manager, or Owner

Malathi Samayan - Distribution Controller

Malathi Samayan
Malathi Samayan

Date 9/18/2021

I certify that all information furnished on this form is true and complete. I understand that anyone who furnishes false or misleading information on this form or who omits material or information requested on the form may be subject to criminal sanctions (including fines and imprisonment) and/or civil sanctions (including civil penalties).

PS Form 3526, July 2014 (Page 3 of 4) PRIVACY NOTICE: See our privacy policy on www.usps.com

Moving?

Make sure your subscription moves with you!

To notify us of your new address, find your **Clinics Account Number** (located on your mailing label above your name), and contact customer service at:

Email: journalscustomerservice-usa@elsevier.com

800-654-2452 (subscribers in the U.S. & Canada)
314-447-8871 (subscribers outside of the U.S. & Canada)

Fax number: 314-447-8029

Elsevier Health Sciences Division
Subscription Customer Service
3251 Riverport Lane
Maryland Heights, MO 63043

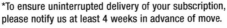

Moving?

Make sure your subscription moves with you!

To notify us of your new address, find your Clinics Account Number (located on your mailing label above your name), and contact customer service at:

Email: journalscustomerservice-usa@elsevier.com

800-654-2452 (subscribers in the U.S. & Canada)
314-447-8871 (subscribers outside of the U.S. & Canada)

Fax number: 314-447-8029

Elsevier Health Sciences Division
Subscription Customer Service
3251 Riverport Lane
Maryland Heights, MO 63043

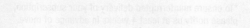

*To ensure uninterrupted delivery of your subscription, please notify us at least 4 weeks in advance of move.

Printed and bound by CPI Group (UK) Ltd, Croydon, CR0 4YY

08/05/2025

01864694-0004